Moving Otherwise

Enjoy reading!.

Victoria

Moving Otherwise

Dance, Violence, and Memory in Buenos Aires

Victoria Fortuna

OXFORD
UNIVERSITY PRESS

OXFORD
UNIVERSITY PRESS

Published in the United States of America by Oxford University Press
198 Madison Avenue, New York, NY 10016, United States of America.

Library of Congress Cataloging-in-Publication Data
Names: Fortuna, Victoria, author.
Title: Moving otherwise : dance, violence, and memory in Buenos Aires / Victoria Fortuna.
Description: New York, NY : Oxford University Press, [2019] |
Includes bibliographical references and index.
Identifiers: LCCN 2018013562 (print) | LCCN 2018034084 (ebook) |
ISBN 9780190627041 (epub) | ISBN 9780190627034 (updf) |
ISBN 9780190627027 (pbk. : alk. paper) | ISBN 9780190627010 (cloth : alk. paper)
Subjects: LCSH: Dance—Argentina—Buenos Aires—History. |
Dance—Political aspects—Argentina—Buenos Aires. |
Dance—Social aspects—Argentina—Buenos Aires.
Classification: LCC GV1636.B84 (ebook) | LCC GV1636.B84 F67 2019 (print) |
DDC 792.80982/11—dc23
LC record available at https://lccn.loc.gov/2018013562

For Hugo, for all the journeys we have taken,
y por todos los que nos esperan.

CONTENTS

Preface   *ix*
Acknowledgments   *xiii*
About the Companion Website   *xvii*

The Dancing Body on the Line: An Introduction   *1*

1. Mobile Bodies   *31*

2. The Revolution Was Danced   *55*

3. Dance as the Art of Survival   *79*

4. Moving Trauma   *109*

5. Common Goods   *139*

Epilogue: The History of Memory   *171*

Notes   *181*
Bibliography   *225*
Index   *241*

PREFACE

Moving Otherwise began in Buenos Aires many years ago, somewhere between my experiences in the city's dance studios and its urban landscapes. I travelled to Buenos Aires for the first time as a US exchange student who wanted to broaden her study of contemporary dance and Latin American literature. To meet the first aspiration, I enrolled in Liliana Toccaceli's course in Jennifer Muller technique at the National University of the Arts (UNA, Universidad Nacional de las Artes), then known as the National University Institute of the Arts (IUNA, Instituto Universitario Nacional del Arte).[1] A former member of the José Limón Dance Company, Muller taught and presented work in Argentina multiple times between 1979 and the early 2000s, and set work on the prestigious Ballet Contemporáneo (Contemporary Ballet) of the General San Martín Municipal Theater (Teatro Municipal General San Martín), with whom Toccaceli had danced professionally.[2] Amid the newness of the city, the unfamiliar particularities of Argentine Spanish, and a decentralized university system, Toccaceli's combinations felt like home. The deep c-curves of the spine, the sense of weight in the arms, and movement originating in the pelvis that characterized everything from the warm-up to center combinations— they all connected immediately with what my body knew through years of training with teachers who were steeped in the same US midcentury modern techniques that Muller's approach drew from and expanded on.

As I pondered the gaps in my understanding of the histories that brought my bodily knowledge, accrued so many thousands of miles away, into close proximity with what we practiced in the IUNA studio, I also experienced a different kind of coordinated bodily movement that departed substantially from my experiences as a white, middle-class woman from suburban Rhode Island. In 2006, Argentina marked the thirtieth anniversary of the military coup that initiated the last military dictatorship, which began with the overthrow of Isabel Martínez de Perón in 1976 and ended in 1983 with the return of constitutional rule. The military government "disappeared" an estimated thirty thousand people accused of political "subversion" during this period. March 24, the anniversary of the 1976 coup, has been officially designated as the National Day of Memory for Truth and Justice (Día Nacional de la Memoria por la Verdad y la Justicia), and in 2006 numerous marches and cultural events took place across the city. Standing on one of the narrow streets leading to the Plaza de Mayo—Buenos Aires's central plaza and home to the government palace—I experienced that year's particularly robust annual human rights march. Thousands of participants carrying banners and chanting slogans moved past me on their way to the plaza, a historic site of activist demonstration and political spectacle alike. As they streamed down the street, the physical presence of those marching honored and called critical attention to those disappeared persons who would never move again. This choreography became one of my enduring reference points for why bodies in motion matter so concretely to calls for justice and recognition in the face of past and present political repression.

My experiences in the IUNA studio and at the march inspired the questions that have driven my research, writing, and dancing over the past twelve years. What relationship did contemporary dance have with Argentina's late-twentieth- and twenty-first-century histories of violence and activism? How did choreographers and dance works respond and/or participate? Why did English-language modern and contemporary dance historiography elide developments in Argentina that took place concurrently—and in conversation—with well-documented US and European dance histories? And why was dance absent from the substantial body of English-language scholarship on histories of cultural resistance in Argentina? In their preliminary forms, these same questions guided my undergraduate and masters theses as well as my doctoral dissertation. As a culmination of my academic and embodied work, *Moving Otherwise* addresses these historiographic gaps and argues for contemporary dance as a powerful mode of enacting politics in contexts of political and economic violence from the mid-1960s to the mid-2010s.

When I first began this project, I repeatedly encountered the notion that contemporary dance is an aesthetic exploration of the body without the same capacity for political critique that is attributed to theater, film, music, and the visual arts—genres that have celebrated histories of resistance in Argentina during the twentieth and twenty-first centuries. Many suggested that my scholarly efforts would be best put to use elsewhere. Others in the field directly or indirectly proposed that contemporary dance simply did not have the representational tools, wide-reaching platform, or even practitioner interest to make the same impact as other artistic traditions. Some also faulted what they saw as contemporary dance's bourgeois history and universalist tendencies. These ideas also emerged with some frequency in interdisciplinary academic forums—despite the insights of dance scholarship that, over the past thirty years, has historicized the construction of concert dance as universal and/or apolitical and analyzed it as a vehicle of social change. I examine this rich body of work in the introduction that follows. However, the dominant message I received as I embarked on this project was that if I was looking for art that "really" engaged with Argentina's histories of political and economic violence, contemporary dance was not it.

One case that seemed to confirm contemporary dance's alleged political shortcomings came up continually across my conversations: the suspended Danza por la Identidad (Dance for Identity) festival. In 2004, the Abuelas de Plaza de Mayo (Grandmothers of the Plaza de Mayo) announced a call for dance works that explored themes related to the memory of political violence. The Abuelas, a well-established activist group, launched an extensive project with the National Genetic Bank to reunite families separated by state violence in the postdictatorship period. The call for concert dance works was part of the expansion of their successful Teatro por la Identidad (Theater for Identity) initiative. Beginning in 2000, the Abuelas partnered with playwrights, actors, and directors on this festival, which featured productions largely (but not exclusively) related to kidnappings that occurred during the dictatorship. Throughout the 2000s, the "por la Identidad" festivals expanded rapidly to include versions that centered on art, music, and even sports. In addition to representatives of the Abuelas organization, the vetting committee for Danza por la Identidad included prestigious contemporary dance figures, such as Ana Kamien, whose early choreographies are at the center of chapter 1. The committee, however, determined that the works submitted for consideration "did not achieve the proposed theme," suggesting that the dances submitted for consideration did not adequately speak to the human rights issues at the center of the Abuelas' work over the past three decades.[3]

Ultimately, the Danza por la Identidad festival-that-was-not turned out to be something of an instructive red herring. It taught me, as critical junctures in the research process so often do, to think again about the central questions that drove my project. While there were likely many reasons the festival did not take place, the fact that multiple members of the dance community remembered and reported it as evidence of dance's political disconnection represented a broader problematic. What do we miss if we look for—and measure—dance's political engagement through the more highly visible repertoires of activist performance that have garnered repeated scholarly attention? To be sure, iconic Argentine activist and performance movements, like the Teatro por la Identidad festival, the Madres (Mothers) and Abuelas de Plaza de Mayo, H.I.J.O.S. ("children" in Spanish, an acronym for Hijos e Hijas por la Identidad y la Justicia contra el Olvido y el Silencio [Sons and Daughters for Identity and Justice Against Forgetting and Silence]), and Teatro Abierto (Open Theater), among others, are outlined throughout this book, as are contemporary dance's intersection with and citation of them. At the same time, however, *Moving Otherwise* is a concerted effort to trace the politics of Buenos Aires-based contemporary dance on its own terms. If the reader finds that *Moving Otherwise* errs toward an emphasis on how dance functions as a resistive force—even as it accounts for dance's replication of normative power dynamics—this is a response, in part, to the notion that dance is somehow less equipped to intervene in histories of violence than are other artistic traditions.

Across my years of research on this project—which combined archival research, interviews, and my own embodied participation with active groups—Buenos Aires-based contemporary dance and dancers taught me to read politics in movements "otherwise." As I detail in the introduction, "moving otherwise" as a concept names how contemporary dance offers alternatives to, and sometimes critiques of, the patterns of movement and bodily comportment that shape everyday life in contexts marked by violence. Over the course of my research, I talked to dancers who drew on their training to navigate the military's surveillance of the public sphere, danced with young people who saw their movement practice as a way of connecting with violent histories they had not personally experienced, and learned of previously undocumented connections between contemporary dance and 1970s leftist political militancy. Through these histories, and many others recounted in this book, a conception of danced politics emerged that addressed a wider range of interventions and exposed the central role of movement within modern state power.

While not always as spectacular in sheer scale and public visibility as the human rights march I witnessed on March 24, 2006, it was precisely these histories of dance that collectively helped me clarify why the movement that characterized the march constituted a kind of politics in and of itself. These dance histories also illuminate—to return to the IUNA classroom—Argentina's role in the global development of contemporary dance. While demonstrating how contemporary dance practices reflected and shaped the politics of movement in quotidian contexts marked by bodily precarity, *Moving Otherwise* aims to both attest to and honor all that dance and dancers do. The final stanza of a poem written by Argentine dancer and choreographer Nora Codina captures this spirit and offers a fitting point of departure. She writes:

> In every ordinary event,
> however insignificant,
> lives the inexhaustible germ of emotion.
> Dance should ignite it into an explosion.[4]

Moving Otherwise aims to illuminate how contemporary dance repeatedly has ignited political critique. It also, in its theoretical and historical approach, aims to ignite new ways of thinking about dance and politics in Argentina and beyond.

ACKNOWLEDGMENTS

This project came to fruition thanks to the generosity, support, and care of an incredible network of mentors, scholars, artists, and friends across the Americas. It all began, as so many dance studies projects do, in the studio. Thank you to Julie Strandberg, Laura Bennett, and Mary Gendreau for creating a space in which modern dance technique, dance history, and an intergenerational dance company not only coexisted but also actively informed one another. Their integration of theory and practice shaped the course of my professional life and continues to guide my approaches to research and teaching. At Brown University, Patricia Ybarra, Esther Whitfield, and Rebecca Schneider were the first to foster the seeds of the ideas developed here as well as my journey into dance scholarship. I am so grateful for their continued guidance and support at every step of my academic career.

As a graduate student in Performance Studies at Northwestern University, I was incredibly fortunate to work with a group of scholars whose mentorship and work continue to inspire and sustain me. Ramón Rivera-Servera's keen insight has shepherded this project for years. He not only taught me to attend acutely to ethnographic detail and render it in language that gives it life on the page, but also generously welcomed me to Chicago the same year as his own arrival at Northwestern. Susan Manning's detailed feedback and vast knowledge have supported and driven this work in profound ways. Her insights on how to best read the gaps fundamentally shaped how I approached this project. Marcela Fuentes also provided invaluable insights during my dissertation defense that I carried with me as I revised this project time and again. I am also deeply grateful to colleagues and friends that I first met through the Northwestern graduate community. Thank you to Kemi Adeyemi, Lisa Biggs, Karima Borni, Andrew Brown, Hilary Cooperman, Meiver De la Cruz, Kareem Khubchandani, Gregory Mitchell, Sage Morgan-Hubbard, Kim Singletary, and Munjulika Tarah for your friendship and ongoing engagement with my work.

I was extremely fortunate to land among the corn and soy fields of northern Ohio following my graduate studies. A Mellon Postdoctoral Fellowship in the Dance Department at Oberlin College provided time and funds to complete additional research toward this project and to envision the leap from doctoral dissertation to book. During my time at Oberlin and since, Ann Cooper

Albright has been an incredible mentor and guiding force. She models how to successfully weave together scholarship, embodiment, pedagogy, and service to the field in ways that I aspire to and thoroughly admire. I thank her for teaching me that there are times for wings and times for claws, and how to discern the difference. The Ohio winters were made far brighter thanks to Myrna García, Evangeline Heiliger, Melanie Huska, Julie Keller, and Julie Kleinman who all offered feedback and nourishing meals at a critical point in this project.

I completed this book in Portland, Oregon, during my first years as an Assistant Professor in the Dance Department at Reed College. Thank you to my colleagues, Carla Mann and Minh Tran, who warmly welcomed me and supported this project as it took its final form. I am deeply indebted to the small but mighty theater, dance, and performance writing group. Kate Bredeson, Kate Duffly, and Elliot Leffler read drafts of every chapter of this book, some twice. They so generously made time to engage with my work amid demanding teaching and production schedules. I am also grateful for Michelle Wang's camaraderie as we navigated our first years as new faculty. I would not have made it to the finish line without them. At Reed I also have been fortunate to work with student research assistants who went above and beyond. Hannah MacKenzie-Margulies conducted thorough secondary source research, Ezra Unterseher and Jack Witcher digitized hours of video that helped to make this book's companion website possible, and Olivia Hasencamp meticulously assembled bibliographic material, formatted endnotes, and proofread. They did so while patiently listening to and challenging my ideas about dance and politics in the ways that great students do. And last but not least, thank you to Nigel Nicholson and the Office of the Dean of Faculty for generous funding that enabled the completion of this book.

This project benefited tremendously from the support of grants and fellowships that allowed me to spend short as well as extended periods of time in Buenos Aires; in particular, a Fulbright facilitated one year of continuous residency in Argentina. A number of seminars and workshops also provided critical forums for feedback on chapters at multiple stages. I am thankful for the insights of members of the Mellon Dance Studies in/and the Humanities community, gained through my participation in the 2012 summer seminar and 2016 publication seminar. Thank you also to the members of the 2015 Alliance to Advance Liberal Arts Colleges "The Age of Unnatural Disasters" workshop as well as the "Human Rights, Political Action, and Performance in the Americas" working group of the American Society for Theatre Research; members of both provided helpful feedback on chapter 5. At Oxford University Press, Norm Hirschy has been a supportive and patient editor, and I am so grateful for his championing of this work. He secured anonymous readers who offered incredibly helpful feedback at multiple points in the project. I also am thankful to

Helen Eby for her work editing my translations, Wendy Weckwerth and Jan A. Maas for their editorial work, and Ana Rivas for transcribing interviews.

I am fortunate to have been welcomed by members of the growing Buenos Aires dance studies community, who have pushed my thinking and circulated my work in the most generous of ways. I am especially grateful to María Eugenia Cadús for her insights on the introduction as well as for her friendship and conference companionship. Patricia Dorin and Juan Ignacio Vallejos graciously opened their classrooms to my work. Thank you also to Carlos Fos of the Documentation Center of the General San Martín Theater for his assistance in locating documents and navigating uneven archival terrain, as well as to librarians and archivists at the Torcuato Di Tella University Library, the National Library of the Argentine Republic, and Memoria Abierta. Thank you also to Nicolás Licera Vidal and Andrés Barragán for their generous assistance procuring the cover image. While so many have lent generous eyes and ears toward the completion of this project, any errors or omissions are of course my own.

This book is most deeply indebted to the choreographers and dancers whose presence lives in these pages and whose artistic and quotidian struggles and successes are the reason for its existence. Throughout my years of research, I never ceased to be amazed by the overwhelming generosity of time and spirit that met my requests for interviews, follow-up interviews, phone calls, archival materials, rehearsal visits, and all the other encounters and re-encounters that make dance research go. Susana Tambutti, whose choreographic work initially inspired this project, first agreed to meet a nervous undergraduate student at the American Dance Festival, and later invited me into her home, classroom, and research community. A brilliant choreographer and committed dance scholar, Susana and her work were quite literally the catalysts for this book. Margarita Bali, Ana Deutsch, Susana Zimmermann, Vivian Luz, Ana Kamien, Silvia Vladimivsky, Alicia Sanguinetti, Nora Codina, and so many others all hosted me in their homes many times and repeatedly opened their private archives, kitchens, and studios to me. I am so grateful to all those that I interviewed, too numerous to list here but all named in the bibliography, for the time they offered to speak with me. I am especially indebted to Aurelia Chillemi, Catherine de la Trinidad, and to the members, past and present, of the Bailarines Toda la Vida (Dancers for Life) community dance project. Performing with this group not only informed chapter 5 but also changed the course of my dancing life. The collective gave me a new perspective on dance, politics, and being together in difference that has given direction and purpose to my work inside and outside of the studio.

Book projects, as we well know, are labors of love not only for authors but also for those closest to them. Thank you to my dear friend Jennifer Schaefer, trusted travel companion, editor extraordinaire, and fellow devotee to dance and all the secrets Buenos Aires's archives hold. I am so grateful for her friendship, which has crossed decades and continents. I am certain that I have run every aspect of this book, small and large, by her at some point. At every step of the process, she reminded me that as scholars the histories we write (and read) are necessarily imperfect, and she also shared document after document from her own carefully compiled research. My parents, Robert Fortuna and Mary Cardillo Fortuna, have been sources of endless support. They never questioned why dance, or why dance scholarship. They have traveled far and wide as our family network grew past the borders of the United States, and they are still coming to see my dance shows (even though now I'm mostly in the wings as a faculty member). During the last year of work on this book, my mother cooked a multitude of meals that quite literally fueled its completion. My dear late grandparents, John and Victoria Cardillo, would be so glad to know that there is finally something to put on the shelf. My mother-in-law Rocio Flores has offered my family gracious support and care from Ecuador during the completion of the book. And finally, my deepest thanks to my partner, Hugo Granja Flores. This book is for him. We met in Buenos Aires as I was starting to sense the beginnings of this project, and he has been there every step of the way. And steps there have been many, across distances and together in the same place, from Argentina, to Ecuador, to Rhode Island, to Illinois, to Ohio, and to Oregon. He is a dancer even if he doesn't want to admit it, and always has been able to describe my work to others more succinctly and clearly than I ever have. There will never quite be the right words to express the extent of my gratitude for his unwavering patience, love, and support.

Finally, I am grateful to those who granted permission to use portions of previously published material. An earlier version of the analysis of Susana Tambutti's *La puñalada* (*The Stab*) featured in chapter 4 first appeared as "A Dance of Many Bodies: Moving Trauma in Susana Tambutti's *La puñalada*" in *Performance Research* 16:1, pages 43–51 (2011). Arguments presented in chapter 5 were first published in "Between the Cultural Center and the *Villa*: Dance, Neoliberalism and Silent Borders in Buenos Aires" from *The Oxford Handbook of Dance and Politics*, edited by Kowal, R. J., Siegmund, G., and Martin, R., pages 371–394, (2017), used with permission of Oxford University Press, USA. Lastly, an earlier version of chapter 5's analysis of Daniel Payero Zaragoza's *Retazos pequeños de nuestra historia más reciente* (*Small Pieces of Our Recent History*) first appeared in "An Enormous Yearning for the Past: Movement/Archive in Two Contemporary Dance Works" in *e-misférica* 9.1–9.2 (2012), http://hemisphericinstitute.org/hemi/en/e-misferica-91/fortuna.

ABOUT THE COMPANION WEBSITE

www.oup.com/us/movingotherwise

Oxford University Press has created a companion website for *Moving Otherwise*, www.oup.com/us/movingotherwise. The website features full-length works or clips from ten of the dances analyzed in this book. Few of these works are publicly accessible, and making them available through this platform aims to support the use of the book in the classroom. These videos not only further illuminate the movement descriptions and arguments presented in the text, but also allow readers to develop their own interpretations of the works under discussion.

Video clips are indicated throughout the book with Oxford's symbol ⊙ and are arranged by chapter and clip number.

The Dancing Body on the Line

An Introduction

On September 22, 2010, I attended a vibrant—and at times contentious—discussion on a proposed National Dance Law (Ley Nacional de Danza) held at the Cooperation Cultural Center (Centro Cultural de la Cooperación) in downtown Buenos Aires. The stakes were high. If passed, the legislation would establish comprehensive state support for dance production in the federal capital of Buenos Aires as well as in Argentina's twenty-three provinces.[1] The *charla*, or presentation, was held as part of a festival presented by the organization Associated Contemporary Choreographers-Independent Dance Theater (Coreógrafos Contemporáneos Asociados-Danza Teatro Independiente). The proposed legislation had developed through a grass-roots movement that members of the independent contemporary dance community initiated in 2008 (echoing earlier efforts stretching back to the 1980s); in the Argentine context, "independent" refers to dance production outside of companies supported by federal and municipal theaters and institutions.[2] Choreographers Mariela Ruggieri, Gabily Anadón, and Eugenia Schvartzman led the discussion, which aimed to capitalize on the festival's attendance to familiarize the contemporary dance community with the legislation and to gather signatures in anticipation of its presentation before Argentina's National Congress.[3]

The air buzzed with questions. First, how did the law define dance? Though the project had gestated among contemporary dancers, the discussion leaders urged attendees to consider the advantages of joining forces with professional practitioners of tango, folklore, African diasporic dance, *murga* (a popular form most visible during Carnival), and ballet. In addition to considering the benefits of creating this kind of coalition, attendees hotly debated the possibility of adding the term "movement" to the title of the law (i.e., National

Dance and Movement Law). For some, "movement" represented inclusive language that rejected implicit genre hierarchies that privilege concert (high art) over social and popular forms (low art). For others, the "movement" question was a debate best kept internal to the dance community, because lawmakers might interpret the term as an attempt to secure state funds for work that did not adhere to standards of artistic rigor, thus endangering the law's passage. This, in turn, led to questions about how to determine funding criteria and to debates around what committees or organizations would be best qualified to administer the law. While debating the language, scope, and structure of the law, the conversation turned to even more fundamental questions: What is (or should be) the relationship between dance production and the state? What does a social movement *for dance* look like? And perhaps most fundamentally, how could legislators be convinced that dance deserves recognition in the eyes of the state? The discussion that day lasted well over three hours.

In the years since the 2010 *charla*, work in support of the National Dance Law developed into a large-scale activist movement. The National Dance Law movement represented a renewed attempt to secure comprehensive federal support for work happening across the provinces, augmenting earlier municipal legislation that had focused exclusively on Buenos Aires where concert dance production had concentrated throughout the twentieth century.[4] In addition to the continued development and revision of the proposed law itself, dancers across Argentina occupied the streets and government chambers to demonstrate their support.[5] Flash mobs, open classes, and other danced demonstrations brought together the dance community on the April 2014 International Day of Dance, when lawmakers introduced the law to Congress.[6] While the Buenos Aires activities occupied the plaza in front of the Congress building (a historic site of political demonstration), social media-savvy organizers asked dancers outside the capital to create "moving postcards" (*postales móviles*). Uploaded to YouTube and shared on Facebook with the tag "I support the National Dance Law," these videos of dancers of all ages and genres moving across studios, stages, and streets established strong virtual connections among supporters and evidenced the breadth and vitality of dance practices across the nation.[7] Mobilization for the law emphasized more than Argentine dance's present; on October 10, 2014 (Argentina's National Day of Dance), organizers held an event in the Congress building to honor seventy influential figures in Argentine dance history and to encourage legislators to discuss the law.[8] The event directly connected prominent dance figures with the interests and responsibilities of the state. Using these embodied and digital tactics, dancers used their moving bodies to call for recognition not only of the dance community as a critical mass but also of dance as a valuable form of cultural labor with a well-established history in Argentina. As the law continued to make its way through Congress, the movement organized ongoing meetings, debates, and demonstrations across the country.[9]

At first glance, the largescale movement for the National Dance Law appears exceptional within Argentine dance history. The law seems to represent an unusual entrance of the dance community into the business of politics traditionally defined: the appeal to and negotiation with the state for recognition, rights, and resources vis-à-vis formally articulated policy and legislative action. The group of contemporary dancers who envisioned and fought for the passage of the law undoubtedly entered unfamiliar territory as they courted federal representatives, learned the convoluted legislative process, worked to mobilize the dance community across genres, and organized mass danced demonstrations. As an activist movement that deployed the tools of direct action, the National Dance Law project visibly aligned the dance community with Argentina's rich history of political and social movements—topics that have garnered considerable scholarly attention.

In my eyes, however, this recent example of Argentine dancers putting their bodies on the line—in this case as advocates for the long-term stability and sustainability of their craft—extended a less-documented tradition. This legislation built on a long, less visible history of Buenos Aires-based dance: one in which contemporary dancers engaged politically on and off the theatrical stage, albeit generally in modes that intersected less explicitly with traditional political processes and activist tactics. *Moving Otherwise* takes up this history, examining how contemporary dance practices enacted politics within climates of political and economic violence from the mid-1960s to the mid-2010s.

Mobilization around the National Dance Law first developed within the relative political stability of President Cristina Fernández de Kirchner's populist, left-wing administration (2007–15). A range of state violence, however, had marked the rise of contemporary dance practice in Buenos Aires during the late twentieth century. During the previous five decades, contemporary dancers and audiences consistently responded to and reimagined the movement landscapes that have accompanied Argentina's volatile political history. From the repression of the military dictatorships of the 1960s, 1970s, and early 1980s to the physical toll exacted by the landscapes of economic inequality that marked the 1990s and 2000s, Argentine bodies consistently faced quotidian choreographies defined by strict control and physical censure. For example, during the period of the last military dictatorship (1976–83), Argentines walking, standing, or otherwise occupying city streets feared kidnapping, forced disappearance, and torture.[10] This brutally repressive regime claimed the lives of an estimated thirty thousand people accused of political "subversion." To control citizen bodies and foreclose mobilization, the government banned mass gatherings in public and private spaces. In that climate, the masses of dancing bodies that flooded the Plaza del Congreso in Buenos Aires and animated *postales móviles* shot on city streets across the nation would have been unthinkable.

Yet, despite the injunction against public gathering, the Buenos Aires dance community found a way to strategically rechoreograph movement through the public sphere and reaffirm the value of dance. In December 1981, hundreds of spectators waited in a line that wrapped around a full city block. Defying fear as well as official government policy, these spectators assembled for ostensibly artistic rather than political reasons. However, as they gathered to attend the Danza Abierta (Open Dance) festival, they also took a boldly political stance against military control. Willing to take on visibility and vulnerability to view a dance festival staged against state violence and censorship, both spectators and dancers involved in Danza Abierta performed inclusion and community in the face of a military regime intent on stilling and separating bodies. Histories such as this one, in which dancers and audiences together disrupt dominant patterns of movement, drive this book.

While the last military dictatorship looms largest in Argentina's recent history, multiple authoritarian governments marked an even earlier period, following populist President Juan Domingo Perón's ousting by the military in 1955. Throughout the late 1950s and 1960s, a series of military governments disassembled the welfare state and began to target the left as part of the ongoing global Cold War. After Perón's brief return to power in 1973 and death in 1974, violence between conservative military factions and right- and left-leaning militant groups grew, culminating in the 1976 military coup d'état. Elected following the return to democracy in 1983, President Raúl Alfonsín made initial motions to address legacies of violence, but the truncation of trials of military leaders made national healing all the more difficult. Following broader trends across the Southern Cone, as the southernmost areas of South America are often termed, neoliberal policies intensified under Carlos Menem's presidency (1989–99) and concentrated class power throughout the 1990s. Violent confrontations between citizens and the state again engulfed Argentina in December 2001 under the presidency of Fernando de la Rúa; the economic ravages left by the dictatorships and compounded by 1990s policies resulted in an unprecedented economic collapse the effects of which are ongoing. As it moves across the decades, *Moving Otherwise* engages a wide range of dance practices that span concert works, community dance initiatives, and the everyday labor that animates dance, including rehearsals, classes, and urban travels to and from theaters and studios. This book demonstrates how these diverse practices represent, resist, and remember violence and engender new forms of mobilization on and off the theatrical stage.

To theorize how dance intervenes politically in contexts of political and economic violence, the book develops the notion of "moving otherwise." Moving otherwise names how concert dance—and its offstage practice and consumption—offers alternatives to, and sometimes critiques, the patterns of movement and bodily comportment that shape everyday life in contexts marked by violence. Dancer Déborah Kalmar's words, offered during our interview, distill how this book develops and invokes the concept of moving otherwise. As she contemplated the relationship between movement practices and repressive governments, Kalmar incisively captured the political stakes of movement in twentieth- and twenty-first-century Argentina: "It's as if someone else, not oneself, is moving. There is a reason why the most explicit, implicit, or covert forms of repression have to do with restraining the body."[11] With this statement, Kalmar's words recall political theorist Hannah Arendt's understanding of the relationship between movement and repression. For Arendt, terror "stabilizes" bodies in order to unleash a totalitarian regime's "law of movement" that seeks out and destroys an "objective enemy," that is, unruly bodies.[12] For both Kalmar and Arendt, disciplinary power functions through movement technologies that regulate (i.e., "stabilize") bodies, while movements otherwise expose their limits.[13]

As Kalmar points out, bodies are "stabilized" through both explicit and implicit repertoires that enforce particular modes of embodying citizenship: performing gender, sexuality, race, and class, and circulating through and occupying public space. While explicit forms of political violence (particularly during periods of military dictatorship) frequently enforced normative "laws of movement" in late twentieth-century Argentina, this book also attends to what Rob Nixon calls "slow violence." Nixon's concept names the "delayed destruction" that neoliberal capitalism inflicts; slow violence is "neither spectacular nor instantaneous, but rather accretive."[14] While Nixon's study focuses on environmentally embedded violence, slow violence also characterizes the attritional nature of the bodily precarity that market conditions produced in the decades leading up to and following the 2001 economic crisis. Across its chapters, *Moving Otherwise* tracks both explicit (forced disappearance, torture) and slow (economic precarity, displacement) forms of violence and argues for how dance practices on and off the stage create opportunities for moving otherwise.

Movements otherwise enact politics that echo and sometimes directly cite the Argentine activist concept *poner el cuerpo* (literally "to put the body," or "to put the body on the line"). Scholars trace the emergence of this phrase to leftist activists in the 1960s.[15] Throughout the second half of the twentieth century, resistance movements repeatedly invoked *poner el cuerpo* as a rallying cry against political and economic violence. As sociologist Barbara Sutton explains in the context of her study of feminist activism following Argentina's 2001 economic crisis:

> *Poner el cuerpo* overlaps somewhat with "to put the body on the line" and to "give the body," but it transcends both notions. With respect to political agency, *poner el cuerpo* means not just to talk, think, or desire but to be really present and involved; to put the whole (embodied) being into action, to be committed to a social cause, and to assume the bodily risks, work, and demands of such a

commitment. *Poner el cuerpo* is part of the vocabulary of resistance in Argentina, and implies the importance of material bodies in the transformation of social relations and history.[16]

As a practice, *poner el cuerpo* values embodied action as central to political and social change, emphasizing the bodily risk and literal physicality involved with direct action. While the efficacy of *poner el cuerpo* at times is measured by juridical or legislative strides (the goal of the National Dance Law movement), the concept's ethics more often emphasize a diverse and situated range of what bodies in motion can affect (e.g., Danza Abierta spectators lining up in defiance of the regime). Though dancers only began to use the term in the early 2000s as a way to connect their work to traditional forms of activism, this book demonstrates how diverse forms of moving otherwise instantiated an ethics of *poner el cuerpo* across the late twentieth and early twenty-first centuries. In response to a range of violent social contexts, dancers engendered alternate steps that facilitated community, critiqued violence, afforded networks of bodily care, embodied cultural memory, supported political movements, and defied gendered and classed norms. This book contends that in a social and political context where the regulation of bodies repeatedly has taken center stage, Argentine contemporary dance history offers a privileged site for understanding the role of corporeality in state politics as well as resistance movements.

In its remaining pages, this introduction moves through an overview of *Moving Otherwise*'s theoretical and historical interventions. It first lays out the concept of moving otherwise, outlining the kinds of political engagement it encompasses as well as how it dialogues with broader conversations in dance and performance studies. It then explains how the category of "contemporary" dance functions in this text, and argues for an approach to the telling of contemporary dance history that decenters the United States and Europe as the original sites and ongoing loci of production. Additionally, it offers a brief overview of the transnational history of modern and contemporary dance in Buenos Aires that situates and previews the breadth of practices of moving otherwise documented in this book. Finally, it details the multiple research methodologies that *Moving Otherwise* employs and offers an overview of the book's chapters.

MOVING OTHERWISE

Throughout this book, the concept of moving otherwise functions both as a way of theorizing the relationship between movement and politics and as an interpretive strategy for reading the political effects of Buenos Aires-based contemporary dance. As a conceptualization of the relationship between movement and politics, moving otherwise maintains that the regulation of bodies in motion—how they move and where they can move—is a central function of modern state power and thus a critical point of negotiating new political possibilities. Michel Foucault, Giorgio Agamben, and Achille Mbembe have demonstrated powerfully how the management of life and death, what Foucault terms "biopolitics," establishes and extends the limits of state power.[17] While violent regimes make the management of citizens' bodies and their movements explicit, movement is also germane to the establishment and maintenance of social orders more broadly. Andrew Hewitt captures this notion in the concept of social choreography; for Hewitt, social orders are instilled in and performed at the level of the body.[18]

Movements otherwise accrue political agency through their negotiation of the normative movement patterns that shape and sustain social orders, or what dance scholar André Lepecki, drawing on Jacques Rancière, terms "choreopolice." In Rancière's theorization, "police" is not limited to law enforcement, but rather names the forces that hold the social order in place. The police maintain what Rancière calls the "partition of the sensible," or the boundary that separates modes of action and being that are sanctioned from those that are not.[19] For Rancière, the police do not hail subjects vis-à-vis the law, as in Louis Althusser's oft-cited formulation, but rather condition bodies to "move along" through sanctioned patterns of circulation. As Rancière writes, "The police is that which says that here, on this street, there's nothing to see and so nothing to do but move along. It asserts that the space for circulating is nothing but the space of circulation."[20] Lepecki understands Rancière's police as a fundamentally kinetic force, and adapts this concept into explicitly choreographic terms.[21] Choreopolicing "imposes a forced ontological fitting between pregiven movements, bodies in conformity, and pre-assigned spaces for circulation."[22] Recall the stakes of moving through public space during the last military dictatorship. Choreopolicing not only accounts for the laws that criminalized gatherings in public and private space, but also for the "pregiven movements" to which citizens adhered for survival.[23] Dancers frequently described how obeying the law was simply not enough. Bodies additionally performed highly codified choreographies of gender, class, sexuality, and loyal citizenship to avoid suspicion of subversion.

The lines outside of Danza Abierta constituted movements otherwise because they instantiated what Lepecki theorizes as a tactical response to choreopolicing: choreopolitics. Choreopolitics "requires a redistribution and reinvention of bodies, affects, and senses through which one may learn how to move politically . . . . It is the dancer who, in the most controlled spaces (say even in the tightest of choreographic scores), has the potential to activate the appearing not necessarily of a subject, but of the highly mobile *political thing*."[24] Following Kalmar's observations, moving otherwise names the emergence of the "highly mobile political thing" within Argentina's particular histories of bodily repression. Political agency, in this sense, is not achieved through a consistent or clearly defined activist and/or aesthetic program. It is, to invoke movement theorist Erin Manning's understanding of embodied politics, "an effect of situated practices."[25] The lines to enter the Danza Abierta performance did not dialogue directly with the everyday business of doing politics (lawmaking, etc.) nor did they deploy recognizable repertoires of political protest; however, as a situated practice, they exemplified a powerful form of political movement in light of the dictatorship's choreopolicing.

By illuminating the centrality of movement to life under authoritarianism, *Moving Otherwise* builds on the robust body of English-language scholarship that employs performance as a lens for understanding the power dynamics of Argentina's last military dictatorship and analyzes theater and performance as sites of political resistance and practices of memory in its wake.[26] Diana Taylor's concept of "percepticide"—which names how visual spectacles of violence resulted in forms of self-blinding that solidified the military's control over Argentines—emphasizes the visual economy of political violence.[27] Likewise, scholarship on resistance movements and initiatives to honor the memory of disappeared persons considers the powerful ways performers and activists have made histories of violence visible nationally and internationally.[28] *Moving Otherwise* extends this scholarship on spectatorship and witnessing to consider the ways in which movement practices and staged choreographies not only illuminate the corporeal machinations of state power, but also provide opportunities for bodily care and connection foreclosed in day-to-day life.

While the examples I have offered so far—the movement for the National Dance Law and Danza Abierta's lines—highlight the political import of offstage choreographies, *Moving Otherwise* is equally invested in the dancing that happens on concert stages and in studios. As an interpretive strategy for reading the political effects of contemporary dance practices, moving otherwise crosses the distinction that frequently shapes discussions of dance and politics: "political dance" versus "the politics of dance."[29] Where "political dance" signals movement practices whose content exposes or critiques past or present injustices and/or aligns itself with a particular cause or activist movement, "the politics of dance" directs critical attention to the political economies, modes of production, institutional affiliations, identitarian positions, and local, national, and transnational linkages that materialize dance. Within the dance and performance studies fields, this book joins a vibrant scholarly conversation that develops the "political" and "politics of" lines of inquiry, and often the intersection of both. Book-length studies on political dance have focused frequently on leftist dance in New York City in the 1930s; the emphasis on forming alliances with workers that characterizes this movement resonates with multiple practices considered in *Moving Otherwise*.[30] Dance scholarship also has explored the relationship between dance production and state politics, analyzed dance as a site for articulating racialized and gendered political identities, examined dance's relationship to political economic frameworks, and probed the philosophical and theoretical dimensions of dance and politics.[31] *Moving Otherwise* joins this scholarly conversation as it calls attention to the centrality of movement to contemporary state power, from military dictatorship to free-market politics.

Moving Otherwise takes up dance works that speak to explicitly political themes, charts Argentine contemporary dance's connections to political movements, and attends to the politics that shaped dance production in Buenos Aires. This book also emphasizes how a breadth of danced movements otherwise intervened, often subtly, in the choreopolicing that marked climates of political and economic violence. At times, dance moved otherwise by deliberately *not* referencing (at least directly) the current political context and taking advantage of dance's presumed distance from the realm of "real" politics and/or resistance. For example, Alejandro Cervera's 1983 *Dirección obligatoria* (*One Way*), which premiered in the ashes of the last military dictatorship, makes no specific reference to the Argentine national context or to explicit violence—a move that protected the choreographer from government attention. The choreography of the piece, however, features dancers restricted to a "one way" movement path from right to the left side of the stage (from the perspective of the viewer). In chapter 3, I argue that the piece instantiated the military dictatorship's grip on bodily movement. In chapter 2, I consider a group of contemporary dancers who were members of leftist militant organizations in the early 1970s. I demonstrate how dance classes organized for fellow political prisoners at the Rawson Penitentiary actually functioned as rehearsals for movement used in a prison break. The prison guards, who ostensibly regarded the dance classes as an innocuous form of exercise, never suspected other motives.

Both subtle and explicit examples of moving otherwise expose not only dance's resistive potential, but also how dance practices and quotidian movements themselves "choreopolice," or maintain normative power relations. As scholar Mark Franko notes, "dance can absorb and retain the effects of political power as well as resist the very effects it appears to incorporate within the same gesture."[32] Throughout its chapters, *Moving Otherwise* marks this simultaneity, maintaining that while movements otherwise rechoreograph normative social orders, they are inevitably imbued with them. The stakes, of course, of adhering to or breaking from the norm are particularly high within climates of political and economic violence, where life and death are quite literally at stake. To read how dance practices both reinscribe political power and move otherwise to it, I follow the nuance and grace of Rachmi Diyah Larasati's *The Dance That Makes You Vanish: Cultural Reconstruction in Post-Genocide Indonesia*. To date, Larasati's text is one of the first studies to take up the relationship between dance and twentieth-century histories of political violence in the global south.[33] Drawing in part on auto-ethnographic accounts of her experiences as a state-employed Indonesian national troupe dancer, Larasati demonstrates how state-patronized dance extended mechanisms of state repression by marketing a harmonious image of national identity. At the same time, the Indonesian national troupe granted dancers forms of social mobility that, in Larasati's view, "can become a powerful form of resistance."[34] Larasati's text, in its delicate and deeply attuned approach to traumatic histories, offers a model for tracking the nuances of contemporary dance's resistive and hegemonic moves across Argentina's periods of dictatorship and economic crisis.

ON THE CATEGORY OF CONTEMPORARY DANCE

Moving Otherwise employs the category of "contemporary" to draw together the diverse group of practices considered in this book. As scholars working across the global north and south aptly have pointed out, "contemporary" is a fraught classification that eludes neat temporal or aesthetic categorization, though it typically signals some relationship to the Western concert tradition. Argentina is no exception, with debates arising around distinctions between contemporary, modern, and dance theater, as well as works that incorporate social and/or folkloric forms. Generally speaking, practitioners, critics, and historians in Argentina use the term "modern" to refer to the early- and mid-twentieth-century modernist techniques developed by influential artists, including Mary Wigman and Martha Graham in Germany and the United States, respectively. During the 1940s and 1950s, *danza moderna* (modern dance) was the term used to describe the development of US and German strands of modern dance in Buenos Aires, though the term persists and is invoked in relationship to some of the practices I examine in this book. However, by *Moving Otherwise*'s point of departure in the 1960s, *danza contemporánea* (contemporary dance) began to appear as a way of naming the increasingly heterogeneous field of nonclassical concert dance production. During this decade, the choreographers I consider explicitly challenged *danza moderna*'s received pedagogical and aesthetic principles, and understood their work as emergent—yet distinct—from *danza moderna*. I have chosen to begin the book in the mid-1960s precisely because of the ways these artistic shifts corresponded with the series of military dictatorships that took root following President Perón's ouster in 1955 and signaled, on the part of the choreographers I analyze, a shift toward understanding their practice as deeply rooted in and responsive to Argentine political and cultural realities.[35]

Use of the term "contemporary" increased throughout the 1970s and 1980s and reached dominance during the 1990s. Contemporary dance now functions as an umbrella term that encompasses a wide range of practices that draw on modern, postmodern, ballet, German expressionism, release technique, dance theater (variously defined), *expresión corporal* (corporeal expression, a practice first developed in Argentina in the 1950s), and conceptual choreography. In some instances, "contemporary" also encompasses engagements with social and folkloric practices—such as the tango, the much-mythologized social dance form that first emerged in Buenos Aires at the turn of the twentieth century. *Moving Otherwise* invokes the term "contemporary" in the pluralistic capacity that marks its current usage. However, throughout the book I am careful to attend to the distinct traditions that inform the practices under discussion. For clarity, I use "modern" when referring to pre-1960s production and "contemporary" in reference to the particular practices and concert works considered here that span from the mid-1960s to the mid-2010s.[36]

In addition to following the term's current use in Argentina, I have also opted for "contemporary" because, as Argentine dance historian Marcelo Isse Moyano points out, the debates about modernism that characterize North American scholarship on US modern versus postmodern dance do not translate cleanly to the Argentine context.[37] Similarly, discussions of the categories of dance theater and contemporary dance in the European context, while helpful for thinking through transnational connections, should not be taken as explanatory frameworks for the Argentine context.[38] Though the category of the contemporary in *Moving Otherwise* does not signal a discrete technique, stylistic tendency, or historical periodization, it produces the conditions of possibility for working through a diverse range of practices that broadly share a common lineage and move otherwise in relationship to Argentine histories of political and economic violence. That is, rather than proposing a temporal or aesthetic definition of "the contemporary," this book considers the critical work the term can do to manifest how a select set of on- and offstage movements embody politics.

As it examines how contemporary dance practices in Argentina move otherwise, this book contributes to both the historiography of modern and contemporary dance as well as the growing field of Argentine critical dance studies. Early histories narrated the development of modern and contemporary dance in Buenos Aires in relationship to the arrival of dancers from the United States and Europe and collected oral histories of prominent figures.[39] In their emphasis on key innovators—particularly those attached to state-funded institutions—these texts often privilege a teleological narrative of artistic advancement. In its focus on politics and consideration of practices outside of what some may consider "professional" (or noteworthy) contemporary dance, *Moving Otherwise* moves away from this line of inquiry and joins recent Spanish-language scholarship that is closely attuned to how dance practices shape and are shaped by broader cultural politics and social relations.[40] More broadly, this book contributes to the developing body of English-language work on concert dance forms in Latin America, which has focused especially on how dance articulates with and diverges from racialized nation-making projects in Mexico, Cuba, and Brazil.[41]

The English-language bibliography on dance in Argentina, however, continues to be dominated by work on tango.[42] Broadly speaking, monographs on dance in Latin America have focused largely on social, popular, ritual, and folkloric dance forms.[43] *Moving Otherwise* draws on these texts' insights around how social and folkloric practices articulate complex histories of race and nation. At the same time, the book extends critiques of the "dance" and "world dance" dichotomy.[44] Within this construction, "dance" (i.e., Westernized concert forms, including contemporary dance) is understood to be racially unmarked, universal, and proper to the global north, where "world dance" (i.e., "ethnic" or "cultural" forms of all varieties) is racialized, culturally particular, and southern. This is the logic, in other words, that champions the tango as emblematic of Argentine culture while historiographically absenting Buenos Aires as a past and present center of concert dance production.

Moving Otherwise examines the complex transnational flows that fomented the development of contemporary dance in Buenos Aires and argues for a globalized approach to the telling of contemporary dance history. It challenges the "dance" versus "world dance" dichotomy and proposes greater attention to (all) dance forms' transnational and colonial histories. In taking a globalized approach to contemporary dance history, *Moving Otherwise* does not define Argentine contemporary dance as a stable category with autochthonous— or universal—characteristics. Rather, it considers how Buenos Aires-based practices articulate complex relationships with national identity as well as the global cultural economy. While I opt for the term "contemporary" for the reasons outlined above, I heed scholar Emily E. Wilcox's call for global dance histories that "see modern and postmodern dance as carrying specific political and cultural values and having global relevance because of place-based histories, not because of their artistic neutrality."[45] In the following section, I chart the transnational flows that shaped, and continue to shape, the history of modern and contemporary dance in Argentina.

TRANSNATIONAL MOVES: A BRIEF HISTORY OF MODERN AND CONTEMPORARY DANCE IN ARGENTINA

Moving Otherwise excavates a history of danced politics that is both national and transnational. While this book's chapters attend carefully to how Buenos Aires-based contemporary dance practices intersect with the particularities of the Argentine nation state, the history of moving otherwise is also one of global exchange—artistic, economic, and political. Dance scholar Susan Manning outlines and advocates for the ongoing shift in dance historiography from research focused on the nation state to transnational paradigms. Throughout this book, I follow Manning's call to "integrate the nuance and detail of nation-state approaches with the sweep and generality of transnational approaches."[46] This section details the transnational artistic and economic networks of exchange that inform the contemporary dance practices I examine in the following chapters. I outline the conditions of possibility that fostered the establishment and growth of modern and later contemporary dance in Buenos Aires and trace how contemporary dance became a site for moving otherwise.

Rather than narrate an overarching history, I offer three particularly illustrative moments when global moves exemplified the "friction" that accompanied transnational exchange. Anthropologist Anna Tsing understands the "friction of global connections" as "the awkward, unequal, unstable, and creative qualities of interconnection across difference."[47] Friction, in other words, attends to the unequal power relations that govern the uneven movements of bodies, ideas, and capital across borders while also making space for the productive possibilities that arise. It accounts for both the hegemonic forces at work in transnational dance circuits as well as dancers' tactical negotiation—their movements otherwise—within global cultural economies. Thus, these cases not only provide a window into the history of modern and contemporary dance in Argentina, but also, in the spirit of this book's theoretical frame, establish how choreographers and dance works themselves historically have commented incisively on their roles as subjects and objects of global exchange.

In the mid-1940s, US-born Miriam Winslow founded the Ballet Winslow, Argentina's first modern dance company. The daughter of a wealthy New England industrialist, Winslow trained with modern dance pioneers Ted Shawn and Ruth St. Denis, among others, and performed with Shawn. In 1930, she opened the Miriam Winslow School of the Dance in Boston, which operated for a decade before she closed the school in order to prioritize her artistic partnership with Foster Fitz-Simons, a member of Shawn's all-male dance troupe.[48] Winslow had attempted to sustain a female performing group, but became frustrated when her dancers continually left for opportunities with larger companies or to start families. While the duo and some of Winslow's solo and group work received notable engagements and positive reviews, Winslow's letters suggest that she never achieved the critical acclaim she desired. As part of an effort to identify new audiences, Winslow first travelled to Buenos Aires with Fitz-Simons when the duo toured South America in 1941.[49] They were the first US modern dancers to perform in Buenos Aires since Isadora Duncan's 1916 performance at the Coliseo Theater. The *New York Times* reported that, after a slow premiere night, the Winslow-Fitz-Simons program was so well received that additional performances were added.[50]

While Winslow and Fitz-Simons may have been the first US dancers to tour Argentina since Duncan, their work resonated with middle- and upper-class audiences already well accustomed to concert dance. Argentina's capital city had an established ballet tradition; Buenos Aires is home to the oldest government supported ballet company in South America. While the Colón Theater Ballet was not founded until 1925, ballet had first gained traction in the late 1800s in the context of cultural and economic debates that figured Europe and the United States as models.[51] In the post-independence period, nation-building texts—most notably President Domingo Faustino Sarmiento's *Facundo o civilización y barbarie en la pampas argentinas* (*Facundo Or Civilization and Barbarism on the Argentine Plains*, 1845)—dreamed of modernizing Argentina's urban center and populating its vast countryside pampas with white, disciplined, and hard-working northern Europeans.[52] European immigration to Argentina boomed during the late nineteenth and early twentieth centuries, though the newly arrived population was largely southern European. Urban development projects, particularly those organized around Argentina's 1910 centennial celebrations, "Europeanized" the city, a process that urban historian Adrián Gorelik locates between the turn of the century and 1930.[53] These development projects went hand in hand with explicit construction of the nation as exceptionally white and European among Latin American nations.[54] Within this climate, the Colón Theater Ballet became tasked with both "nationalizing" ballet and supporting the broader project of constructing Argentina as part of Western modernity.[55]

Winslow and Fitz-Simons's visit also coincided roughly with the arrival—both as migrants and on tours—of prestigious performers and companies linked to German expressionism. World War I and its aftermath created a global diaspora of German and Eastern European choreographers and dancers working in the expressionist tradition, with many artists seeking refuge in Argentina and other South American countries.[56] Renate Schottelius, Margarete Wallmann, and Otto Werberg, all influential figures in the development of modern dance in Argentina with links to Mary Wigman, arrived in Buenos Aires in the 1930s. Notable tours during these years included the Ballets Jooss and multiple visits by Clotilde von Derp and Alexander Sakharoff, who later lived in Buenos Aires. This is to say that Winslow and Fitz-Simons's 1941 performances took place in a city that had become further invested in concert dance as it was marked by the forced migrations spurred by conflict in Europe. This trajectory meant that Buenos Aires was already a key nexus in the circulation of global modernisms.[57] While *Moving Otherwise* focuses on histories of political and economic violence during the late twentieth and early twenty-first centuries, the transnational flows that intersected with Winslow and Fitz-Simons's arrival demonstrate dance histories—and histories of state terror—to be always already global.

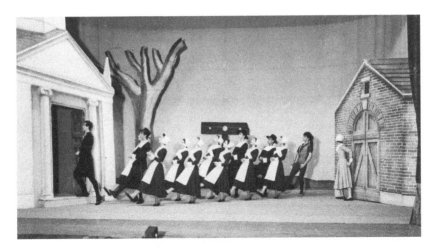

Figure I.1 Ballet Winslow in *The Scarlet Letter*, ca. 1945. Courtesy of the TWU Libraries Woman's Collection, Texas Woman's University, Denton, TX.

In 1943, without Fitz-Simons, Winslow returned to Buenos Aires, where she established and self-funded the Ballet Winslow soon after.[58] As dance historian Jody Weber points out, Winslow's choice to move to Buenos Aires likely had "complex personal and professional roots," though it seems probable that Winslow saw in Buenos Aires an untapped market.[59] That is, the city offered opportunities to work with dancers she selected (she offered a stable salary) and perform at venues of her choice to a theater-going, cosmopolitan public intrigued by the new form, possibly making up for some of the frustrations she encountered in the United States.[60] Winslow was able to secure a regular performance schedule for the Ballet Winslow, and her nationality and dance pedigree likely legitimized her role as an "ambassador" of modern dance in the eyes of Argentine critics, whose responses were largely favorable to the company's work.[61]

Notably, Winslow's letters indicate that her ultimate desire was to bring the Ballet Winslow back to the United States.[62] She felt the work she created in Argentina was her best.[63] Ballet Winslow's repertory explored "American" themes (her work based on Hawthorne's *The Scarlet Letter* was frequently performed) as well as "South American" ones (figure I.1). Photographs of *Andean Impressions*, for example, feature Winslow clad in a shawl and cotton skirt characteristic of those worn by Andean indigenous women (figure I.2). Winslow, it seems, extended a tradition of white, US-born female modern dance "mothers" whose leadership as choreographers challenged gender norms at the same time that their choreographic work essentialized racial difference through primitivized representations of non-white others, a move that reinforced their own whiteness as it fostered career mobility.[64] Ultimately, Winslow was unable to secure financing for a US tour—traveling such a great

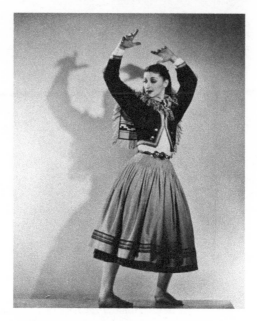

Figure I.2 Miriam Winslow in *Andean Impressions*. Photograph by Marcus Blechman. Courtesy of the Trustees of the Boston Public Library.

distance with her large company was simply too costly. Winslow eventually moved back to the United States, disappointed that her work in Argentina would not be recognized in her home country. Even if Winslow found satisfaction in her role as a modern dance "pioneer" in Argentina, she sought the legitimization of her work before a US audience as the true arbiters of her artistry. Though friction impeded Winslow's recognition on the other side of the hemisphere, members of her company would go on to be central figures in the development of modern dance in Buenos Aires. Schottelius, Paulina Ossona, Cecilia Ingenieros, Luisa Grinberg, Élide Locardi, Rodolfo Dantón, Ana Itelman, and others pursued successful professional careers and became influential teachers.[65] While their choreographic works (save for Schottelius's) lie outside of the scope of this project, their pedagogical and artistic legacies resonate throughout *Moving Otherwise*.

As the twentieth century progressed, the modern dance community expanded and began to find institutional homes in theaters and cultural centers across Buenos Aires. As dance scholar María Eugenia Cadús demonstrates, classical ballet as well as the consolidating modern dance movement embodied the tensions within the cultural politics of President Perón's first two consecutive terms (1946–55), which oscillated between privileging the universality attached to both forms and staunch cultural nationalism that favored folkloric music and dance.[66] At the same time dancers worked to establish infrastructure to support the growing local dance community training and touring abroad—by choice or through exile during Argentina's periods of dictatorship—became central to dance careers. While Winslow (backed by her family's fortune) worked in Argentina with the hope of ultimately legitimizing herself as a choreographer in the United States, later generations of Argentine-born dancers brokered the embodied capital they earned during time spent training and performing in northern "centers" into successful local careers. They also began to use the concert stage to thematize the political and repre-sentational economies that shaped their global moves.

During the late 1980s and 1990s, Susana Tambutti and Margarita Bali's prominent contemporary dance group, Nucleodanza, toured extensively throughout the United States, Europe, and Asia. Nucleodanza formed in 1974 and developed their early work during the height of repression under the last military dictatorship, an experience recounted in chapter 3. Realized through support from private and corporate organizations as well as the na-tional government, these tours put Nucleodanza on the global dance map and created an operating model for up-and-coming independent groups. In par-ticular, Bali and Tambutti both identify their participation in the prestigious American Dance Festival's international programs as key to the company's growth and continued success.[67] While this international approach reinforces constructions of the global north as the site of "legitimate" modern and con-temporary dance, groups like Nucleodanza also used the concert stage as a site for critically engaging with the friction of global movement. Tambutti's 1989 *Patagonia Song and Dance Team*, later titled *Patagonia trío* (*Patagonia Trio*), grew explicitly out of Nucleodanza's experiences touring. It exemplifies the tensions of transnational work that shape contemporary dance production in Argentina as well as its histories of political engagement.

Tambutti's trio critically engages with dance center-periphery relations, parodically deflects global-north audiences' expectation of the folkloric or ex-otic of a South American dance group, and generally pokes fun at touring as an enterprise linked to financial and cultural capital. *Patagonia*'s title playfully responds to Eurocentric designations of Argentina as the "bottom" or "end" of the world by naming the nation's southernmost region.[68] Set to a series of pop-ular songs, the piece mixes contemporary dance vocabularies with clowning and improvisation to hyperbolize "iconic" elements of the tourist imaginary. The dancers wear ponchos and *bombachas* (or gaucho pants, traditionally worn by the rugged men of the pampas), one of the female dancers attempts a strip-tease that summons the stereotype of the Latina femme fatale, and all three perform "serious" choreographies and tableau vivants with soccer balls, the much-publicized Argentine national sport (figure I.3, video clip I.1 ⏵).[69] The piece also targets regional and national identity narratives: The performers' costumes were in part inspired by the Podestá brothers' *circo criollo*. Started in the 1870s by the children of Italian immigrants who moved back and forth

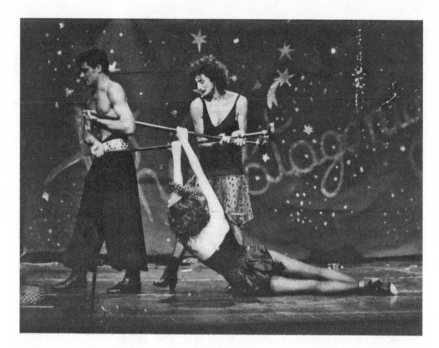

Figure I.3 Gustavo Lesgart (left), Laura Hanson (floor), and Inés Sanguinetti (back) in *Patagonia trío*. Photograph: Andrés Barragán. Courtesy of Susana Tambutti.

between Buenos Aires and Montevideo, Uruguay, the "creole circus's" skits often satirized the challenges of migrant life.[70] In one of the final scenes, the performers attempt to perform a song in French, and their failure to properly pronounce words and convincingly execute the act pokes fun at Argentine discourses that privilege European—and specifically French—cultural production.[71]

In one of our conversations, Tambutti described the impetus behind creating the piece:

> The idea for *Patagonia trío* appeared when I was in Europe and it seemed, I don't know if *funny* is the word, that lots of South American people (I see them now too) played the *quena* (Andean flute) in Saint-Michel Square [in Paris]. That is, the idea of the South American artist that tries as hard as possible to give a dignified show, but in reality is the antihero, trying to sell folklore from a tourist point of view. Even the idea of giving the piece an English name on purpose, *The Patagonia Song and Dance Team*, [was meant to be ironic] . . . afterwards it ended up being *Patagonia trío* because we were afraid that when we did the piece here [in Argentina] people would think that we put the title in English because we did a lot of touring and they would criticize us like, "oh look, they title their works in *English*."[72]

The street performers prompted Tambutti to question and choreographically probe the repertoires that "sell" Latin American artists on the global market and the politics framing artists' decisions to self-exoticize. The company's concerns about the title—whether the English version would signal arrogance before an Argentine audience despite its intended critique of Eurocentric desire for the exotic—demonstrate the group's navigation of strategic legibility and translation for viewing publics on both sides of the north/south axis. While *Patagonia* caricatured the international mandate that an Argentine group display stereotypical markers like gaucho culture, hypersexuality, and soccer, it also took to task national histories that reinforced colonial logics by privileging European economic and cultural models. Additionally, the piece rejected what Ananya Chatterjea has identified as the homogenizing tendencies of contemporary choreography as a commodity on the global dance market. Writing about the category of "contemporary" as it is deployed in Asian dance, Chatterjea notes that in some cases, "Asian 'contemporary' dance is a kind of ventriloquism, where contemporary Asia finds its voice through the signifiers of the Euro-American modern/postmodern, the latter passing once again as the neutral universal, which is able to contain all difference."[73]

Patagonia, however, does not contain difference vis-à-vis elements of the Euro-American concert tradition. Rather, it purposefully questions the politics that mark and unmark certain bodies and forms on the global stage, and perhaps most critically, humorously challenges the stability of these categories in and of themselves. In not allowing the category of the contemporary to "pass once again as the neutral universal," the piece calls attention to contemporary dance, influenced as it is by a myriad of traditions and local realities, as a complex and contested global practice. Decades following Miriam Winslow's north-south negotiations (and flirtation with the marketability of cultural particulars in *Andean Impressions*), *Patagonia* demonstrates how contemporary dance itself had come to function as a powerful site for critiquing the representational politics that shape global connection. While here *Patagonia* illustrates the politics that accompanied Nucleodanza and other groups' entrance onto the global dance scene in the 1980s, *Moving Otherwise* returns to Nucleodanza across its pages: Chapter 3 takes up the company's experiences forming in the midst of the last military dictatorship and chapter 4 examines how Tambutti's 1985 *La puñalada* (*The Stab*) approaches traumatic cultural memory in the wake of this period.

Nucleodanza was one of the first independent Argentine companies to both garner international acclaim and use the concert stage to flesh out the politics of dancing difference. However, later groups continued to rigorously question the cultural and economic state of the Argentine dancer, particularly in the wake of the neoliberal reforms that marked the 1990s. In 2013, Luciana Acuña and Alejo Moguillansky directed and performed *Por el dinero* (*For the Money*), a piece that, like *Patagonia*, creatively illuminates the friction of global movement. Acuña is a highly acclaimed and accomplished performer and choreographer who formed part of the well-known experimental collective Grupo Krapp. The group formed in 2000 and extended the theatrical and parodical elements that characterized Nucleodanza's work while also incorporating conceptual approaches often associated with European dance theater, elements that marked a number of groups that emerged in the 1990s and early 2000s.[74] Moguillansky is an award-winning independent filmmaker, as well as Acuña's personal and sometimes professional partner. Their interdisciplinary, evening-length piece follows in *Patagonia*'s genre-crossing steps, spanning contemporary dance, personal narrative, and documentary theater. In the creators' words, "*Por el dinero* is a study or analysis, perhaps a festive portrait, of the financial life of our country's artists and the absurd role of the artist in the market. It is also a portrait of the perverse relationship between European funding structures and artists in the periphery."[75] In addition to Argentine-born Acuña and Moguillansky, the piece also features Matthieu Perpoint, a French dancer and former member of Maguy Marin's company. Perpoint and his partner, Argentine dancer Agustina Sario, danced together with the French company before deciding to settle and raise their family in Buenos Aires (figure I.4).

The three performers' personal and economic narratives are at the center of the performance. The audience experiences these stories, at times partially fictionalized, through spoken text. Confusing any sense of stable narrative,

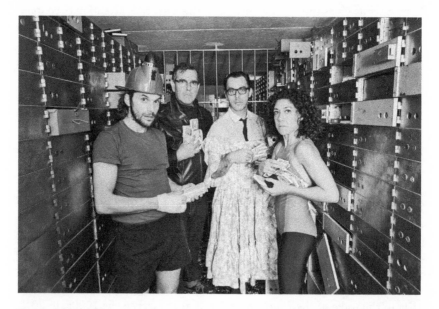

Figure I.4 Matthieu Perpoint, Gabriel Chwojnik, Alejo Moguillansky, and Luciana Acuña (from left to right) in *Por el dinero*. Photograph: Sebastián Arpesella. Courtesy of Luciana Acuña.

onstage speakers read stories that are often not their own, and which alternate between first and second person. Among other things, we learn that Acuña completed undergraduate degrees in dance and psychology ("just in case"), and used a scholarship plus money she earned from a successful international tour to fund her participation in a series of expensive dance workshops in France. A friend tells her that with the cost of two of those workshops, she could have bought a car in Buenos Aires. At the beginning of the show, spectators watch a video of a King's College London economist comparing Acuña's personal income over the past decade—uneven due to sporadic grants and residencies—to fluctuations in the Argentine GDP over the same time period. At one point, Acuña reads her partner Moguillansky's recollection of a time the two found a folkloric dance manual in her parent's home, and she wondered what her life might have been like if she danced folklore for a living.[76] This story is immediately followed by Acuña's frantic pas de deux with Perpoint set to music reminiscent of a circus theme (video clip I.2 ▶). Moguillansky reads a narrative that addresses Perpoint's biography, which includes discovering contact improvisation through a girlfriend and making a relatively quick transition to professional dancer with a prestigious company (Marin's), a period that represented the greatest income stability in his life. He now teaches dance and language classes in Buenos Aires.[77]

Perhaps the most cutting narrative, however, belongs to Moguillansky. Through a series of emails read by Acuña and Perpoint, we hear Moguillansky's communications with a Danish film festival and the Tate Modern about funding for a film project. After the Danish festival representative is unable to secure supplemental funding needed to complete the project, she offers Moguillansky the opportunity to participate in Icelandic-Danish artist Olafur Eliasson's Little Sun project. The Little Sun is a portable solar lamp that Eliasson designed for use in areas without access to electricity. To celebrate the project's launch, the Tate Modern asked fifteen filmmakers in "off-grid" areas—a euphemism for filmmakers from Africa, Asia, the Middle East, and South America—to film thirty minutes of footage lit by the Little Sun, in exchange for a stipend of one thousand euros. Moguillansky, having exhausted other funding and with filming for his project already underway, agreed. The lamp, however, is detained in Argentine customs. This detail in particular elicited laughter from the Buenos Aires audience when I saw the piece in 2014; President Cristina Fernández de Kirchner's state-centered government of the time imposed high import taxes, which meant that packages sent from abroad frequently were held in customs until the recipient paid a tariff. Moguillansky ultimately sent footage filmed without the Little Sun, which featured grazing cows. He shot the footage, using daylight, in the rural setting of his film. The curators loved the footage of the cows—Argentina is frequently associated with its meat-heavy cuisine and cattle industry—and invited him to attend the Little Sun launch in London. They agreed to reimburse his travel expenses; however, due to a series of miscommunications, delays, and hefty taxes imposed on international bank transactions, months later Moguillansky was still waiting to receive the money to cover the trip as well as the one thousand euro stipend from the Little Sun project. The trip, we learn, cost more than his young daughter's yearly private school tuition.[78]

Por el dinero exposes the friction of the global cultural economy in all of its maddening detail. While the question of funding structures shaped Winslow and Nucleodanza's experiences—the former's private wealth allowed her to form her Argentine company, but was not enough to bring the company to the United States, while the latter's tours were made possible by combining public and private funding—*Por el dinero* makes money the central theme of the work itself. The piece emphasizes not only the uneven flow of global capital (the cost of French dance workshops and European trips are translated into the living expenses that they represent in Argentina), but also how funding structures replicate and perpetuate colonial frameworks that continue to racialize, exoticize, and provincialize South American artists. Acuña wonders what her career would have been like had she been a folklore dancer as she frantically demonstrates her embodied knowledge of classical ballet, asking the audience to contemplate its worth. In Moguillansky's case, we are faced with the bitter irony that he was only able to secure modest funding for his film by fitting into a project predicated on the fetishization of difference. Ultimately, *Por el dinero* echoes Marta Savigliano's question: "Under what conditions would World[ing] Dance undo the obsession with the otherness of the other?"[79]

A view of the development of modern and contemporary dance in Argentina through these cases moves toward a transnational history. These three moments challenge facile conceptions of uninhibited cultural flow from "center" to "periphery" across the twentieth and twenty-first centuries and expose complex relationships rooted in the politics of difference in dancing. They explicitly challenge conceptions and applications of modern and contemporary dance as culturally, socially, and politically neutral. These cases not only demonstrate Argentine modern and contemporary dance as the product of intercultural encounters, but also expose the conditions of possibility that fostered contemporary dance as a site of moving otherwise from the 1940s onward.

While north-south circuits of exchange, like those highlighted above, are critical to understanding how Buenos Aires contemporary dance moves otherwise across the following chapters, this book also attends to the importance of the regional flow of political vanguards. For example, between the late 1960s and 1970s the choreographers and dance practices that I consider repeatedly invoked revolutionary concepts linked to the Cuban Revolution as well as to the broader leftist movements that spread throughout Latin America in its wake. Inevitably, however, multiple networks fall outside of the scope of this project. The relationship between Buenos Aires contemporary dance and other Latin American urban centers and sites across the global south promises to be a rich site for investigation.[80] And though Buenos Aires is undoubtedly the historical and current center of dance production in Argentina, *Moving Otherwise* compounds scholarly overemphasis on cultural production in Argentina's capital city. As the National Dance Law mobilization made clear, the prolific dance production happening across Argentina's provinces deserves future scholarly attention. It is my hope, however, that *Moving Otherwise* joins Argentine dance scholarship in starting the conversation.

ON METHODS

Moving Otherwise sits at the intersection of dance, performance, and cultural studies scholarship and draws on the insights of critical theory and political economy to understand danced politics as movements otherwise. In step with recent publications in the field of dance studies, this book employs an inter-disciplinary methodology that moves between archival research, interviews with dancers and choreographers, close analyses of dance works, and my own embodied experience as a collaborator and performer with active groups.[81] This approach not only most richly illuminates how Buenos Aires-based contemporary dance practices move otherwise, but also was necessary in the face of limited archival resources and uneven documentation practices. Aside from the Documentation Center of the San Martín Theater, which primarily documents the activity of artists affiliated with that theater, there are no comprehensive institutional archives in Argentina dedicated to modern and contemporary dance. And, as mentioned previously, published texts and collections of oral histories primarily focus on prominent figures considered artistic innovators, whose narratives provide an important but partial view of contemporary dance's past and present. Thus, it is necessarily in the connections among performance analysis, the insights of interlocutors, archival documents, my own dancing, and quotidian choreographies that glimpses of moving otherwise emerge.

Given the decentralized nature of archival materials, my research took place in official as well as "unofficial" collections. I conducted a widespread search for materials related to dance in print, photographic, and audio-visual collections contained in municipal, federal, and institutional archives. However, the material that most strongly grounds this book comes from the private collections of the artists this study analyzes—and to whom this book is deeply indebted. I examined material from the private collections of more than twenty-five artists and critics. In its integration of selected materials from these collections, *Moving Otherwise* embraces the embodied nature of archival encounters, particularly "unofficial" ones.[82] As a temporary presence in the living rooms, studies, and storage rooms of many of my interlocutors' homes, I developed personal relationships that deeply shape how I read the traces that make up dance's afterlife. Archival work in private homes took on an intimacy marked by afternoon coffee and *chisme* (gossip); rambunctious grandchildren upsetting neatly sorted piles of documents; curious, allergy-inducing cats; and the formation of mutual investments in a research project that led to a joyful sense of shared ownership across my weekly or monthly visits. The informal conversations with my interlocutors that accompanied the sorting, digitization, and review of photographs, programs, reviews, published profiles, performance documentation, ticket stubs, and production bills brought these documents to life.

Moving Otherwise combines the insights gained from archival research with those of ethnographic encounters more traditionally conceived. The book draws on fifty-three personal interviews conducted with dancers, choreographers, and other figures in the field. These conversations both illuminated the archival material I gathered and provided a wealth of insight beyond them. Across the book's chapters, I cite my interlocutors' words as a method as well as an object of analysis. In the book, their words do not simply offer "evidence." Rather, their nuanced reflections on what it means to practice dance and travel through the city in particular times and places guide my understanding of moving otherwise, providing grounded theoretical frameworks alongside academic concepts. The concept of moving otherwise itself, inspired as it is by my interview with dancer Déborah Kalmar, exemplifies how this book deploys my interlocutors' words *as* theory. In addition to drawing on dancers and choreographers' insights into their own work as well as contemporary dance's history, I also frequently highlight what performance ethnographer D. Soyini Madison thinks of as "small stories." In her book *Acts of Activism: Human Rights as Radical Performance*, Madison advocates for attention to how the personal, day-to-day narratives of struggle and hope that accompany performance making and political mobilization contain "macro forces" of history and political economy "ingrained within their plots."[83] These small stories—which evidence the power dynamics and political possibilities at play in seemingly inconsequential moments—are central to *Moving Otherwise*.

In addition to formal interviews, *Moving Otherwise* also draws from my ongoing participation in the Buenos Aires contemporary dance community as an interlocutor at events ranging from rehearsals, performances, and academic events to gatherings such as the National Dance Law discussion that opened this introduction. Performance ethnography, or critical assessment of my danced participation with active groups and choreographers, also informs the text. As a dancer trained in modern and contemporary techniques, I share embodied knowledge of many of the movement practices considered throughout. I have danced on and off in Buenos Aires since 2006, as both a student and a performer. In 2011, I danced for nearly a year with

Bailarines Toda la Vida (Dancers for Life), the community dance collective at the center of chapter 5. I continue to collaborate with the company during research trips to Buenos Aires and as an artistic associate at large. My embodied experience of their collective creation method fundamentally shapes how I analyze their work. I also studied in a long-term capacity with Vivian Luz, a dancer whose testimony informs chapter 2, and danced briefly with Oduduwá Danza Afroamericana (Oduduwá Afro-American Dance). In March 2011, I joined Oduduwá during their participation in the march that commemorates the coup that began the last military dictatorship, an experience that structures the book's epilogue. In addition to these formal movement repertoires, *Moving Otherwise* draws on and critically attends to my physical experiences of moving through the city of Buenos Aires during short- and long-term research residencies between 2007 and 2016. Just as these embodied experiences deeply inform my arguments, so too does my position as a US scholar who considers herself a grateful guest within the Buenos Aires dance community.

CHARTING MOVEMENTS OTHERWISE

While the following chapters proceed chronologically, *Moving Otherwise* does not trace a comprehensive history of Argentine contemporary dance. Rather, each of the five chapters focus on how a select set of practices moved otherwise along the following axes: mobility, militancy, survival, trauma, and cooperation. The first chapter, "Mobile Bodies" examines how contemporary dance enabled new and intersecting forms of artistic, social, and political mobility during the 1960s. During the early portion of the decade, a new network of cultural institutions helped establish contemporary dance on the Buenos Aires artistic scene and fostered the emergence of dance vanguards attuned to the nation's political climate. Socially, dance practices allowed dancers and choreographers to challenge gendered and classed norms sustained at the national and familial levels, all of which were in flux nationally as well as globally. By the mid-1960s, however, the climate of cultural vitality that marked life in Buenos Aires shifted dramatically. In 1966, a military coup known as the "Argentine Revolution" (1966–70) installed General Juan Carlos Onganía and ushered in a period of government repression that retracted civil rights and enforced conservative, Catholic values. Civil uprisings, right- and left-wing organizations, and politicized art movements alike responded to the regime. This chapter demonstrates how influential choreographers Ana Kamien and Susana Zimmermann translated the artistic and social mobilities that dance afforded in the first half of the decade into critique of Onganía's repressive government in their concert works and innovative creation processes in the late 1960s.

Chapter 2, "The Revolution Was Danced," examines contemporary dance's intersection with militant politics during the late 1960s and early 1970s. Armed leftist militant organizations grew concurrently with the tightening of military control over social expression under the military governments between 1966 and 1973. This chapter demonstrates how contemporary dance "put the body" in quotidian militant acts as well as in staged choreographies that explored militant themes. I examine testimony from Silvia Hodgers and Alicia Sanguinetti that highlights how their dance training informed their embodied participation in militant groups, especially during periods of incarceration in federal prisons. I go on to analyze how dance served as a ploy to distract guards in the 1972 Rawson Penitentiary prison escape plot organized by militant groups that included Hodgers and Sanguinetti. The initiative ended tragically with the execution of sixteen of the political prisoners, an event known as the Trelew Massacre. I discuss contemporaneous concert works by Cuca Taburelli and Estela Maris; the former memorializes the Trelew Massacre while the latter invites comparison between late-twentieth-century militant women and Juana Azurduy, the mestiza independence-era guerrilla military leader. This chapter argues that these cases of militants dancing and dances about militants underscore contemporary dance's intersections with explicitly political repertoires and make visible bodies committed to revolutionary causes on the contemporary dance stage. It challenges the dominant historical narrative that masculinizes leftist militant activity and marginalizes the role of cultural production generally, and dance practice specifically, within histories of militant activity.

The leftist political fervor of the late 1960s and early 1970s withered following the 1976 coup d'état that began the last military dictatorship. Chapter 3, "Dance as the Art of Survival" demonstrates how contemporary dance provided relatively protected spaces in studios, schools, and professional companies for negotiating bodily autonomy while dictatorial terror restricted quotidian movement and took bodies at will. During the last military dictatorship, contemporary dance moved otherwise as a strategy of survival. In interviews, dancers Ana Kamien, Alicia Muñoz, Déborah Kalmar, Ana María Stekelman, and Susana Tambutti all testified to the role of the contemporary dance studio as a safe haven within a city literally stagnated by terror. The chapter also examines the rise of *expresión corporal*, a movement practice that experienced increased institutional presence (in private studios as well as secondary and higher education) during the dictatorship. Based on exercises designed to access individuals' creative potential, *expresión corporal* valorized and celebrated the body as bodies were literally disappeared from streets and homes. Outside of the studio, I consider how the Danza Abierta festival—which was open to anyone who wanted to participate, regardless of professional trajectory—staged community, cohesion, and endurance during the waning years of the dictatorship. And finally, the chapter examines concert works by Renate Schottelius and Alejandro Cervera that premiered on the highly visible stage of the San Martín Theater in the later years of the dictatorship. Both addressed the military dictatorship's grip on bodily movement over the past years as well as the grief that often accompanies survival.

The last military dictatorship's nationalistic and economic failures led to re-democratization in 1983. Elected in the same year, President Raúl Alfonsín made initial actions to address state violence. However, the 1986 Full Stop Law set an end date for the investigation and prosecution of human rights violations by high-ranking military officials, and the 1987 Law of Due Obedience declared that subordinate military officers were simply following orders. Chapter 4, "Moving Trauma," explores how postdictatorship dance works moved otherwise to government imperatives to move on and forget the painful past. The chapter focuses on the prominence of tango themes—Argentina's much-mythologized national dance—within contemporary dances that engage the dictatorial past. I examine Tambutti's *La puñalada* (1985), a work presented by Nucleodanza in the immediate wake of the last military dictatorship. I also take up works by and documentary films on Silvia Vladimivsky and Silvia Hodgers, whose tango-inflected dances engaged dictatorship violence in the late 1990s and early 2000s. The chapter argues that, in these works, tango functions as an embodied paradigm for approaching the collective and individual trauma of political violence. Their dances critically positioned themselves relative to tango as a global signifier of Argentine national identity while exploring how the form's historical relationship to violence and exclusion offered an embodied rubric for exploring trauma and possibilities for healing.

Violent confrontations between citizens and the state once again engulfed Argentina in December 2001 when the economic ravages left by the last military dictatorship and compounded by 1990s neoliberal reforms resulted in unprecedented economic collapse. The crisis grew out of years of neoliberal reforms that championed privatization, free trade, and flexible labor. In the midst of bloody riots and widespread police violence following currency devaluation and an attempted run on the banks, workers, artists, and middle-class professionals alike turned toward cooperative politics not only as a means of sustaining themselves, but also to contest neoliberal emphases on individual achievement and financial gain. In an effort to make the corporeal effects of the crisis legible within broader histories of national trauma, social movements identified a new generation of *desaparecidos* (disappeared persons): the economic disappeared.

Chapter 5, "Common Goods," examines how post-2001 contemporary dance embraced cooperative politics and moved otherwise to economic exclusion. It considers two initiatives that share explicit ties to labor movements, both of which rejected neoliberal emphases on worker dispensability, working instead toward sustainable structures that supported cooperative creative and administrative action. I begin by considering the 2007-8 labor dispute at the San Martín Theater that gave rise to the Bailarines Organizados (Organized Dancers) labor-rights group and the Compañía Nacional de Danza Contemporánea (National Contemporary Dance Company, CNDC), a company whose repertory initially focused on social justice issues generally and the last military dictatorship specifically. The chapter then turns to Bailarines Toda la Vida, a community dance troupe that practices collaborative creation and rehearsed weekly for fifteen years in a breadstick factory reopened by a workers' labor cooperative following the factory's closure during the 2001 crisis. Like the CNDC, their repertory emphasizes works based on the last military dictatorship. Through an analysis of their work on and off the stage, the chapter demonstrates how Bailarines Organizados, the CNDC, and Bailarines Toda la Vida forged and have maintained cooperative structures by linking histories of political and economic disappearance.

The epilogue turns to a scene of mass dance in the streets of downtown Buenos Aires: the March 2011 human-rights march commemorating the coup that began the last military dictatorship. That year, I participated in the march with Oduduwá Danza Afroamericana, a group that between 2005 and 2012 brought together hundreds of volunteers to perform choreography based in Orishá dance. As I recount my experience as a dancer in the march, I reflect on the possibilities of the transnational and transhistorical memory to which Oduduwá aspired, returning to the questions of transnational exchange that shaped this introduction's approach to Argentine contemporary dance history. Orishá dance's origins in Yoruban culture and practice throughout the African diaspora (most notably in Cuba, Haiti, and Brazil) made it an unexpected addition to a march commemorating Argentine national trauma. Despite significant work by indigenous and Afro-Argentine groups to recuperate histories of racial difference, the Argentine population continues to imagine itself as predominantly white. Oduduwá, however, strove to make an embodied connection between Orishá dance's link to the violence of the trans-Atlantic slave trade and Argentina's history of political disappearance, as well as the country's own practices of racial erasure. Their project opens up complex questions about how memories travel with dances, where they travel, and to what ends. As a point of conclusion, the march reiterates the importance of taking dance seriously as a political practice and as a site for unpacking the corporeal logics of political and economic violence from national and transnational perspectives.

Charting movements otherwise in relationship to mobility, militancy, survival, trauma, and cooperation inevitably involved difficult decisions around omitting projects and practices that ultimately fell outside the scope of this book. While some related cases have received separate treatment elsewhere, *Moving Otherwise* does not (and could not) chronicle all of Buenos Aires-based contemporary dance's engagements with Argentina's histories of political and economic violence between the 1960s and the 2010s.[84] Furthermore, the focus on violence and memory of it that defines this book's chapters also means that several notable threads that emerge throughout are deserving of more sustained analysis than I am able to offer. For example, a significant number of dancers and choreographers centered in this book identify as Jewish. While I examine two works that cite the Holocaust as a way of speaking to Argentine histories of violence— Susana Zimmermann's *Polymorphias* (1969) and Renate Schottelius's *Paisaje de gritos* (*Landscape of Screams*, 1981)—I also analyze the works and experiences of a number of other Jewish dancers and choreographers that do not necessarily center this aspect of their identity. Additionally, while the vast majority of the dancers and choreographers that I highlight are women, and my claims around moving otherwise are often rooted in the analysis of gendered power dynamics, I do not take up how Buenos Aires contemporary dance intersected with feminist movements throughout the timeperiod under consideration. And lastly, much remains to be researched and written about the role that concert dance has played in both constructing and challenging Argentine racial exceptionalism, a focus of future research. However, it is my hope that the numerous and diverse histories of moving otherwise documented here prompt discussion not only around *how* contemporary dance enacted politics in contexts marked by political and economic violence, but also inspire future research.

CHAPTER 1

Mobile Bodies

The story of the 1960s is a familiar one. As we know from abundant popular and scholarly narratives, the decade brought sweeping cultural, social, economic, political, and scientific changes that profoundly transformed the global landscape. Within dance history, some of the most familiar references are the oft-celebrated innovations of the dancers associated with the Judson Memorial Church in New York City; their rejection of virtuosity and concert dance conventions echoed broader countercultural movements in the United States. Artistic innovation in the context of rapid social change likewise marked contemporary dance in 1960s Buenos Aires, and this book's story of moving otherwise begins here. As it traces a set of less-documented artistic histories, this chapter evidences how contemporary dance in Buenos Aires came to be an incisive site of political critique. It also works to decenter dance history's consistent alignment of 1960s experimentalism with the United States and Europe.

Throughout the 1960s, Buenos Aires contemporary dance enabled new and intersecting forms of artistic, social, and political mobility. These "mobilities" refer to dancers' options for moving in, between, and beyond established dance genres, class and gender norms, and political stances. Artistically, this decade marked the emergence of dance vanguards within new public and private cultural organizations and institutions, including the Friends of Dance Association (AADA, Asociación Amigos de la Danza, 1962–72), the famed Torcuato Di Tella Institute (Instituto Torcuato Di Tella, 1958–70), and later the General San Martín Cultural Center (CCGSM, Centro Cultural General San Martín, 1970–).[1] These organizations and institutions arose as part of the cultural growth that marked the early 1960s. Socially, dance practices allowed dancers and choreographers to challenge gendered and classed norms sustained at the national, neighborhood, and familial levels, all of which were in flux nationally as well as globally. By the mid-1960s, however, the climate of cultural vitality that marked life in Buenos Aires shifted dramatically. In 1966, a military coup known as the "Argentine Revolution" (1966–70) installed General Juan Carlos Onganía as de facto president and ushered in a period of government repression. Civil uprisings, right- and left-wing organizations, and politicized art movements responded to the regime's retraction of civil rights and enforcement of conservative, Catholic values. This chapter demonstrates how influential choreographers Ana Kamien and Susana Zimmermann translated the artistic and social mobilities that dance afforded in the first half of the decade into critique of Onganía's repressive government in their concert works and innovative creation processes in the late 1960s.

Throughout the chapter, I draw on personal and published interviews with the choreographers, their writings, and archival material from institutional and private collections to reconstruct their experiences and artistic works. While Kamien and Zimmermann are two among many figures who shaped the dance field during this decade, their trajectories illuminate, with particular clarity, the shift from artistic and social experimentation to political resistance that marked the 1960s. As first-generation daughters of Eastern European Jewish immigrants, both Kamien and Zimmermann negotiated working- and middle-class women's changing roles in the public sphere as they established careers as choreographers in the early 1960s and later created concert works that grappled directly with the repression of Onganía's dictatorship. Additionally, Kamien and Zimmermann are central figures within the genealogy of moving otherwise traced in this book. Chapter 2 examines dancers and choreographers linked to leftist militant groups who had performed with Zimmermann's collective. Likewise, chapter 3 examines Kamien and Zimmermann's continued movements otherwise in the context of the last military dictatorship, as well as the interventions of dancers they taught and mentored.

This discussion first explores how contemporary dance provided Kamien and Zimmermann with the literal steps for attaining social mobility in the early 1960s. Both challenged gender and class norms—in and outside of the dance community—as they built their careers as choreographers in the midst of Buenos Aires's flourishing cultural landscape. New cultural institutions not only provided a "home" for their work, but also facilitated artistic mobility that allowed Kamien and Zimmermann to challenge the bounds of modern dance as it was practiced at the time. The artistic and social mobilities that materialized through their dance careers emerged in the context of modernization projects that marked the post-Peronist period. Following the fall of the populist Peronist government in 1955, a series of civilian and military governments dismantled the welfare state and advocated for capitalist development based on foreign investment. They also celebrated a Western, cosmopolitan nationalism that privileged the Buenos Aires middle classes in particular.[2]

Beginning in the late 1950s, middle-class consumption patterns changed with economic policies, including expanded ownership of cars, television sets, and home appliances, as well as increased participation in leisure activities.[3] Influenced by trends in the business world, a crop of cultural institutions including theaters, cultural centers, art galleries, bookstores, music halls, and publishing houses in Buenos Aires "elaborated new cultural values and promoted new urban sensibilities."[4] As a 1966 *Panorama* article put it: "While the economists talked about illiquidity and retraction in the market, we Argentines made culture an important consumer good."[5] During the early 1960s, consuming and producing culture became an integral part of attaining and maintaining a cosmopolitan, middle-class lifestyle. As Valeria Manzano explains in her study of young women, gender, and sexuality in 1960s Argentina, shifting cultural practices affected young women in particular. Thousands of urban middle- and lower-middle-class young women like Zimmermann and Kamien began to "leave home" in unprecedented numbers to participate in an expanded horizon of leisure activities, to study at universities and training schools, and to enter and remain in the labor force.[6] Further contesting the traditional equation of womanhood with domestic space, wifehood, and motherhood, shifting perceptions around sexuality meant that women increasingly challenged courtship conventions, publicly acknowledged practicing premarital sex, and married later in life.[7]

The climate of violence and control that marked the later portion of the decade shifted the terms of moving otherwise. Onganía's June 1966 military coup extended socioeconomic modernization projects rooted in liberalism while also waging a morality campaign in the name of rescuing the country's Western Catholic values from a supposedly degenerate, leftist youth culture. Onganía intensified the military's political control by suspending political parties, challenging university autonomy, and limiting labor movements. Anticommunist policies and censorship—which specifically targeted intellectuals and artists—further tightened control on social expression. The Night of the Long Sticks (La Noche de los Bastones Largos), a violent military intervention at the University of Buenos Aires on July 29, 1966, established a pervasive environment of fear. Legislation also doubled down on "traditional" gender and sexual values that had been challenged during the early 1960s. For example, the 1969 "Name Law" mandated that married women take their husband's last name.[8]

The second portion of this chapter examines how Zimmermann's and Kamien's work responded to the climate of repression under Onganía. As Onganía's government aimed to still the possibilities for artistic and social mobility that marked the earlier portion of the decade, Kamien's and Zimmermann's post-1966 works expressed political mobility in their critique of the regime. I first consider Zimmermann's Laboratorio de Danza (Dance Laboratory) project at the Di Tella, which was launched in the late 1960s.

I examine the group's political and creative agenda and demonstrate how their 1969 work *Polymorphias* turned to Zimmermann's Jewish heritage to simultaneously memorialize the victims of the Holocaust and sound a "state of alert" around the current national climate.[9] Lastly, the chapter takes up Kamien's eponymous *Ana Kamien*, which premiered in 1970 at the newly opened CCGSM. Following the closure of the Di Tella in 1970 and the dissolution of AADA in 1972, the CCGSM emerged as one of the few remaining spaces for independent dance production. *Ana Kamien* explicitly critiqued military violence at the same time that it asserted dance as a form of (now endangered) cultural labor.[10] Both works echo politicized art and activist movements of their moment, including the rise of leftist militant groups whose ideologies drew on internationally circulating currents of Marxism-Leninism, Maoism, Guevarism, and Trotskyism, as well as nationally based Peronism. Scholars frequently point to the *Tucumán Arde* (*Tucumán Is Burning*) exhibition as exemplary of the unification of revolutionary politics with artistic production. This collective multimedia exhibition held in Buenos Aires and the province of Rosario in 1968 critiqued the working conditions in sugar mills in the northern province of Tucumán and denounced the government's censorship of artistic production.[11]

By highlighting Kamien's and Zimmermann's work during the 1960s, this chapter aims not only to demonstrate the breadth of mobilities that dance practices enabled but also to integrate contemporary dance into an otherwise well-documented period of Argentine cultural history. While Argentine dance historiography has emphasized dance's institutional history during this period, and particularly the role of AADA in developing Argentine concert dance, focusing on Kamien and Zimmermann illuminates a genealogy of moving otherwise within contemporary dance's early history. Their dance careers and concert works not only indexed the rapid social, cultural, and political shifts that shaped bodily life in the 1960s, but actively instantiated new modes of moving as women and as dancers on Buenos Aires stages and streets.

DANCING SOCIAL AND ARTISTIC MOBILITY

Kamien's and Zimmermann's training as dancers and choreographers in the 1950s and early 1960s reflects the confluence of movement styles circulating in Buenos Aires at the time. Both first trained in classical ballet at a young age with Colón Theater dancers; Kamien with Lida Martinoli at her neighborhood social club and Zimmermann with Mercedes Quintana. By the late 1950s, however, Kamien and Zimmermann had begun to focus their training in modern dance and were exposed to a breadth of global modernisms. Both studied with Renate Schottelius, the noted German-born dancer who taught techniques and composition methods associated with US midcentury modernist choreographers, particularly Martha Graham and José Limón.[12] Schottelius had been a member of Miriam Winslow's company (discussed briefly in the introduction), and her pedagogy emphasized the repetition of set exercises and structured approaches to creating choreographic work.[13] As part of her training, Kamien also studied with María Fux, whose classes at the University of Buenos Aires took a decidedly different approach by focusing on individualized, free-form improvisation.[14] Dore Hoyer—the former Mary Wigman dancer who led a series of workshops based on expressionist principles and improvisation methods at the La Plata Argentine Theater (Teatro Argentino de La Plata) in 1960—deeply shaped Zimmermann's artistic development in particular.[15] Many up-and-coming dancers and choreographers participated in Hoyer's highly influential classes; Kamien also attended, though only briefly.[16] Zimmermann's interest in German expressionism solidified that same year when she saw the Chilean National Ballet perform Kurt Jooss's *The Green Table* (1932) in Buenos Aires, a work that depicts the futility and destruction of war. Inspired by the iconic work's blend of political critique and expressionist movement, Zimmermann applied for and received a grant to study with Jooss at the Folkwang Schule in Germany in 1961.[17]

While Kamien's and Zimmermann's Buenos Aires-based teachers formed part of an earlier generation of choreographers who helped introduce and disseminate modern dance in the city, both built their careers as choreographers within the new public and private cultural institutions that emerged in the early 1960s and offered unprecedented visibility and infrastructure for dance. Some of these sites primarily supported choreographers working in the relatively established midcentury modernisms that marked their training, while other institutions took an explicitly vanguard stance. Zimmermann's early career articulated with the former, while Kamien's aligned with the latter. Zimmermann's early works *Huis Clos* (*No Exit*, choreographed with Ana Labat, 1964) and *Amor humano* (*Human Love*, 1965) premiered at the then recently inaugurated San Martín Theater. Though the San Martín Theater originally opened in 1944, reconstruction of a new, state-of-the-art facility began in 1954. Following its inauguration in May 1960, the downtown space quickly became one of the most prominent performing arts centers in the city.[18] The presentation of *Huis Clos* and *Amor humano* was the product of cooperation between the theater and the Friends of Dance Association (AADA). An independent consortium of ballet and modern dancers, AADA was founded by prominent figures including Schottelius, Tamara Grigorieva (a former Ballets Russes dancer who settled in Argentina in 1950), Amalia Lozano, Ekaterina de Galanta, and Roberto Giachero. AADA aimed to professionalize the Buenos Aires dance community and produce new work. On Monday evenings when the San Martín Theater had no regular programming scheduled, AADA presented programs (usually composed of works by three choreographers) on the theater's main stage.

Across its years of activity, AADA helped establish a broader public for modern dance and cultivated ballet spectatorship outside of the Colón Theater. By presenting ballet and modern dance together, AADA created a forum for enduring local debates around the differences and similarities between modern dance and ballet, a frequent subject of press coverage at the time.[19] In our interview, Zimmermann emphasized the significance of jointly programming work from multiple genres, which she described as encompassing "classical, neoclassical, [and] modern, not an ultra innovative modern, but modern."[20] Classical dance pieces featured selections from well-known ballets as well as original choreographies. The consortium often presented modern dance works rooted in midcentury techniques.[21] These works tended toward universalized and classical themes that, in line with Clare Croft's definition of dance modernism, framed "bodies as forms in motion, not necessarily as people, and, even more so, not as people who [come] to the stage to share movements from specific historical, cultural, or geographic circumstances."[22]

AADA's participation in the construction of ballet and modern dance as universal (i.e., Western and culturally unmarked) thus constituted a substantial part of its effort to advance Argentine dance. This echoed 1960s government discourses that, in their rejection of Perón's state-centered populism, equated national modernization with US and European economic and cultural models themselves imagined as universal. Furthermore, AADA's prioritization of neutral universals took place within a broader Cold War context where the US State Department actively promoted dance modernism as part of its effort to contain communism and promote US interests in the global south, including Argentina.[23] Dance scholars Rebekah Kowal and Clare Croft have demonstrated how the equation of universalist abstraction with US cultural values of freedom and democracy vis-à-vis cultural diplomacy, though a seemingly odd pairing, in fact worked in tandem: "if dance modernism could be universally accessible around the globe *and* be marked as American, that would help establish an argument that indeed what was American was possible for—and even good for—the rest of the world."[24]

Zimmermann's "not an ultra innovative modern, but modern" designation also hints at a perceived aesthetic traditionalism in AADA's modernist tendencies. Kamien elaborated this point in a published interview, asserting that AADA works "danced the grand themes of humanity. Anguish, pain, suffering—it was a post-War thing. They danced to Bach, Vivaldi. They were grand themes, grand gestures, grand choreographies . . . . We began to want to knock all of that down and do something else. For me, in part, because I didn't have access to that world."[25] The "we" in Kamien's statement includes frequent collaborator Marilú Marini. The "postwar" "grand themes of humanity" that marked many AADA works struck Kamien as dated and disconnected from current social and cultural trends in Buenos Aires.[26] For Kamien, the "grandness" of AADA works also indexed an artistic elitism that, despite her training with prominent figures like Schottelius, appeared inaccessible. Unlike Zimmermann, work demands kept her from pursuing training opportunities in Europe or the United States, a form of cultural capital within an organization like AADA that emphasized technical mastery. The daughter of a textile worker, Kamien grew up in the working-class Parque Patricios neighborhood and, following her graduation from secondary school in the late 1950s, found work at a bank that allowed her to help support her family.[27] While Zimmermann found a "home" in AADA, class difference shaped Kamien's more limited access to the organization.

For Zimmermann, AADA's public reach and emphasis on rigorous technical and artistic standards made it an important site of artistic and social mobility.[28] Artistically, AADA provided a critical professional platform for launching and legitimizing her career, and those of many others, by centralizing, investing in, and valorizing Buenos Aires-based dance production. Socially, it allowed her to circumvent acceptable paths of middle-class womanhood. Like many middle-class women in the 1950s, after completing secondary school Zimmermann enrolled in a professional school to pursue a career as a secondary-school teacher.[29] While Zimmermann ostensibly focused her study in philosophy and psychology, in our interview she recounted how she applied her pedagogical training to dance classes that she taught at one of her first teaching jobs, out of the desire "to concretize in action something of what I had studied."[30] For Zimmermann, presenting her early works at AADA was instrumental in transitioning from a conventional job into a full-time career as a choreographer. As an organization, AADA modeled female leadership (women consistently composed the majority of the executive board) and heavily featured female-authored choreographies, placing it at the forefront of shifting gender roles and women's increasing visibility as artists in Buenos Aires.

While artistically AADA took "not an ultra innovative modern, but modern" approach, the Di Tella multidisciplinary art center, where Kamien launched her career, was explicitly experimental. Located alongside galleries, cafés, and bookstores on a downtown block referred to as "the crazy block" (*la manzana loca*), the Di Tella fostered a vibrant new generation of avant-garde artists working in the visual and performing arts who challenged artistic conventions and engaged in genre-crossing work.[31] As a choreographer, Kamien was interested in deconstructing her training in classical and modern dance techniques and exploring the relationship between dance, popular culture, and the visual arts. Kamien's choreographic vision aligned strongly with the Di Tella's mission, which did not value the same kind of pedigree and approach to making dances as AADA. The entrepreneurial Di Tella family established the institute with the purpose of advancing Argentine cultural production at home and promoting it abroad. The Di Tella's financial structure was philanthropic as opposed to patronage based; the relationship between the Di Tella business enterprise and artistic production was not direct, but rather mediated by the cultural center's autonomous management.[32] Though the Di Tella and AADA differed in their aesthetic tendencies, both advocated for artistic advancement through dialogue with US and European vanguards (Di Tella) and traditions (AADA), echoing the government's rejection of the perceived economic and cultural isolationism of the Peronist era. The center boasted visual, audiovisual (which included theater and dance), and music departments as well as a performance space equipped with state-of-the-art lighting, sound, and video technology financially inaccessible for public theaters—even the new San Martín Theater.[33] Well-known conceptual artists associated with the Di Tella include Marta Minujín, known for happenings that blended visual art and performance, and León Ferrari. Ferrari's work in protest of the Vietnam War, *La civilización occidental y cristiana* (*Western Christian Civilization*), depicted Christ crucified on a fighter plane in place of a cross and caused a highly publicized controversy when displayed at the Di Tella in 1965.

At the same time that the Di Tella became known for happenings and installations that transgressed aesthetic, social, and cultural norms, it also created space for quotidian subversions. Over tea in her Buenos Aires apartment, Kamien smiled when she told me that she used to wait until she arrived to change into her miniskirt.[34] She did not dare to wear the new fashion on public transportation or in her household. The Di Tella, she explained, was ready for new things not yet acceptable in broader social and cultural spaces. Men with long hair and women wearing miniskirts—Kamien included—circulated through the so-called crazy block around the Di Tella, making it as much a place for stylish young *porteños* (Buenos Aires dwellers) to see and be seen as it was a space for showcasing experimental art.[35] Through her association with the Di Tella, Kamien became a protagonist in the latest cultural modernity.

Dance began to figure regularly on the Di Tella Audiovisual Experimentation Center's programming following the premiere on September 23, 1965, of Kamien and Marini's *Danse Bouquet* (*Dance Bouquet*), a work that parodied the artistic elitism the choreographers felt marked other sectors of the Buenos Aires concert dance scene.[36] I address Zimmermann's work at the Di Tella following the 1966 coup in the following section, but here I highlight *Danse Bouquet* as an example of how Kamien's work at the Di Tella explicitly transgressed the norms of concert dance production and challenged offstage gender norms during the early 1960s. As stated on the program, *Danse Bouquet* aimed "to avoid all the affectations: those of classical dance and those of modern dance."[37] Rather than pursuing the "grandness" that Kamien believed characterized AADA's programming, *Danse Bouquet* followed a sketch-based, variety-show structure and embraced popular culture.[38] The piece sought inspiration in and cited comics, fashion magazines, and the *Goldfinger* James Bond movie (1964)—a stark departure from AADA artists' frequent engagement with high-art music, poetry, and literature. Kamien and Marini's interests in these materials reflected the emergence of leisure activities, like movie going and magazine reading, as central to the performance of being young and modern in 1960s Buenos Aires.

To build their movement vocabulary, Kamien and Marini poked fun at the perceived grandeur of established movement genres and explored quotidian movement vocabularies. For example, in one sketch Kamien reconstructed choreography from the opera *Aida* that she originally learned from Martinoli as a young student. She set the movement to music from *La Traviata* (a different Verdi opera) and performed in a baroque-style red dress so voluminous that it barely allowed her to move (figure 1.1).[39] Other episodes of the piece targeted offstage gender norms, such as Marini's *Vestida de novia* (*Dressed as a Bride*) sketch set to popular singer Palito Ortega's love ballad of the same name.[40] The song tells the melodramatic story of a woman who dies before her wedding day and is laid to rest in her wedding dress. *Danse Bouquet* parodied the hyperbole of popular romance narratives exemplified in the song, engaging unabashedly in the "cheesy," as Marini put it in *Primera Plana* magazine's write-up of the piece.[41] Marini played the bride in the sketch, dressed in a white wedding gown replete with layered tulle sleeves and veil. Photographic documentation of the piece features her flanked by bridesmaids who wear simpler white dresses and floral crowns. In one image, she looks

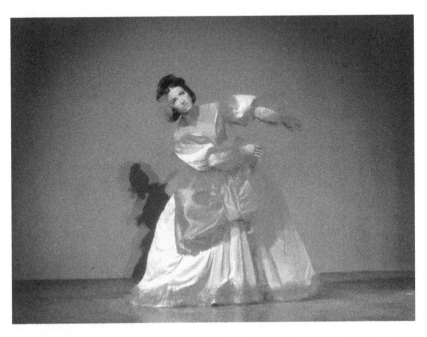

Figure 1.1 Ana Kamien in *Danse Bouquet*, Di Tella Institute, 1965. Photograph: Leone Sonnino. Courtesy of photographer.

piously skyward as if in prayer, suggesting the chastity expected of unmarried women and symbolized by the white wedding dress.[42] The sketch not only pointed to the "cheesy" nature of a popular love song, but also took aim at the notion that a woman's greatest destiny in life was wifehood and motherhood. *Danse Bouquet* moved otherwise to the perpetuation and reinforcement of gender and sexual principles in popular culture, norms that women like Kamien were already challenging offstage by pursuing lives as choreographers and marrying later in life, if at all.

Kamien's subsequent works at the Di Tella included *La fiesta* (*The Party,* 1966, with Marini) and *Oh! Casta Diva* (1967, after Italian composer Vincenzo Bellini's nineteenth-century aria). Like *Danse Bouquet*, these interdisciplinary works followed episodic structures, incorporated found objects and visual elements, and worked with pedestrian gesture and parodies of both classical ballet and modern dance.[43] These choreographic strategies echoed and took place congruently with the well-documented challenges to virtuosity, originality, and cohesive narrative that characterized 1960s US postmodern dance, particularly work associated with the Judson Memorial Church.[44] Within a national context, Kamien's work articulated with the rise of conceptual art that the Di Tella fostered. As part of this broader vanguard art movement, the Di Tella introduced experimental dance to a larger art-consuming public, both at the center itself and through coverage in prestigious publications like *Primera Plana* that followed the Di Tella's activities closely. At the same time that Kamien's works dialogued with other art disciplines and reached broader audiences, they also helped open an explicitly vanguard line of aesthetic inquiry within Buenos Aires concert dance. For Kamien, the Di Tella facilitated a questioning of aesthetic and gendered norms and a performance of cultural modernity onstage and off that constituted forms of artistic and social mobility. Though Kamien perceived AADA as inaccessibly elite, her oppositional work at the Di Tella ultimately secured her membership in an unquestionably elite, if irreverent, institution.

Within the new cultural institutions that developed across the early to mid-1960s, Kamien and Zimmermann moved otherwise to gendered, classed, and artistic norms and built their professional careers in dance at the same time that these institutions' missions, and the broader embrace of dance modernism, also reinforced the government's emphasis on Western cultural and economic development. However, Onganía's 1966 coup and its subsequent restrictions on the possibilities of personal and artistic expression fundamentally shifted the climate at the Di Tella and in Argentina broadly. In the wake of the coup, both Kamien and Zimmermann translated the social and artistic mobilities they gained in the early 1960s into dance projects that incisively critiqued the political climate. In the following section, I consider Zimmermann's work at the Di Tella in the wake of Onganía's coup. I demonstrate how her Laboratorio de Danza, and specifically the work *Polymorphias*

(1969), responded to the military government's tightening stranglehold on public life and spoke to the building political movements that interpolated cultural production into revolutionary projects. While Kamien's earlier choreographies at the Di Tella took aim at bourgeois gendered norms and questioned the authority of established dance forms, this same site offered Zimmermann the possibility to explore a movement methodology rooted in an explicitly political consciousness.[45]

MOVEMENT AS A STATE OF ALERT: EL LABORATORIO DE DANZA AND *POLYMORPHIAS* (1969)

Following her early engagements with AADA, Zimmermann began to explore improvisation as a creation technique in the studio as well as on the concert stage. She developed a work based on structured improvisation called *Danza ya* (*Dance Now*, 1967) with a group of dancers, actors, musicians, poets, and visual artists. The work unfolded through a series of prompts (based in formal concerns as well as everyday life) that changed with every presentation, and the piece ended with an invitation for the audience to join the performance.[46] For Zimmermann, the Di Tella was unquestionably the place to show such experimental work that did not feature set choreography and encouraged audience participation. As she writes, the Di Tella was "the place" of the moment and "it would not have occurred to me to present it [*Danza ya*] through the Friends of Dance Association, which was a shrine in which the [movement] language was more formal."[47] Furthermore, the Di Tella's audiences were familiar with experimental dance works through earlier programming, and the popular happenings had primed them for improvisational performances that involved audience participation. Likely for these reasons, Roberto Villanueva (director of the Audiovisual Experimentation Center) agreed to present the work from September to November 1967.

Zimmermann's arrival at the Di Tella in 1967, however, corresponded to political shifts that impacted the possibilities for artistic and social transgression that had inspired Kamien earlier in the decade. Onganía's government identified the Di Tella as a "corrupting influence" against its vision of a modernity rooted in conservative Catholic values and modes of social conduct.[48] Throughout the late 1960s, conservative groups and publications associated the Di Tella with a constellation of alleged corruption, including communism, political militancy, hippies, drug use, and dissident sexuality.[49] The "crazy block" became a specific target of police surveillance. The unconventional fashions and self-styling that marked bodies as part of the Di Tella's cultural vanguard now brought repercussions in the form of police harassment and arrest.[50] The Di Tella experienced direct censorship for the first time in 1968 when the government shut down Roberto Plate's *Baño* (*Bathroom*), which was part of the larger *Experiencias 68* (*Experiences 68*) exhibition.[51] The installation featured simulated bathrooms—one for men and one for women—and invited viewers to use the walls for graffiti. The installation played on public restrooms as simultaneously public and private spaces charged with the possibility of communicating anonymous confessions and denunciations. When a criticism of the Onganía regime appeared on the walls of the installation, the government ordered it to close.[52]

Within this charged climate, Villanueva offered Zimmermann the opportunity to establish an ongoing dance project, the Laboratorio de Danza, which further developed *Danza ya*'s experimental principles.[53] Zimmermann chose the term "laboratory" because of its emphasis on experimentation. As she writes in *El laboratorio de danza y movimiento creativo* (*The Dance Laboratory and Creative Movement*), her 1983 book that explains the methodologies first developed in the 1960s, the laboratory "is a place where one tries things out, experiments, analyzes, transforms and ultimately creates new essences, new subject matter."[54] In the same text, Zimmermann elaborates the practices she employed to lead a "profound exploration of the body," including techniques for relaxation and concentration; isolated explorations of different body parts as well as focused investigation of the relationship between them; improvisations based on the senses, emotions, objects, rhythms, vocalizations, and space; and finally exercises designed to foster an interconnected group dynamic.[55] The Laboratorio de Danza shared several principles with Kamien's earlier work at the Di Tella, including the rejection of virtuosity, incorporation of theatrical elements like the spoken word and character development, and work with pedestrian movement and everyday objects.[56] Zimmermann's Laboratorio de Danza also emphasized group creation, creative process over staged product, and audience participation.[57] Through the Laboratorio de Danza, Zimmermann synthesized her interest in German expressionism's emotional interiority (through exercises that strove to uncover emotional "essences") with the spirit of experimentalism (e.g., audience interaction and pedestrian movement) that the Di Tella was known for.[58] If AADA first helped secure Zimmermann's place within the elite circuit of artists working in the modern dance traditions that marked her training, then the Di Tella allowed her to devise an experimental project that challenged established modes of making dance.

While Kamien's work at the Di Tella enabled challenges to concert dance traditions and quotidian gendered norms—both onstage and off— Zimmermann's Laboratorio de Danza introduced an explicitly social and political frame to the Di Tella's dance programming. For Zimmermann, the Laboratorio de Danza's creative agenda had an "ethical-political commitment."[59] The group's 1969 *Polymorphias* program states that the Laboratorio de Danza aimed to "recuperate the capacity for human creation, breaking the traditional schema: choreographer, performer, audience as three separate entities and integrating these three elements in a new dynamic performance . . . we propose to create-together-a-new-language-for-a-new-man."[60] While Zimmermann's later publications do not include the "new man" language, its presence on the 1969 program is noteworthy.

The notion of the "new man" echoes Argentine revolutionary Ernesto "Che" Guevara's writing on the anticipated emergence of new subjectivities following the installation of the socialist project in Cuba.[61] Among other factors, Guevara's death in Bolivia in 1967 contributed to the spread of leftist movements across Latin America. In the late 1960s, Argentine youth (particularly students) became politicized across a spectrum that, in its most revolutionary instantiations, included the rise of national armed guerrilla groups. As noted in the introduction, during these years the concept *poner el cuerpo* (to put the body on the line) gained traction, naming embodied action as central to political and social change. Though not explicitly aligned with militant movements, Zimmermann's connection of dance practice to the social transformation of a "new man" echoed this developing political vanguard, and imagined a danced ethics of *poner el cuerpo*.[62] The incorporation of the "new man" phrase into the *Polymorphias* program's description of the Laboratorio de Danza reflected, as historian Andrea Andújar notes, how "concepts and words such as revolution, socialism in its different varieties, unity of action, liberation, victory, among others, were incorporated in a definitive manner into the language of the era."[63] Chapter 2 tells the story of two artists connected to the Laboratorio de Danza, Silvia Hodgers and Alicia Sanguinetti, who participated directly in militant movements. Both were members of the People's Revolutionary Army (Ejército Revolucionario del Pueblo, ERP), the armed branch of the Marxist-Leninist Workers' Revolutionary Party (Partido Revolucionario de los Trabajadores, PRT).

The Laboratorio de Danza's politicized project mirrored a broader movement that sought to unite artistic vanguards with growing leftist movements committed to working-class revolution.[64] Where the artistic vanguard of the early to mid-1960s (centered at the Di Tella) emphasized radical breaks with artistic tradition, the late 1960s saw "an urgency to create collective art that impacted directly on reality and denounced political, social, and economic situations that troubled the country."[65] Art historians Ana Longoni and Mariano Mestman note that this "new work" aimed to support the "transformation of society (inscribing it in the revolutionary wave) as well as the artistic field (destroying the bourgeois myth of art, the concept of art as only for personal enjoyment, etc.)."[66] The Laboratorio de Danza's studio practices and stage works were not as explicitly oppositional (and certainly not as widely publicized and debated) as better-known projects, such as the *Tucumán Arde* exhibition; however, they merit consideration within what Longoni and Mestman term the "revolutionary wave."[67] The Laboratorio de Danza's collective creations rejected the single-authorship model of choreography, investing instead in the dialogic potential of group decision-making and unified action. Furthermore, the Laboratorio de Danza did not conceive of their stage works as finite, consumable end products, but rather as experiences that aimed to foster a "better relationship with oneself and the other" through embodied political consciousness.[68] As the military government increasingly employed violent force to demonstrate its authority, compel the performance of "traditional" Christian values in its citizens, and censor dissent in the institution that the project called home, the Laboratorio de Danza's commitment to exploring movement-based communication with oneself and others offered a powerful form of moving otherwise.

Among the Laboratorio de Danza's stage works, *Polymorphias* in particular exemplifies how the group's work imagined a movement-based politics. In 1968, Zimmermann received a scholarship from the Belgian Embassy and the National Arts Fund to study with French choreographer Maurice Béjart, an experience that catalyzed the creation of *Polymorphias* the following year. While Zimmermann was studying with him, Béjart denounced Prime Minister António de Oliveira Salazar's dictatorship during a concert in Portugal following a tribute to the recently assassinated Robert Kennedy. As a result, Béjart was asked to leave the country. Deeply impacted by a prestigious choreographer taking a vocal stand against authoritarianism, Zimmermann returned to the Laboratorio de Danza invested in exploring histories of political violence and inequality.[69] For the musical score, Zimmermann selected Polish composer Krzysztof Penderecki's *Polymorphia* (1961) and the haunting *Dies Irae* (1967), which is dedicated to the victims of the Auschwitz concentration camp.

Polymorphias blended structured improvisation with set choreography. Reviews emphasized the choreography's group genesis, emotional charge, and pedestrian quality.[70] Existing video documentation of the work is limited to brief clips from a 1981 restaging, so here I also draw on Zimmermann's description of the work in her original 1969 score, photographs from the Di Tella premiere, and reviews, in conjunction with my interviews with Zimmermann. Scenographically, the work featured a scaffold-like structure that the dancers assemble at the beginning of the work and disassemble at the end. *Polymorphias* unfolds in two primary sections, each named after Penderecki's music. "Polymorphia" explores group dynamics and confrontation, or, as the score describes it, "the history of communication—lack of communication."[71]

The opening features the cast huddled together in a tight cluster. Some dancers are standing while others lie at their feet. The dancers' heads drape toward the floor, resting on nearby limbs or the stage. This "anonymous mass," as the score refers to it, begins to undulate in unison as if it were a collective, breathing body.[72] The dancers elongate their spines and raise their faces toward the sky on the "inhale," and the mass collapses inward again at the bottom of each collective "exhale."[73] The mass gradually fractures throughout the course of the first section; the group divides into factions, exploring tensions around leadership, agency, and individual versus group identity (figure 1.2).[74] The second section, "Dies Irae," honors the score's dedication to the victims of Auschwitz. Dressed in street clothes, terror-stricken dancers climb on and hang from the scaffolding—its bars come to symbolize the concentration camp itself.[75] According to the *Polymorphias* score, the group attempts to band together in an appeal to a common sense of humanity, but is ultimately torn apart by "hunger, thirst, or fear."[76]

The piece culminates in the performers' interaction with the audience. Breaking the fourth wall, the dancers enter the audience and stand before randomly selected spectators and invite contact through an extended hand.[77] By literally asking for a hand, the piece extends its interrogation of the possibilities for bodily connection off the theatrical stage. For Zimmermann, this interactive component sealed the "ethical-political" commitment of the group's work. Following a choreographic exploration of the trauma of Auschwitz, the final moments of the piece ask the audience members to become physically accountable—to "put" the body on the line vis-à-vis grasped hands—for the well-being of other bodies in the face of violence, destruction, and death.

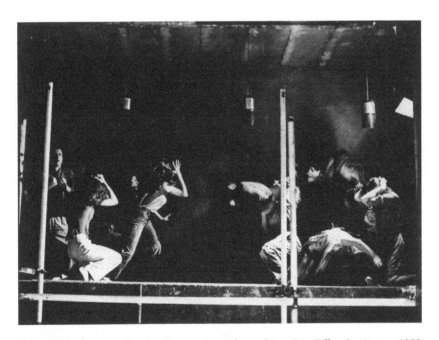

Figure 1.2 Laboratorio de Danza in *Polymorphias*, Di Tella Institute, 1969. Choreography: Susana Zimmermann. Music: Krzysztof Penderecki. Photographer unknown. Courtesy of Susana Zimmermann.

During our discussion about *Polymorphias*, Zimmermann shared an anonymous letter she received following the work's premiere that addressed these final moments. Though anecdotal in the sense it describes only one spectator's response, the letter offers a way to parse the politics of the final scene. On a yellowed piece of paper dated 1969, the anonymous viewer writes:

> In the end, in "Dies Irae," when they come down and join us and ask for help, something very strange happened to me. One of the male performers came into my row and moved down it very slowly. It was distressing to see him with his hands outstretched, demanding another hand . . . . A guy in a gray suit, tie, and polished shoes with his fat wife was next to me. The performer stopped in front of the guy . . . . The man in the grey suit looked at them and lowered his eyes, his hands were trembling . . . . He was livid, he would have done anything to be a million kilometers away. He couldn't take it anymore. I reached out my hand and the performer grabbed it firmly . . . . I had to help him, because if I didn't, he, everyone, and myself, we were going to fall to pieces.[78]

The letter depicts the man in the gray suit, tie, and polished shoes as the stereotypical bourgeois art consumer. In the anonymous viewer's interpretation, he experiences tremendous discomfort in the face of *Polymorphias*'s challenge to a passive audience-performer relationship. Within the context of the piece's invocation of Holocaust violence, the resistant viewer's refusal to touch the dancer or make eye contact indexes not only discomfort, but also an unwillingness to put his own body on the line to "help" the dancer. Alternately, the author expresses her or his own significant investment in the ethical contract that this touch implies. She or he equates the act of grasping the performer's hand with the possibility of a different (nonviolent) future. The sense that the audience's collective future depended on that physical connection points, at least in the case of this spectator, to *Polymorphias*'s ability to foster critical reflection on the need for empathetic social contracts between bodies outside of the theater.

What, then, did *Polymorphias*'s exploration of relational dynamics (audience members included) and the invocation of concentration camps mean in the context of Onganía's dictatorship, particularly considering the government's record of censorship and repression of public criticism? The piece did not draw any explicit parallels between the Third Reich and the current Argentine political situation. Rather it sounded, as the score suggestively states, a "state of alert" from a safe thematic difference.[79] In other words, *Polymorphias* referenced the horror of Holocaust violence to attune viewers to the dangers of the local authoritarian present without actually naming Onganía, or even referencing the Argentine national context. As an allegory, this representational move invokes what Michael Rothberg understands as the "multidirectionality" of memory. For Rothberg, invoking historically and culturally specific traumatic histories like the Holocaust to make sense of violence in different times and places evidences "the convoluted, sometimes historically unjustified, back-and-forth movement of seemingly distant collective memories . . . [that] traverse sacrosanct borders of ethnicity and era."[80] Within a climate marked by censorship, *Polymorphias* asked performers and audience members to move otherwise by joining together in the face of past (the Holocaust) and present (Onganía's dictatorship) violence and repression.

While out of place in terms of nation and era, the citation of the Holocaust in Zimmermann's piece is not "historically unjustified" considering Argentina's significant Jewish population and the critical role Jewish dancers, Zimmermann and Kamien included, played in the development of concert dance in Buenos Aires. While *Polymorphias* "directs" Holocaust memory to call attention to a present Argentine dictatorship, the work's artistic lineage and choreographer are part of the Jewish diaspora. A decade later, the piece accrued additional meaning in Argentina in light of another and far more repressive government. Following its run at the Di Tella, *Polymorphias* was not presented again in Buenos Aires until 1981, when Zimmermann returned briefly from her self-imposed exile in Italy during the last military dictatorship (1976–83).[81]

Following *Polymorphias*, the Laboratorio de Danza presented a final piece titled *Ceremonias*. Loosely inspired by the activism of May 1968 in France, *Ceremonias* extended the Laboratorio de Danza's interest in catalyzing and sustaining group action.[82] The piece premiered in May 1970, the same month that the Di Tella permanently closed its doors. The exact reasons for the closure were never fully disclosed, though some attributed it to the falling profit margins of the Di Tella family's industries. Media coverage also questioned whether government and conservative pressure played a role. In a 1970 *Panorama* article reporting on the Di Tella's closure, former director of the Visual Arts Center and noted art critic Jorge Romero Brest highlighted these doubts: "The issues have been proposed on the economic level, and analyzing them in that light, they are correct. Analyzing things at a cultural level, I don't know if consciously or not, the elimination of Florida [referring to the Di Tella's street address] implies the destruction of a way of life."[83] Romero Brest's comment emphasizes that the closure represented not only the end of a decade of artistic experimentation, but also the "elimination" of a space that facilitated movements otherwise in everyday life. The days of the crazy block's miniskirts, unconventional fashions, and long hair were over.

By 1970, dance had also found itself largely displaced from the San Martín Theater; AADA's heyday had passed and the organization permanently dissolved in 1972. However, a new center of dance activity developed briefly at the recently opened General San Martín Cultural Center (CCGSM, 1970–present), located adjacent to the San Martín Theater. Juan Falzone organized the dance programming between 1970 and 1973. Many dance artists previously affiliated with AADA as well as the Di Tella presented work and participated in meetings and roundtables at the center, creating a forum for debating the cultural politics of dance practice and production in Buenos Aires. Within the context of these debates, Kamien presented a work that, like *Polymorphias*, called attention to government repression and moved otherwise to the re-entrenchment of conservative values and devaluation of the arts.

"MY OWN MODERNITY": THE GENERAL SAN MARTÍN CULTURAL CENTER AND *ANA KAMIEN* (1970)

Ana Kamien's eponymous solo work premiered in May 1970 as part of the "Expodanza" programming at the CCGSM. The CCGSM was not as well resourced or technically equipped as the Di Tella or the San Martín Theater. The fifth-floor space often used for dance performances featured exposed brick and a distinctive staircase against the upstage wall.[84] The space's capacity (two hundred persons) could not accommodate the now substantial public that had grown with dance's institutional presence during the 1960s.[85] In interviews, Kamien as well as dancers Estela Maris and Silvia Kaehler all recalled the cramped quarters of the performance space and their frustration that it could not accommodate all who wanted to see their work.[86]

Kamien's solo shared some characteristics with her earlier work at the Di Tella. Like her Di Tella works, *Ana Kamien* was structured episodically, referenced her background in classical ballet, and featured a musical score that sampled popular music and news broadcasts, among other sources. In this sense, the solo extended her iconoclastic vision; in her words, *Ana Kamien* was "my own modernity, that language, not made from Graham."[87] Kamien's statement distinguishes her work from the familiar modern dance referent and boldly delinks danced modernity from Europe and the United States. In our interview she also pointed out that she self-titled the piece because she felt it was her debut before the "other dance world."[88] This was Kamien's first time presenting work alongside AADA-associated artists and before a public more familiar with that organization's strand of modern dance.

Where Kamien's earlier works at the Di Tella evidenced social and artistic mobility through their challenges to gendered expectations and parodies of artistic elitism, *Ana Kamien* moved toward an explicitly political stance as it reflected the dictatorship's restriction of labor rights and civil liberties. The work premiered in the wake of the 1969 Cordobazo (May) and Rosariazo (May–September) civil uprisings, which were named for the cities where they took place (Córdoba and Rosario). Student organizations and labor unions led these popular insurrections in protest of dictatorship policies that curtailed political participation and privileged the interests of large companies and the economic elite over labor conditions and wage protections. Violent riots erupted when the military and police response resulted in multiple protestors' deaths. *Ana Kamien* echoed these events on two levels. On one hand, the piece examined labor politics from the perspective of the dance community and in light of the drastic retraction of institutional support. On the other, the dance called explicit attention to military violence and repression.

While there is no video and limited photographic documentation of the work, Kamien described the action of the piece to me in vivid detail, dancing out pieces of the choreography as we spoke together in her living room. She explained how the piece began with her slow descent down the set of stairs that formed part of the performance space. Carrying a broom with a large rectangular head, she carefully swept each step and then the stage itself. As she swept, the score played snippets of the recording of a 1970 round table inaugurating the CCGSM dance programming. The round table featured Falzone, Ricardo Freixá (then Buenos Aires's secretary of culture), and choreographer María Fux, among others, discussing the state of the dance field. It covered topics ranging from the difficulties of attaining ongoing institutional support for dance to frustration with the "piecework" nature of dance training in Buenos Aires.[89] As Kamien descended the stairs, the audience heard Falzone thank the secretary of culture for the surprising bureaucratic ease with which the office implemented his programming. He also highlighted Freixá's willingness to assist with humble activities such as arranging audience chairs.[90] The score then skipped to Freixá's statement that, "Unfortunately, what I know is that ever since I became the secretary of culture, I actually have no time for culture."[91] Freixá's statement suggested that administrative responsibilities, as opposed to artistic concerns, monopolized his time.

By pairing the sweeping action with the recording of the roundtable, *Ana Kamien* highlights the administrative and physical labor that both facilitates and impedes dance production. In the midst of the retraction of private and public support, *Ana Kamien* asked its audience to see this work as dance *and* to see dance as work.[92] It transformed debate about the dance field and references to the preparation of a performance space (sweeping, setting up chairs) into the event itself, placing the labor politics of dance center stage. Additionally, upon arrival spectators were presented with a blank piece of paper in lieu of a program, which as one review put it, functioned as a "symbol of the resources put at her [Kamien's] disposal."[93] With the sweeping choreography and blank program, the opening moments of *Ana Kamien* called attention both to shrinking resources under a repressive dictatorship as well as to choreographers' resilience. The juxtaposition of the sweeping with the roundtable discussion also emphasized what Kamien saw as the contradiction of the panelists "complaints" given that they had gathered to inaugurate a new program.[94] *Ana Kamien*, then, was both a call to action (what can we do with what we have?) and an acknowledgment of the changing artistic and political landscape. Although the piece did not directly reference fights for worker rights at the center of the recent anti-Onganía Cordobazo and Rosariazo uprisings, *Ana Kamien* asked the audience to consider the dancing body within a broader national conversation about labor rights. On a personal level, the opening also echoed the important role Kamien's own working-class background and employment history played in navigating her early dance career.

The dance's opening gave way to a series of movement episodes with vocabularies that traversed Kamien's dance background. After she finished sweeping, Kamien moved a chair to center stage as the score switched to the harp cadenza of Tchaikovsky's *Swan Lake*. Employing the chair as her "partner," Kamien performed a pas de deux based in classical ballet vocabulary. As a technique, ballet conditions the body to hide the signs of its own labor—a stark contrast to the opening's emphasis on performance as labor. While this episode echoed Kamien's earlier citations of classical ballet in her Di Tella works, parody is noticeably absent. In fact, the empty chair itself marks a void, perhaps the one left by the Di Tella's closure. This absence not only meant the retraction of resources, but also the removal of possibilities for artistic and social transgressions. However, other episodes of the piece did revisit the experimentation characteristic of Kamien's Di Tella works. In one moment of the piece, Kamien inserted herself into a body stocking made of stretch material and moved to the sound of an Italian broadcast reporting the first moon landing.[95]

While earlier portions of the piece explored movement genres and labor politics particular to dance, the closing episode turned its attention to military violence. For the music score, Kamien chose selections from Beethoven's "Funeral March" and The Doors' "Unknown Soldier." Beethoven's composition first set a somber tone, while "Unknown Soldier" invoked one of protest. Released in 1968 in the midst of the Vietnam War, "Unknown Soldier" was emblematic of antiwar music in the United States.[96] The lyrics juxtapose the death of a soldier with desensitization to US news coverage of violence and war. The song features the sounds of military marching, drumming, and a firing squad, elements that were central to Kamien's movement. Her description of her choreography that accompanied the song bears extended citation:

> I take the broom and I put it here [under my arm] and I walk around as if I were a guard doing rounds around a military camp. And after that I point the bristles of the broom behind me and I turn to the audience and the handle becomes a weapon. All of this to the "Funeral March" . . . . At a certain point I leave it [the broom] in the middle of the stage. I sit down and I begin to march like that again, but seated on the floor with my legs extended as in the goose step and I circle around the broom that is there, upright. I begin to move faster and when I arrive at the center where the broom is, it ties my hands like this [the broom stick interlaced with wrists behind the back]. It was a broom, it was a weapon, and it

was my cross. With my hands interlaced with the broomstick, I turn my back to the audience and I move toward the back of the stage. And as I advance you hear the loading and cocking of guns, and "fire" [from "Unknown Soldier"]! Then blackout, and they fire and execute me. I cannot escape.[97]

Re-employing the broom as a transformational object, the scene began with citations of military choreography. Kamien first assumed the role of the soldier, purposing the broom handle as a weapon. Before beginning her seated march, she also briefly used the broom as a crutch to invoke wounds suffered in battle. The "goose step" refers to a kind of military march in which the legs are extended without a bend at the knee. Upon grasping the broom for a second time, however, Kamien's body became the object of violence. Her bound wrists invoked arrest and detainment, and as Kamien pointed out, also suggested crucifixion (figure 1.3). In the closing moment of the piece, her slumped and motionless body indexed the death and destruction wrought by military action.

Ana Kamien, like *Polymorphias*, sounded a state of alert around the repressive climate of Onganía's military dictatorship. This commentary was not lost on critics; as one write-up noted, "the most celebrated object that accompanied Kamien in her steps was the broom that she brandished—cross, rifle, crutch, maybe even symbol of authoritarian rulers—in her Expodanza show."[98] The

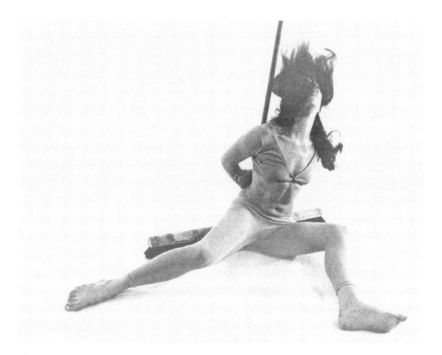

Figure 1.3 Ana Kamien in *Ana Kamien*, 1970. Photograph: Leone Sonnino. Courtesy of photographer.

piece, however, also accrued new meaning just days following its premiere. On May 29, 1970, the Peronist Montoneros militant group, as their inaugural act, kidnapped and later executed former President Pedro Eugenio Aramburu. Aramburu was a principal figure behind the 1955 military coup that removed Perón from power. The Montoneros conceived of Aramburu's execution as an act of revolutionary justice for Perón's ousting. They also held his body as a bargaining chip for the recuperation of the corpse of Perón's late wife, Eva Perón, who passed away in 1952.[99] Aramburu had helped orchestrate the "disappearance" of her corpse, which was held in Argentina for several years before it was sent to Italy. The corpse then traveled to Spain, where Perón spent part of his exile, before it was ultimately interred at the Recoleta cemetery in Buenos Aires in 1976.[100] The Montoneros conceived the execution, quite literally, as a body-for-a-body transaction. Aramburu's execution coupled with the lasting effects of the Cordobazo and Rosariazo uprisings rapidly destabilized Onganía's government. In early June, the military deposed Onganía in an internal coup d'état, appointing general Roberto M. Levingston as de facto president. The temporal collision of the execution in Kamien's piece with the Montoneros' pivotal offstage act highlights the work's incisive critique of the body as political currency and battleground amid escalating conflict between the military and militant groups of various ideological banners.

Ana Kamien boldly introduced the choreographer to the broader Buenos Aires dance community—a public that Kamien felt was inaccessible at the start of the decade. As Kamien's own "modernity," the piece shared the iconoclastic spirit of her earlier Di Tella works. The work's thematization of dance as labor and its representation of militarism used the dancing body to call attention to multiple forms of violence affecting Argentine bodies offstage. Within the context of rapidly retracting institutional support and government censorship, the very act of remaining committed to a professional career in dance constituted a form of moving otherwise. And perhaps most critically, like *Polymorphias*, *Ana Kamien* signaled dance as a site of political critique that both engaged with the political vanguards of the late 1960s and employed the concert stage as a site for expressing dissent.

REVOLUTIONARY PATHWAYS

This chapter has demonstrated how, during the fast-changing decade of the 1960s, Ana Kamien and Susana Zimmermann moved within, between, and beyond established dance genres, class and gender norms, and political stances. The social and artistic mobilities they negotiated in the first half of the decade translated into danced critiques of Onganía's repressive dictatorship in the second half of the decade. In the early 1960s, AADA and the Di Tella helped Zimmermann and Kamien, respectively, occupy artistic roles marked by leadership, authorship, and "modern" lifestyles. These organizations allowed them to circumvent expected career paths for middle- and working-class women, like Zimmermann's initial training as a secondary-school teacher and Kamien's early bank job, and facilitated movements otherwise even as aspects of the organizations and concert dance practices themselves echoed government modernization projects. While Zimmermann first worked within the relatively established modernisms of AADA, Kamien built her professional career from the start in the Di Tella, an organization at the vanguard of performance in Buenos Aires. Following the 1966 installation of Onganía's dictatorship—which restricted civil rights, actively policed gender and sexuality, violently repressed protest, and openly censored artistic works—both artists used their dance practice as a means of moving otherwise. Zimmermann's Laboratorio de Danza and stage work *Polymorphias*, both created as the Di Tella became a direct target of government repression, modeled cooperative, empathetic modes of relationality in contexts of violence. *Ana Kamien*, which premiered at one of the only remaining institutional footholds for dance at the time, aligned dance with broader struggles for labor rights and against the military.

More broadly, this chapter's attention to Kamien's and Zimmermann's 1960s activities establishes a genealogy of moving otherwise within the early history of contemporary dance in Buenos Aires. As mentioned previously, both went on to train and work with a number of dancers whose work populates the chapters to follow. As *Ana Kamien* and *Polymorphias* spoke to the repression of Onganía's "Argentine Revolution"—his regime's official name—a very different revolution was brewing. Leftist militant movements, whose whispers were audible in the Laboratorio de Danza's echo of Guevara's "new man" and whose indignation materialized in the startling resonances between *Ana Kamien*'s execution scene and the Montoneros' literal execution of Aramburu, steadily grew in strength and public visibility. In the next chapter, I turn to a group of female dancers and choreographers—several of whom worked with Zimmermann's Laboratorio de Danza—whose dancing intersected with and informed their political militancy in the early 1970s. I also consider a series of dance works that reflected revolutionary themes on the concert stage.

CHAPTER 2

The Revolution Was Danced

"What is the face of the Argentine left?" asked a 1972 cover of the widely circulated magazine *Panorama*, a weekly publication that reported on culture and politics.[1] The question appeared inside the faceless silhouette of a blue, distinctly masculine figure. In the corner, diagonally printed text announced "the guerrilla's new offensive."[2] The cover articulated middle-class anxiety around a growing climate of violence between armed militant groups and the military government of de facto president Alejandro Agustín Lanusse (1971–73)—the leader of the latest in a string of short-lived military dictatorships and military-instituted civilian governments that marked the 1960s and early 1970s.[3] The rugged, fatigue-clad images of iconic revolutionaries like Ernesto "Che" Guevara and Fidel Castro ghost *Panorama*'s cover silhouette. At the same time, however, the title and blank face worry over whether the "new offensive" might look different than anticipated—a tactical advantage against the Argentine authorities. This chapter explores one, perhaps surprising, answer to *Panorama*'s questioning headline: female contemporary dancers. Widespread press coverage of political organizations during the early 1970s helped foment panic around militancy, though dance—unlike movements in theater, music, and the visual arts—was not broadly associated with political activity. In the following pages, I examine how previously undocumented intersections between Argentine contemporary dancers and political militancy in the early 1970s moved otherwise both to normative images and practices of militancy as well as to the violent repression of political dissidence that took place under Lanusse's military dictatorship.

As mentioned in the previous chapter, in the late 1960s and early 1970s Latin American leftist movements developed in the context of the ongoing Cold War, the conflict in Vietnam, and decolonization movements—as well as regional events, including the success of the Cuban Revolution in 1959, the death of student protestors in Mexico City's 1968 Tlatelolco massacre, and the rise and fall of socialist President Salvador Allende in Chile between 1970 and 1973. In Argentina, leftist movements drew on internationally circulating currents of Marxism-Leninism, Maoism, Guevarism, and Trotskyism, and nationally based Peronism. All of the Argentine leftist groups expressed opposition to the series of right-wing military governments that followed Juan Carlos Onganía's "Argentine Revolution" (1966–70), and many dedicated their efforts to fostering working-class revolution.

Many Argentines, especially artists, workers, intellectuals, and university students circulated through the political left, including through parties associated with armed factions. Prominent armed organizations included the People's Revolutionary Army (ERP, Ejército Revolucionario del Pueblo), the armed branch of the Marxist-Leninist Worker's Revolutionary Party (PRT, Partido Revolucionario de los Trabajadores); the Peronist Montoneros; the Peronist Armed Forces (FAP, Fuerzas Armadas Peronistas); and the Revolutionary Armed Forces (FAR, Fuerzas Armadas Revolucionarias). However, membership in armed militant organizations was clandestine, and participation or even affiliation with members could bring harsh reprisals such as torture, incarceration, and in many cases, death. Secrecy shrouded, and continues to shroud, discussions of militancy. In my interviews with dancers and choreographers, compulsory forgetting and partial knowledge frequently blurred recollections of who, or whose partner, participated in militant organizations. In its moment, the *Panorama* cover captured the fear of the unidentified militant body that gripped the Argentine middle classes. Today the image also resonates for researchers who are struggling to piece together traces of pasts purposefully shaded from public view, by both militant organizations themselves as well as the government. In short, Argentine history is still asking, "What is the face of the Argentine left?"

During the early years of my research, choreographers, scholars, and archivists assured me that, to the best of their knowledge, no members of the Buenos Aires contemporary dance community participated in armed militancy. I initially did not push too hard past that universal answer; for reasons I will explore in greater detail, militancy is an especially sensitive topic. The dictatorships of the 1970s justified their violent repression as a response to militant operations that targeted government officials, an explanation that glossed over the scale of the state's human rights violations and the obvious power differential between the government and political opposition.[4] Argentine historian Hugo Vezzetti has demonstrated compellingly how, in response to the government's identification of militant violence as justification for state violence, scholarly texts—as well as human rights groups and state-sponsored memory projects—struggle to represent revolutionary violence within the history of state violence, either absenting or idealizing it.[5] Within this fraught terrain, I initially accepted assertions that contemporary dancers did not "militate," in the sense of being active with, armed factions.[6]

This chapter begins with a consideration of how the dance archive revealed the stories of women who led separate lives as contemporary dancers and political militants. I explain how these materials led me to several women who linked the supposedly separate spheres of contemporary dance and militancy: Silvia Hodgers, María Elena Maucieri, and Alicia Sanguinetti. Hodgers, Sanguinetti, and Maucieri all militated with the PRT-ERP. All three experienced periods of incarceration, sometimes together, throughout the 1970s. Their stories, pieced together from personal and published interviews as well as archival documents, demonstrate how the dance archive makes visible histories of militancy otherwise obscured by secrecy as well as dance's presumed distance from revolutionary politics. The next section of the chapter focuses specifically on Hodgers's and Sanguinetti's incarceration at the Rawson Penitentiary in 1972. It examines how these dancers' accounts bring to light the unexpected role that dance and movement played in creating and sustaining community among incarcerated political prisoners with a range of affiliations. In particular, I analyze the key role of dancing in the escape plot that prisoners planned and executed that year. At Rawson, dance quite literally served as the prelude to and pretext for revolt. The initiative, however, ended tragically with the military's execution of sixteen political prisoners, an event known as the Trelew Massacre.

My journey into learning about dancers who militated also led me to question if two 1973 dance works might also be productively considered "militant": Cuca Taburelli's *Preludio para un final* (*Prelude for an Ending*), which explicitly takes up the Trelew Massacre, and Estela Maris's *Juana Azurduy*. The final section of the chapter analyzes these two dances, both of which take up militant themes, in relationship to offstage repertoires of militancy. Although neither choreographer militated, I follow Argentine theater historian Lorena Verzero's call for an expansion of the term "militant" beyond actors or theater groups with explicit party affiliations to include "related cultural experiences in their social or revolutionary ideology."[7] While this chapter begins by discussing how dancers acted politically outside of the studio and theater, my analysis of these two works demonstrates how concert dance itself functioned as a site for imagining and debating political futures and possibilities. By questioning the relationship between gendered militant bodies, revolutionary politics, and the political potential of dance, these works extended the revolution onto the concert stage.

I argue that these cases of militants dancing and dances about militancy reconfigure the normative choreographies of both repertoires; they underscore contemporary dance's role in explicitly political repertoires and make visible bodies committed to the leftist cause on the contemporary dance stage. At its core, the chapter takes up a question that, as Vezzetti notes, deeply preoccupied militant groups (and echoes *Panorama*'s headline): "what acts, behaviors, decisions, and passions should be legitimately considered a militant revolutionary work or act?"[8] I argue that the blurred lines between dancing and militating considered here offer dance as an unexpected answer to this question. This response intervenes not only in Argentine dance historiography, but also in a dominant historical narrative that masculinizes leftist militant activity and marginalizes the role of cultural production generally, and dance practice specifically, within legacies of political struggle.

READING THE GAPS

This story begins where the previous chapter left off—with noted choreographer Susana Zimmermann. As examined in the previous chapter, the creative agenda of Zimmermann's Laboratorio de Danza (1967–70), based at the Di Tella Institute, reflected the leftist political movements and politicized art projects of the late 1960s. The 1969 work *Polymorphias* simultaneously memorialized the victims of the Holocaust and sounded a state of alert around the social and political repression that took place under de facto president Juan Carlos Onganía's military dictatorship. However, it was my work with archival materials related to the group's 1967 production of *Danza ya* (*Dance Now*) that led me to the interconnected stories of three cast and production team members' journeys through the worlds of contemporary dance and political militancy. I knew through other published sources that Alicia Sanguinetti, a well-known dance photographer who created the slides projected in *Danza ya*, had militated in the 1970s. Subsequent research into others credited on the *Danza ya* program revealed that cast members Silvia Hodgers and María Elena Maucieri did as well. Though Zimmermann herself never militated, it makes sense that *Danza ya* would have attracted people who formed part of, or would ultimately join, leftist organizations. *Danza ya*'s emphasis on collective decision-making departed from traditional dance creation methods where authorial power rests solely with the choreographer. This collaborative, egalitarian approach fit with the revolutionary ideologies that were influencing art makers not only to create work that commented on social and political realities, but also to critically assess the politics of their own production methods.[9]

All of the dancers whose lives intersect in the following narrative ultimately lost partners or close friends to government practices of forced disappearance. Several experienced torture. With the weight of these traumas ever present, the reconstruction of events that follows is my attempt to shed light on how the dance archive—in this case a single program—excavates a select history of militancy that will always, necessarily, remain partially in the shadows. As state repression escalated throughout the 1970s, dancers had to exercise practices of self-protection, policing, and censorship in an atmosphere where even ostensibly nonmilitant association with suspected militants could result in death. This atmosphere of fear and clandestine knowledge became further intensified following the increasing state terror after 1974 that would culminate in Argentina's last military dictatorship in 1976. While our research takes place in different contexts marked by violence, Rachmi Diyah Larasati's reflection on her study of dance in post-genocide Indonesia resonates with my approach here. Like Larasati, I am acutely aware that "at stake are difficult decisions as to which parts of this long journey it is possible to mention specifically or describe in detail in order to support my arguments in this book while minimizing the potential to cause harm or put others at risk."[10] I am deeply grateful to Hodgers and Sanguinetti for authorizing the inclusion of their stories in considerable detail here, and to the multiple others who confidentially shared stories that fundamentally shaped my understanding of contemporary dance's crossings with 1970s militancy.

At the time of *Danza ya*'s development in 1967, Sanguinetti already had experience with organized political activity. From a young age, art and leftist politics mixed in Sanguinetti's home; Sanguinetti's mother is the well-known photographer, political activist, and German émigré Annemarie Heinrich.[11] As early as secondary school, Sanguinetti participated briefly in the youth sector of the Communist Party.[12] She trained in ballet with María Ruanova (one of the first Argentine-born ballet dancers to gain international acclaim), but chose to dedicate her career to dance photography, working out of her mother's Recoleta studio. Sanguinetti worked closely with choreographers presenting work at the Di Tella and through the Friends of Dance Association (AADA) throughout the 1960s. She designed the slides used in *Danza ya* as well as *Polymorphias* (1969) and *Ceremonias* (1970), Zimmermann's other productions at the Di Tella. On the activist front, Sanguinetti became involved with the Cultural Workers Anti-Imperialist Front (FATRAC, Frente Antiimperialista de Trabajadores de la Cultura) following the initiative's emergence in 1968.[13] Composed of artists and intellectuals, the FATRAC was linked to the PRT. According to scholars Ana Longoni and Mariano Mestman, the group understood itself as a recruitment tool for the party and as an activist organization in and of itself.[14]

After working with the FATRAC for a brief period, Sanguinetti affiliated with the PRT-ERP following the formation of the armed branch.[15] In one of our interviews, Sanguinetti noted that, because of the clandestine nature of militancy (complicated by the frequent use of pseudonyms), in the early years she never really knew who in her artistic circuit was also involved. She did express that she often had a sense of who might be a militant or perhaps sympathetic to the leftist cause based on the way they spoke about or reacted to current events.[16] By 1971, however, Sanguinetti would have known that María Elena Maucieri—another *Danza ya* cast member—was also a member of the PRT-ERP. It is unclear when Maucieri joined; however, Sanguinetti's testimony coupled with archival documents confirms that both were involved in an operation slated for July 9, 1971—Independence Day.[17] Sanguinetti and Maucieri, along with Martín Marco, Pedro Cazes Camarero, Eduardo Streger, and Mario Rodriguez, reportedly planned to commandeer a gas truck and destroy the stage where President Lanusse, along with Uruguayan President Jorge Pacheco Areco, would view the annual military parade.[18] According to Sanguinetti, the group was discussing the plan in a café when police overheard the conversation and took them in for questioning.[19] After passing through the local precinct and federal custody, Sanguinetti and Maucieri were transferred to the women's unit of the Villa Devoto prison in Buenos Aires (now called the Complejo Penitenciario Federal de la C.A.B.A., or the Federal Penitentiary Complex of the Autonomous City of Buenos Aires).

Silvia Hodgers worked in a different branch of the PRT-ERP. However, through an unrelated series of events, she was also detained and transferred to Villa Devoto in 1971. Upon arrival, she was reunited with her fellow *Danza ya* production mates—and learned of Sanguinetti's militant affiliation for the first time.[20] As a dancer, Hodgers began her training in Buenos Aires at a young age, and studied modern dance and ballet with prominent figures including Renate Schottelius and, like Sanguinetti, María Ruanova.[21] During the 1960s, Hodgers performed in works by prominent choreographer Oscar Araiz as well as Zimmermann. However, Hodgers's first direct contact with leftist organizations did not happen through Zimmermann's group, or in Buenos Aires. Rather, the impetus for her political involvement occurred during her time training and performing in Europe. In 1968, Hodgers traveled to England, where she studied as a scholarship student at the London Contemporary Dance School before working briefly with Maurice Béjart's company in Brussels. Zimmermann also studied with Béjart around this time (recall from chapter 1 that his 1968 denunciation of Prime Minister António de Oliveira Salazar's dictatorship during a concert in Portugal inspired her work *Polymorphias*). Following Hodgers's time with Béjart, she moved to Paris and began working with Peruvian theater maker Emilio Galli. Hodgers identifies Galli's politicized work as a turning point in her artistic career. Galli had close connections with the Peruvian left, and through him Hodgers met Peruvian economist Hilda Gadea (Ernesto "Che" Guevara's first wife). Hodgers's performance work with Galli and friendship with Gadea catalyzed her interest in creating politically committed art and joining the armed struggle.[22]

Following her return to Buenos Aires in late 1970, Hodgers joined the PRT-ERP. In September 1971, only a few months following the botched Independence Day plan, federal police arrested Hodgers when they found arms and police uniforms in her apartment.[23] Her PRT-ERP superiors had asked her to store these items, though she had no knowledge of the specific operation in which they were to be used. Before her transfer to Villa Devoto, federal police tortured Hodgers, resulting in permanent damage to her eardrums. Federal police and military officials frequently tortured political prisoners during this period, a practice that anticipated the intensification of state violence in the mid-1970s. In our interview, Hodgers recounted the harrowing way in which she (narrowly) escaped the sexual assault frequently inflicted on female political prisoners. Hodgers's father called a nephew who had a position of authority within the federal police and requested: "if you have to torture her, torture her, but don't rape her."[24] Hodgers's father's comment directly acknowledges the incorporation of rape into torture practices at the same time that his appeal both authorizes physical violence against political prisoners and implicitly affirms a patriarchal view of female sexual propriety as a measure of worth.

Following their detainment at Villa Devoto, Hodgers and Sanguinetti were both transferred to the Rawson Penitentiary in 1972.[25] In the following section, I turn to the unexpected role of dance at Rawson leading up to—and during—the now infamous prison break in August of the same year. Hodgers, Sanguinetti, and Maucieri's intersecting journeys through the worlds of contemporary dance and militancy recounted in this section unveil, in powerful and unexpected ways, how the dance archive allows for a reconstruction of militant histories. Embedded in cast lists and production credits, these archival traces beckon with the possibility of rediscovery. Some stories, however, will (and should) remain partially told. This incompleteness not only maps the continued struggle to write militant bodies into history, but also the responsibility of the researcher to remain vigilant about the point at which telling the story of painful pasts, or even asking questions about it, might do more harm than good.

"THE CROUCHED-DOWN MARCH": DANCING THE PRISON BREAK

Hodgers and Sanguinetti were two of many political prisoners who were transferred to the Rawson Penitentiary from Villa Devoto and other prisons in 1972. Rawson is located near Trelew, a city in Argentina's southern Chubut Province in the Patagonia region (figure 2.1). The military considered the prison an ideal location to house political prisoners given its isolated location. Rawson's location might have been remote, but testimonies suggest that the collective presence of so many members of the armed left—from a range of parties and including prominent leaders—in fact fostered a sense of community and renewed energy around the revolutionary cause. Prisoners used their time at Rawson to continue their militancy by studying (primarily through reading and discussing contraband texts) and preparing for future operations outside—and inside—the prison.[26] Here I consider the role of another activity at Rawson: dancing. Drawing on my interviews with Hodgers and Sanguinetti, as well as other published testimonies and accounts, I examine how dance

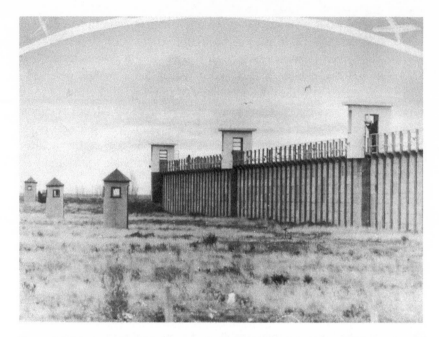

Figure 2.1 Exterior walls of the Rawson Penitentiary, *Diario La Razón*, 1972. Courtesy of the Documentation and Research Center of Leftist Cultures (CeDInCI).

helped create community in the prison—and played a key role in the preparation for and execution of the August 15 escape plan that coordinated over one hundred political prisoners, allied prison guard Carmelo Facio, and several Trelew locals. While the content of the *Danza ya* program demonstrated how dance histories illuminate militant histories, accounts from the Rawson Penitentiary suggest that dance also constituted part of the repertoire of militancy itself.

In our interviews, as well as in testimony featured in the documentary *Trelew: La fuga que fue masacre (Trelew: The Jailbreak That Was a Massacre)*, Hodgers and Sanguinetti recall that Rawson danced in two ways: folkloric dance performed to pass the time and *gimnasia* (physical exercise) classes that Hodgers offered to keep herself and her unit mates in good physical shape.[27] In order to execute both kinds of movement, political prisoners interacted tactically with the architecture of the prison and had to remain vigilant about guards' watchful eyes and ears. In ex-prisoners' recollections, political prisoners were distributed across multiple floors; each floor of the prison had parallel rows of individual cells with a hallway between them.[28] The floors of the cells featured thick glass bricks set in cement. In the *Trelew* documentary, multiple ex-prisoners report that they were able to chip away at the glass, forming a hole that grew larger over time and allowed prisoners to see and communicate with each other between floors. The communication and sight lines through the glass not only facilitated escape planning, but also fostered a network of care among prisoners that allowed them to sustain romantic partnerships and comfort those struggling with the conditions of incarceration.[29]

Hodgers and Sanguinetti both recalled that Mario Roberto Santucho—the founder and leader of the PRT-ERP—would dance in his cell while prisoners watched through the hole in the glass, performances that helped to raise the spirits of his imprisoned comrades. Sanguinetti identified his movement as *chacarera*, a folkloric form characteristic of the northern Argentine provinces, while Hodgers remembered it as *malambo*, another folkloric dance associated with the rural pampas.[30] *Chacarera* is a partner-based form, while the *malambo* is historically performed by men and features fast-paced footwork. Santucho's solo performance might have linked the dance with *malambo* in Hodgers's mind, though *chacarera* is equally likely; Santucho is from Santiago del Estero, a city closely associated with *chacarera*'s historical development and contemporary practice. Ultimately, which folkloric form Santucho performed is less important than the national sentiments and imaginary that both imply. *Malambo* and *chacarera* not only signal regional identity, but also summon a national identity rooted in nostalgic celebrations of rural farm life and the rugged gauchos (cowboys) of the eighteenth and nineteenth centuries, which evoke strong associations with criollo (creole) culture. For the prisoners watching Santucho, then, his dance not only established a sense of community within a disciplinary architecture specifically designed to foreclose connection, but also invoked the legacy of the patria (homeland) that these militant groups understood themselves to be fighting for.

Folkloric music was also an important aspect of the prisoners' community building and consolidation around their political mandate. Carlos Astudillo, a FAR member, reportedly liked to sing the *zamba* "Luis Burela."[31] The song memorializes the independence-era military hero who began the "Gaucho War" in the northwest city of Salta. When colonial forces invaded Salta, Burela's guerrilla group successfully disarmed them. Faces pressed up against the bars of their cells, the Rawson political prisoners would listen to Astudillo and sing along to the lines: "'And with what arms will we fight, sir? With the ones that we take from them,' they say he yelled."[32]

Ultimately, the folkloric dancing and singing that created community and raised (militant) spirits among political prisoners across a range of affiliations became scripted into the escape plan itself. In the *Trelew* documentary, ex-Montonero leader Fernando Vaca Narvaja explains how the inmates wagered that these established practices would create a festive—and distracting—environment in which to initiate the plan:

> We had to generate certain kinds of movement in the prison that would not attract the particular attention of the inside guards. So we began doing things

that we hadn't done normally, like *peñas* (dances), guitar-playing sessions, and songs. This way, when we did the escape, it would seem normal that the prison was filled with noise, singing, and movement.[33]

Ostensibly "entertainment," folkloric dance and music functioned contiguously in the prison as community-building practices—breathing life into a space constructed to stifle it—and as the mobilizing strategy for the escape plan. Militant action depended on political prisoners' (including famous ones like Santucho's) embodied knowledge of dance, something normally considered peripheral to revolutionary activity. Dance as pretext and prelude to revolt at Rawson echoes culturally and geographically distinct histories that linked dance and rebellion. In her study of the history of black social dance forms in the United States, Katrina Hazzard-Gordon notes that "ample evidence indicates that slave insurrections were either plotted at dances or scheduled to take place on occasions that involved dancing," a phenomenon that she links more broadly to "war dances, or dances in which preparation for battle was the central theme."[34] I am not suggesting that the political prisoners' incarceration and chattel slavery are equivalent circumstances; rather, both contexts point to how social dancing has consistently moved otherwise within contexts aimed at disciplining and controlling bodies.

Just as folkloric dance and music became part of the plan, so too did Hodgers's *gimnasia* classes. During her time at Rawson, Hodgers taught classes in the hall between the cells on her floor. These sessions combined balance, strength, flexibility, and alignment exercises that drew on her contemporary dance training and background in yoga.[35] However, as Sanguinetti put it, Hodgers's classes were not just "common exercise"—in two senses.[36] On the one hand, Sanguinetti felt Hodgers's exercises had aesthetic and kinesthetic qualities marked by the principles of modern and contemporary dance. On the other hand, they were not simply intended as recreation or creative expression—these classes kept the women in action-ready shape. The primary prison-break planners saw the opportunity in these classes for training for the escape itself, and asked Hodgers to choreograph and rehearse movement that would allow the female prisoners to pass stealthily through the prison's hallways toward the arms room and prison exit.[37] While Hodgers's *gimnasia* exercises could be dismissed as "common exercise" by the guards, the women had to be careful to rehearse the choreography for the break itself— what Hodgers called "the crouched-down march"—in secret.[38] The crouched-down march meant advancing single file, quickly and quietly, in a squatted position—sitting bones to heels. The low position allowed the women to duck below the windows that lined the hallways; by hugging the walls as they marched along, they would be out of the guards' lines of sight.

Given the stakes of properly performing the crouched-down march, Hodgers's *gimnasia* classes were hardly "common exercise." To sustain this movement for any period of time required core and thigh strength as well as flexibility in the hips—not to mention healthy knee and ankle joints and full concentration. Hodgers drew on her embodied knowledge, garnered from years spent training as a dancer, to condition and rehearse bodies for specific militant action. Hodgers's pedagogical approach, based as it was in repetition, emphasized that this movement training itself exercised discipline over the prisoners' bodies, even as it was conceived as a strategy of moving otherwise within the disciplinary architecture of the prison. Hodgers's choreographic labor, as well as the militants' uses of folkloric dance and music, instantiated a politicized relationship between movement practice and militant action otherwise obscured by their respective historiographies. The Rawson prison revolt was, quite literally, choreographed. Where the names in the *Danza ya* program helped uncover parallel histories of dance and militancy, the events at Rawson reveal a story of dance and movement *as* militant action. By taking advantage of assumptions that movement practices are merely "entertainment" or "common exercise," the break was rehearsed as dance.

Notably, dancing among political prisoners appeared in other penitentiaries as well. Another contemporary dancer who was incarcerated at the Villa Devoto prison in the 1970s recounted teaching dance and *gimnasia* classes for other female inmates during recreation periods, albeit outside of the context of a prison break. In addition to teaching classes, she gave short dance performances for fellow prisoners in the shower room, which she remembered as one of the only spaces where the prisoners could talk, debate, and pass time together in relative freedom.[39] These classes and shower-room performances evidence, like the narrative of dance's role at Rawson, how dance created and sustained community during periods of incarceration, moving otherwise within a context specifically designed to foreclose it.

On the day of the Rawson escape, the *peña* and "crouched-down march" succeeded and the prisoners successfully took control of the prison. According to the account given in the book *Detenidos-aparecidos: presas y presos políticos desde Trelew a la dictadura (Re-appeared Detainees: Political Prisoners from Trelew to the Dictatorship)*, charismatic singer Astudillo in fact signaled the start of the plan with the militants' favorite lines from "Luis Burela": "'And with what arms will we fight, sir? With the ones that we take from them,' they say he yelled."[40] The lyrics no longer just invoked a sense of revolutionary camaraderie among militants—they literally described what was about to take place. The plan reportedly began when Marcos Osatinsky (FAR) pulled a pistol on a guard from inside his cell and demanded the guard's keys. Allied guard Carmelo Facio had allowed the weapon to pass through prison security.[41]

The inmates then went on to capture the prison unit by unit by dressing in guards' uniforms and using confiscated weapons and found objects that had been turned into weapons in the weeks prior to the escape.[42] Despite the successful orchestration of the internal plan—save the death of guard

Juan Gregorio Valenzuela—the escape plan ultimately failed. According to testimonies outlining the escape published by journalist and poet Francisco Urondo in *La patria fusilada (The Executed Nation)*, in the original plan, escapees planned to enter vehicles waiting outside that would transport them to the nearby airport. There they would hijack a flight and divert it to Chile, where they hoped socialist President Salvador Allende would offer immunity, with the goal of continuing on to Cuba. Only one vehicle, carrying six prisoners, made it to the airport. Back at the prison, one of the other drivers misinterpreted a signal, and additional anticipated transportation never arrived. At this point, nineteen prisoners decided to call taxis to take them to the airport; however, they arrived after the plane had taken off.[43] Hodgers and Sanguinetti were among those who remained at Rawson, where military personal regained control of the facility and initiated a lockdown.[44]

In preparation for confrontation with the military, the escapees who made it out of Rawson took control of the airport. They took hostages and called journalists, holding a press conference to draw public attention in hopes of securing their safety.[45] In negotiations, Captain Luis Emilio Sosa of the military indicated that the escapees would be allowed to enter military custody with legal counsel. However, Sosa prevented the lawyer from boarding the bus carrying the prisoners and took them to the nearby naval base in Trelew, where they were interrogated and tortured for six days.[46] During the early hours of August 22, Sosa and several officers abruptly awoke the prisoners and forced them into a corridor between the cells.[47] Sixteen prisoners were shot and killed, and three others were injured but survived. In the official narrative circulated by Lanusse's government, the military was forced to return fire when one of the prisoners apprehended Sosa's gun. In *La patria fusilada*, the three survivors María Antonia Berger (FAR), Alberto Miguel Camps (FAR), and Ricardo René Haidar (Montoneros) indicate that there was no such action on the part of the prisoners.[48] Following the Trelew escape, lockdown, and massacre, Hodgers and Sanguinetti, among others, were transferred back to Villa Devoto.

Government justification of the Trelew killings generated public backlash against the military, widespread protests in Buenos Aires, and broad national recognition of the militant left. Increased guerrilla activity and military reprisals against suspected collaborators ensued and destabilized Lanusse's government. As Lanusse's government faltered, he set in action a course of events that allowed for democratic elections. In a last-ditch effort to keep former President Perón from running, Lanusse instituted residency requirements that disqualified Perón based on his continued exile in Spain. Perón's "personal delegate" Héctor José Cámpora was elected president in March 1973 and assumed the office on May 25. That same day, he ordered the release of all political prisoners, which included Hodgers and Sanguinetti. The day before the release, Sanguinetti's brother Ricardo visited his sister and, given the more relaxed control in the prison in anticipation of the return to democratic governance, Ricardo was able to sneak in a camera.[49] He left the camera with his sister, who documented her final hours in Villa Devoto. Collected in the publication *El Devotazo*, the photographs show the prisoners gathered in common spaces, hard at work making armbands, flyers, and banners in anticipation of their release (figure 2.2). Even though their release would not be confirmed until the following day, the photographs capture a sense of renewed purpose in their cause and evidence how the militants continued to organize in prison, directly challenging it as a disciplinary space.

Cámpora's presidency offered a brief period of openness for leftist groups. This changed quickly, however, when Perón returned to Argentina on June 20, 1973. As Peronists from both the right and left wings of the movement gathered in a field near the Buenos Aires Ezeiza Airport to welcome Perón, right-wing Peronists opened fire on left-wing groups. Known as the Ezeiza Massacre, the event left an estimated thirteen dead and more than three hundred wounded in its immediate aftermath.[50] The following month, Cámpora resigned from the presidency to allow for Perón's democratic election in September 1973. Over the next year, the effects of the Ezeiza Massacre provoked bitter divisions and further violence as the Peronist left, which had militated and mobilized to enable Perón's return, accused him of betrayal. Perón's minister of social welfare, José López Rega, formed the Argentine Anti-Communist Alliance (Alianza Anticomunista Argentina, known as the

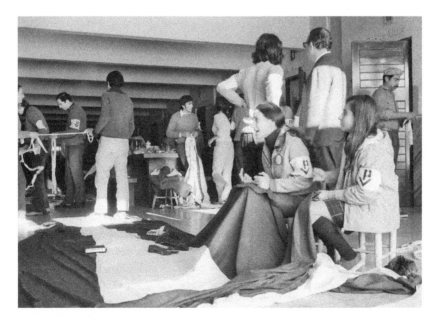

Figure 2.2 Militants making banners inside the Villa Devoto prison in anticipation of their release on May 25, 1973. Photograph: Alicia Sanguinetti. Courtesy of photographer.

Triple A), an extra-official death squad composed of military and police that targeted leftist organizations, including Peronist ones. While the term *desaparecido*, or disappeared person, does not emerge as an official historical category until after the 1976 coup that began the last military dictatorship, targeted government killings of activists first began through the Triple A. It is within this context of rapid political shifts that the two works considered in the next section—Estela Maris's *Juana Azurduy* (June 1973) and Cuca Taburelli's *Preludio para un final* (November 1973)—invoked militant themes and grappled with violence on the concert dance stage.

Following their release from Villa Devoto, Hodgers and Sanguinetti continued to militate through the mid-1970s, though both pulled back from their participation in the Buenos Aires dance community and eventually went into exile following the disappearance of their partners. Sanguinetti's partner, PRT-ERP member Alberto José Munarriz—who had also been at Rawson during the escape—was disappeared in 1974. Following the 1976 coup, Sanguinetti and her young son went into "internal" exile, living under assumed names in the interior of the country.[51] She reentered public life following the 1983 return to democracy and reassumed her prominent place in cultural circles and political organizing alike. Following her release in 1973, Hodgers continued to work with the PRT-ERP until she fled Argentina with her son following the May 1976 disappearance of her partner Héctor Fernández Baños, a University of Buenos Aires law professor and PRT-ERP member.[52] Hodgers had continued to teach and perform briefly in Buenos Aires under an assumed name following her release from prison in 1973; however, she did not resume full-time work in the dance field until the early 1980s when she settled in Geneva, where she continues to live today. In chapter 4, *Moving Otherwise* returns to Hodgers and considers her choreographic work, created in the late 1990s, that reflects on her experiences of torture, detainment, and loss during the 1970s.

REVOLUTION ON THE CONCERT STAGE: *PRELUDIO PARA UN FINAL* (1973) AND *JUANA AZURDUY* (1973)

In the wake of the Trelew Massacre and in the midst of the events that surrounded Cámpora's resignation and Perón's return to the Argentine presidency, two dance works premiered that portrayed revolutionary themes. Cuca Taburelli's *Preludio para un final* (*Prelude to an Ending*, 1973) directly responded to the Trelew Massacre and staged text and movement that expressed solidarity with the leftist cause. Estela Maris's *Juana Azurduy* (1973) embodied the eponymous mestiza (indigenous and Spanish descent) who fought alongside her husband in Argentine independence campaigns (1810–18). Though Maris's piece does not explicitly reference contemporaneous militancy, it employed a representational strategy common among 1970s militant groups: it invoked an independence-era hero to give meaning to current political struggles. Though neither Taburelli nor Maris were members of political organizations, these works evidence how contemporary dance extended leftist revolutionary movements to the concert stage. They constituted, to re-cite Verzero's expanded conception of the term "militant," "related cultural experiences in their social or revolutionary ideology."[53] Both works are relatively unknown and have limited documentation, so in the following discussion I rely primarily on the memories of the choreographers and dancers involved in their production.

Preludio was the first and only piece created and performed by Cuca Taburelli's short-lived collective Pulso Cinco Danza Teatro (Five Pulse Dance Theater). Although Pulso Cinco was only active for a brief time in the early 1970s, all members went on to, or continued, successful careers in dance and other arts in Argentina and abroad.[54] Notably, member Milka Truol performed in Ana Kamien and Marilú Marini's Di Tella Institute works mentioned in the previous chapter, including *Danse bouquet* (1965) and *La fiesta* (1966), as well as Kamien's *Oh! Casta Diva* (1967). As Pulso Cinco member Vivian Luz recalled in our interview, the five-member group grew out of a desire to address political concerns and support broader leftist movements through dance, bringing Pulso Cinco in line with the work of the FATRAC and other explicitly leftist artistic collectives of the time.[55] In Luz's words, "five people between the ages of twenty and thirty got together to express the concerns we had in that moment, which had to do with Yankee [US] imperialism, the Vietnam War—all the concerns of our generation, which we were filled with."[56]

In Taburelli's account, *Preludio* aimed to both memorialize the Trelew killings and serve as a site of "rebirth."[57] In this context, rebirth is open to a dual meaning: dance as a practice of life in the face of violent death, and as a site for giving new life to the ideas for which the militants were fighting. The piece, Taburelli recounted, included spoken text drawn from Guevara's speeches and writings, materials that signaled a clear connection to militant ideologies.[58] While the exact details of the choreography escaped the memories of the choreographer as well as the dancers I was able to interview, Truol did recall the importance of prioritizing content over form in the group's creative process.[59] Photographs from the production suggest that the work used stylized choreography and quotidian gesture to denounce the Trelew Massacre and signal defiance. Clad in leotards and tights, the dancers' bodies are charged with tension, particularly through the upper body. In several photographs, arms bent at sharp right angles that end in clawed fingers transmit a spirit of struggle (figure 2.3).[60] The program design additionally supports the dancers' and choreographer's recollections of the work's militant spirit. It features five silhouettes holding hands; three female and two male figures reflect the gender composition of the cast.[61] The figures on the end

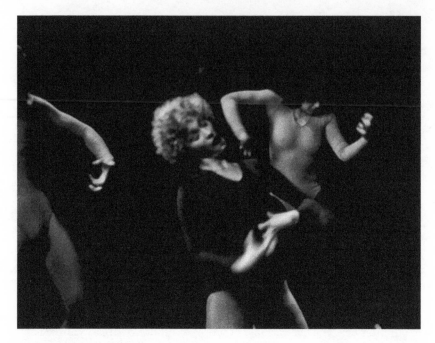

Figure 2.3 Pulso Cinco Danza Teatro (Vivian Luz, front) in *Preludio para un final*, 1973. Photograph: Aldo Delport. Courtesy of Cuca Taburelli.

make fists, echoing an iconic gesture of protest. Their bold stance captured the sense of resistance and hope reportedly embodied in the choreography and verbalized in the spoken text.

While material on *Preludio* is relatively scant, the work (and the Pulso Cinco project more broadly) registers a notable engagement with revolutionary politics as it aimed to honor those lost in the Trelew Massacre and support the principles that drove militant politics. The work's mix of stylized movement and politicized text instantiates connections between the contemporary dance stage and militancy absent from existing historiographies. Similar to my first encounter with crossings between dance and militancy through *Danza ya* archival materials, I first learned about *Preludio* and Pulso Cinco when working with documents from Luz's private collection. Knowing my interests, she pointed out the piece and connected me with Taburelli well before I knew that contemporary dancers had even taken part in the Trelew escape plan. When I shared Hodgers and Sanguinetti's stories with both Taburelli and Luz, they were surprised to hear of this unexpected crossing between a choreographic representation and the historical event itself.

While the *Preludio* production received no direct government censure, a growing climate of violence and fear deeply affected all members in the years to come. Asking my interlocutors to "stir up the past," as Taburelli put it, ultimately highlighted the extension of state repression to Argentines with and without official membership in political organizations.[62] Following the 1976 coup, Taburelli self-exiled to Bogotá, Colombia, where she established a successful dance career. Taburelli restaged *Preludio* there—albeit a much different version—in 1981.[63] Like Sanguinetti and Hodgers, Truol also experienced the tragedy of losing her partner to forced disappearance in the early years of the last military dictatorship. Her husband, José Miguel Pais, an architect, was disappeared in 1976.[64]

Estela Maris's *Juana Azurduy* offers another example of revolutionary politics on the contemporary dance stage. Though Maris is widely recognized as an accomplished performer, teacher, and choreographer, this solo is a lesser-known work. Maris began performing in the 1950s and gained notoriety through AADA in the 1960s; she performed in works by Araiz, Schottelius, and others, and presented a number of her own works on AADA's programs as well as in other venues.[65] *Juana Azurduy* premiered in June 1973 in the third-floor space of the General San Martín Cultural Center as part of Juan Falzone's dance programming—the same space where Kamien premiered *Ana Kamien* in 1970, as discussed in the previous chapter. The work was part of Maris's evening-length program titled *Perfiles* (*Profiles*); however, *Juana Azurduy* was also presented as a stand-alone piece that same year.[66]

Over lunch in the apartment Maris shares with dancer Marta Sol Bendahan in Mar del Plata, a coastal city several hours south of Buenos Aires, Maris shared that she wanted to dance Azurduy's story because she considers her "the most exemplary woman in our history."[67] Of mestiza descent, Azurduy was born in what is now Sucre, Bolivia. Azurduy married the Spanish descendant Manuel Padilla, with whom she had four sons and one daughter. Together with her husband, she joined the independence struggle, fighting primarily in the Upper Peru region—present-day Bolivia and northern Argentina. Padilla and Azurduy became revolutionary leaders; at one point Azurduy commanded an estimated six thousand troops composed largely of indigenous soldiers. Indigenous guerrilla fighters followed rural caudillos, or leaders, like Azurduy and Padilla in the South American wars of independence and national consolidation. Azurduy also trained a group of female soldiers, known as the Amazonas (Amazons), who fought alongside her.[68] Around the same time royalist forces captured and executed Padilla, Argentine independence leader General Manuel Belgrano named Azurduy a lieutenant colonel based on reports of her physical prowess in combat and exemplary leadership skills. After Padilla's death, Azurduy fought under Martín Miguel de Güemes in northwest Argentina until his death in 1821. Azurduy was promoted to the rank of colonel once Bolivia became an independent nation in 1825; however, the small pension she was granted was not enough to survive, and she reportedly lived the rest of her life in poverty.[69] All four of Azurduy's sons died fighting in the war, though she was eventually reunited with her daughter.

As a result of her centrality in key battles for independence, Azurduy came to figure prominently, though centuries later, in Argentine as well as Bolivian historical imaginaries. She was awarded the rank of general in the Argentine army in 2009, and between July 2015 and September 2017 her statue (a gift from Bolivia) replaced that of Christopher Columbus outside of the Argentine presidential palace.[70]

Maris based her interpretation of Azurduy's life on Argentine playwright Andrés Lizárraga's 1960 *Santa Juana de América* (*Saint Juana of America*).[71] The three-act play depicts Azurduy's life in different moments of the independence struggle, emphasizing her advocacy for indigenous populations before powerful landowners, her impressive military leadership, and the tragedy of her ultimate death in poverty. In collaboration with Marta Inés Talia, Maris adapted the play's portrayal of Azurduy's life into choreography that drew on modern dance vocabularies.[72] She did not include the play's other characters through the use of additional cast members, opting instead to focus attention exclusively on Azurduy. While there is no video documentation of the piece, a single photograph from Maris's private collection depicts Maris costumed in a gray, long-sleeved dress, apron, and headscarf. She is crouched on the floor with an outstretched arm, her mournful gaze cast downward (figure 2.4).[73] Notably, the costuming does not invoke the iconic red military jacket in which Azurduy is so frequently depicted, along with her sword, in portraits. Instead, Maris's costuming emphasizes Azurduy's humble beginnings and end rather than her time on the battlefield.

While there are limited traces of Maris's production, Lizárraga's play offers insight into the representation of Azurduy that Maris drew on and contextualizes the relationship between the dance and 1970s revolutionary ideologies. In his analysis of Lizárraga's play, scholar Fernando de Toro considers *Santa Juana* an example of Brechtian epic theater that represents past events in order to comment on contemporary political issues—in this case, the class struggles and anti-imperialist movements that galvanized leftist movements across Latin America in the wake of the Cuban Revolution.[74] De Toro demonstrates how *Santa Juana* constructs the independence struggle as unfinished. The play points to Azurduy's poverty-stricken end as evidence of how colonial ties and class power reconsolidated in the years following independence. Lizárraga's Azurduy, however despondent, does not give up. Her final lines in the play are, "this war is not finished!"[75] The play, de Toro argues, calls contemporary leftist movements to arms through Azurduy's example: "it directly incites armed action as the only revolutionary channel."[76] Notably, the play received the prestigious Casa de las Américas theater award in 1960. (The well-known Cuban publishing house had only recently been established in 1959 following the revolution.)

By invoking the wars of independence as continuous with the political movements of the 1960s and 1970s, Lizárraga's play foreshadowed the myriad

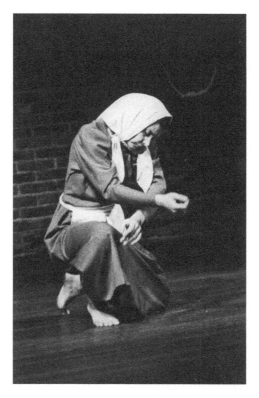

Figure 2.4 Estela Maris in *Juana Azurduy*, 1973. Photographer unknown. Courtesy of Estela Maris.

ways Argentine militants invoked independence-era heroes to mobilize—and legitimize—their use of force. In fact, the Peronist Montoneros of the 1960s and 1970s drew inspiration and their name from the *montoneros* of the nineteenth century. *Montonero* was the elite's pejorative term for the rural followers of caudillos like Azurduy and Padilla. Here we might also recall how the song "Luis Burela," which memorializes the independence hero who began the "Gaucho War" in the northwest city of Salta, reportedly became the literal battle cry for the Rawson prison revolt. While the heroic stories of male figures like Belgrano and José de San Martín appeared regularly in militant group's publications, an edition of *Estrella Roja* (*Red Star*), the internal publication of the PRT-ERP, specifically narrates Azurduy and Padilla's story as part of a shared history of struggle.[77] By dancing the life of Azurduy—and specifically Lizárraga's interpretation of Azurduy—Maris's work reflected the historical imaginary of 1970s militant movements that understood themselves, in part, to be completing the unfinished business of independence.[78]

Even as Maris's *Juana Azurduy* articulates with the militant groups' celebration of independence-era figures, the piece also invites comparison between the gender politics at play in historical representations of Azurduy and those of women who militated in the 1970s. A tension between masculinized bravery in battle versus feminized dedication to her husband and children characterize different strains of Azurduy mythology. In her study of women in the Upper Peruvian revolutionary forces, Argentine historian Berta Wexler notes that early biographies of Azurduy worked to "justify her masculine character" by detailing an early interest in playing with boys' toys and reading accounts of male saint soldiers during her time living in a convent as a child.[79] She also notes that nineteenth- and early-twentieth-century visual depictions of Azurduy consistently represent her with masculinized features, including an angular chin and faint mustache—an effort to make her legible within gender norms that assign military leadership roles to male bodies.[80] Wexler marks a transition in representations of Azurduy following the 1960 Bolivian national celebration of the centennial of her death and subsequent consecration as a hero—and hemispheric "mother." No longer a masculinized anomaly within historical narratives of male independence heroes, Azurduy emerged as "Juana of the Americas." As Wexler writes, "this official incorporation, and the incorporation of 'mother earth' as Pachamama, imagines a 'we' through the figure of the mother."[81] The refeminized incorporation of Azurduy into the historical imaginary of the Americas hinged on Azurduy's heteronormative gendering as suffering wife and mother.

Lizárraga's play, on the other hand, privileges what we might call the "militant" Azurduy. In its emphasis on Azurduy's dedication to armed revolution, Lizárraga's play reiterates the belief among 1970s militant groups that gender issues were secondary to achieving political-economic revolution, which, if realized, was expected to deliver gender equality.[82] While women sometimes held leadership positions in organizations, Marta Vassallo notes that the intense valorization of the militant couple as the "'basic cell' of action and affection" ultimately reinscribed gender hierarchies and compulsory heteronormativity.[83] Militant groups affirmed normative codes of "sexual morality," as Isabella Cosse puts it, which painted as heroic the supporting roles of wife and girlfriend and "established a direct relationship between political loyalty (understood as sacrificing one's life for a cause) and fidelity to one's spouse or partner."[84]

Militant motherhood, according to Cosse, was a point of particular tension. While some groups argued that raising children was part of women's revolutionary work, female militants also pushed back on gendered divisions of domestic labor.[85] Self-presentation functioned as a site for negotiating gendered power dynamics; testimonies suggest that some women embraced a "masculinized" wardrobe (jeans, men's shirts) and short hairstyles in an effort to be taken more seriously within organizations.[86] Female militants subsequently found themselves in gendered binds similar to the ones that mark Azurduy's depictions along a politicized spectrum of masculinity and femininity. They embodied a masculinized repertoire of armed action that broke from traditional gender norms at the same time that they tactically negotiated organizations' gendered ideals for militant women's behavior as loyal spouses, partners, and mothers.[87]

Maris's *Juana Azurduy* proposed a danced conversation about female militancy, past and present. Maris's choice to stage this historic female revolutionary not only participated in militant organizations' celebration of independence heroes as part of a shared history of struggle, but also offered a space for reflecting on the conflicted role of women in this "new" revolution. As a solo performance, Maris's choreographic memorialization of Azurduy's life on the contemporary dance stage celebrated the role of women in defining revolutionary action independent of their relationships with men. Even as the piece draws on the revolutionary message of Lizárraga's play, Maris's choice to jettison the other characters literally gives Azurduy's story—and by extension those of 1970s female militants— the floor. Maris attests that her choreography indeed depicted the painful loss of Azurduy's husband and children as central parts of her life; however, their physical absence helps interrupt the ways in which the militant couple, as the "'basic cell' of action and affection," reified male privilege and heteronormative desire.[88] Additionally, the costuming's notable de-militarization of Azurduy—recall that Maris wears a plain gray dress and headscarf rather than military garb—also suggests an attempt to hybridize masculinized/militarized images of Azurduy with later representations that emphasized her femininity, paralleling female militants' negotiations of multiple gendered codes. Ultimately, *Juana Azurduy* attempts to stay faithful to the choreographer's admiration of Azurduy as "the most exemplary woman in our history," honoring Azurduy's militancy and linking it to contemporary movements without pitting femininity against military prowess or reducing her role to spouse or mother.[89] *Juana Azurduy*'s celebration of this independence figure on the concert stage, then, not only moved otherwise to escalating government repression but also to the normative offstage gendered choreographies that leftist groups themselves enforced.

Though little-known works, *Juana Azurduy* and *Preludio para un final* (as well as the broader Pulso Cinco project) provide examples of concert works that extended the spirit of militant revolutionary projects to the concert stage in the early 1970s. While *Preludio* took up a recent event—the Trelew Massacre—*Juana Azurduy* looked to a female independence leader, ultimately commenting on the gendered codes negotiated by women in militant organizations more than a century later. By drawing attention to both of these works, and considering them under the rubric of "militancy," this chapter connects dance to the broader scholarly conversation about 1970s revolutionary projects.

THE MEMORY OF WHAT WAS NOT IN THE SHADOW OF WHAT WAS TO COME

This chapter has demonstrated how dance practices—in prisons and on stages—constituted militant revolutionary works and acts. Dancers like Hodgers and Sanguinetti *were* the faces of the Argentine left, to recall the *Panorama* magazine cover that opened this chapter. At the Rawson Penitentiary in Trelew, dance practices not only established community among a diverse population of militants but also became central to the prison break plan itself, functioning as both a decoy to distract the guards and the literal choreography of escape. And though Pulso Cinco Danza Teatro and Estela Maris were not affiliated with official parties, their early 1970s stage works resonated with, and in Maris's case also challenged, militant ideologies. *Preludio para un final* memorialized the lives lost at Trelew and aimed to keep the spirit of revolution alive in the wake of the highly publicized killings. In choreographing the story of an independence-era hero, *Juana Azurduy* both highlighted one of the militant groups' imagined political ancestors and called attention to their reification of gender norms. Militants who danced and dancers who danced about past and present militants contribute to histories of revolutionary artistic movements—and challenge narratives that render culture, and dance in particular, secondary to political action. In this chapter, the dance archive itself moves otherwise to existing historiographies to reveal a history of militancy in motion.

Following Vezzetti's call for deeper critical attention to militant histories, this chapter illuminates details of the unfinished political projects—including violent operations—that drove 1970s militant actions.[90] The joined hands and raised fists on *Preludio*'s program cover and Sanguinetti's photographs capturing the fervent work of making armbands, flyers, and banners on the day prior to the release of Villa Devoto's political prisoners provide glimpses into a project that, in 1973, still seemed viable. While for some groups Perón's return to the presidency had signaled possibility, the interventions of the Triple A death squad quickly began to dispel hope. The Triple A's actions intensified following Perón's unexpected death on July 1, 1974, and the ascension of his third wife and vice president, María Estela Martínez de Perón, to the presidency. As the next chapter considers, the coup d'état that deposed Martínez de Perón on March 24, 1976, installed a junta of leaders—including Jorge Rafael Videla (army), Emilio Massera (navy), and Orlando Ramón Agosti (air force). Extending and amplifying the practices of the Triple A, authorities began to detain citizens with any connections or history of activity that broadly could be construed as leftist. They pursued the practice of extra-official execution with unprecedented vigor.

The notion of recuperating unfinished projects, however, might also be extended to the broader experience of the Buenos Aires dance community during these years. The dance activity considered in this chapter and the previous one itself constituted, to some degree, an interrupted project. As evidenced in many of the narratives traced in this chapter, escalating repression and the retraction of the artistic scene throughout the mid-1970s prompted many dancers, such as Taburelli and Hodgers, to seek exile abroad. Zimmermann, whose work *Danza ya* connects the militant dancers considered in this chapter, also chose to self-exile in 1976 when she was offered the opportunity to work in Italy.[91] Dancer Alicia Muñoz's 1976 *Clarín* article, titled "For the Disappearance of Almost All of Their Groups, the Dancers Ask for Help," chronicled the loss of institutional footholds, consistent programming, and prominent artists, and lamented the lack of opportunity for current and future generations of Argentine dancers.[92] The retraction of the artistic sphere, particularly with the onset of the last military dictatorship, was indeed dramatic. However, dance, like the political ideologies considered here, did not disappear completely. Rather, as the early and most repressive years of the dictatorship set in, dancers gathered in unprecedented numbers in dance studios and schools across the city. The next chapter demonstrates how, while not always visible on prominent stages, Buenos Aires contemporary dance did not disappear but rather moved otherwise from the margins.

CHAPTER 3

Dance as the Art of Survival

One afternoon in the *hemeroteca* (newspapers and periodicals collection) housed in the basement of Argentina's National Library, I came across a striking image in the midst of a search for press coverage of dance during the early years of the last military dictatorship (1976–83). I paused on a 1977 *Gente* article entitled "The Fantastic War of the Human Body Against Its Enemies."[1] The article described the body's immunological responses to disease and infection through a militarized metaphor of war and defense. In the illustration, small colorful soldiers occupied the interior space of the outline of a masculine body. The colors of the soldiers' uniforms corresponded to the formation and response of different antibodies. The numerous soldiers were in motion, their legs raised in a determined march, arms gripping rifles. They all faced the same direction and appeared on the brink of colliding with the figure's skin and compelling the body into motion.[2] The article was ostensibly about the body's immunological response; however, I was immediately struck by how the illustration also rendered, with painful concision, the military's insidious hold over citizens' bodies and movements during the last military dictatorship. The image, as it turns out, also illuminates this chapter's central question: What were the options for movement in the context of a dictatorship that tightly scripted how the body should look and act, and that clandestinely practiced torture and murder as punishment for misperformed citizenship?

During the National Reorganization Process, as its leaders called it, the military government launched a brutal campaign against citizens that they deemed "subversive"—generally construed as leftist or anti-Argentine. An estimated thirty thousand people experienced forced disappearance, torture, and murder in clandestine detention centers.[3] Military discourse repeatedly and explicitly characterized political subversion as a disease that threatened the health of the national body. In August 1976, foreign minister César Augusto Guzzetti stated before the United Nations that, "when the social body of the country has been contaminated by a disease that corrodes its entrails, it forms antibodies . . . . As the government controls and destroys the guerrilla, the action of the antibody will disappear, as is already happening. It is only a natural reaction to the sick body."[4] In Guzzetti's statement, the metaphor of disease justifies state violence as an "antibiotic" response. Though Guzzetti implies that state terrorism was waning at the time of his speech, in fact the mid- to late 1970s marked the height of forced disappearances.

At the same time that the military deployed "antibodies," it also compelled the performance of "healthy" citizenship through pamphlets, public speeches, and decrees disseminated throughout the educational system and other media outlets that outlined how the proper citizen should look (conservative clothing, neat haircuts) and move (erect bodily posture, folded hands, and crossed feet). Citizens were also encouraged to remain vigilant of embodied signs of subversion (a disheveled appearance, activities such as handing out flyers) in their fellow Argentines. To further control citizen bodies and foreclose collective mobilization, the regime banned mass gatherings in public and private spaces and suspended all political activity. Military police and artillery became a regular presence in public space, and officers routinely asked citizens on the street to produce identification.[5] Under the dictatorship's omniscient gaze, the internalization of terror and suspicion extended into all aspects of bodily comportment. As choreographer Ana María Stekelman incisively describes, "It's the kind of fear that gets in through the pores."[6] Stekelman's statement emphasizes how fear literally enters and takes up residence in the body, accruing through the body's interaction with displays of military power as well as repeated performances of state-sanctioned forms of citizenship, settling into muscles and joints like so many tiny soldiers. Outlined in *Disappearing Acts: Spectacles of Gender and Nationalism in Argentina's "Dirty War,"* performance scholar Diana Taylor's concept of "percepticide" names how visual spectacles of violence resulted in forms of self-blinding that consolidated military power.[7] Stekelman's statement, however, signals how discipline was also learned and executed directly through embodied knowledge during this period.

This chapter demonstrates how, in the midst of the militarized siege of Argentine bodies, contemporary dance offered strategies for survival by preserving the *possibility* of movement outside of the choreographies that the military government established and actively policed. Survival, here, refers both to staying alive as well as carrying out artistic projects and maintaining communities that gave life meaning and purpose, acting on possibilities for strategic critique and situated resistance, and imagining alternate futures. The stories and archival materials my interlocutors so generously shared and that drive the arguments in this chapter were frankly matters of life and death. As with my discussion of militancy in the previous chapter, I am acutely aware of the stakes of stirring up traumatic experiences, including the need to not disclose certain histories in order to minimize extending additional harm—even when those histories both support and/or point to the limits of the arguments developed here. I am deeply grateful for the willingness of my interlocutors, some named here and others not, to return to this painful past and for their guidance as I searched for the cracks of light that danced in during this period. I hope that this chapter serves as an act of witness to their myriad movements otherwise.

The chapter first considers how studios, schools, professional companies, and festivals provided relatively protected spaces for negotiating bodily autonomy as dictatorial terror restricted everyday movement. Dancers including Ana Kamien, Alicia Muñoz, Déborah Kalmar, Ana María Stekelman, and Susana Tambutti all testified to the role of multiple spaces as havens for moving otherwise. These spaces included private studios, public schools, and municipally funded theaters, pointing to the limits of the dictatorship's attempts at totalizing control across privately and publicly managed sites. The last military dictatorship also marked the expansion of *expresión corporal* (corporeal expression), a practice considered in the chapter's second section. Based on exercises designed to access dancers' unique creative potential, *expresión corporal* valorized and celebrated the body even as citizens' bodies were literally disappeared from streets and homes.

The last two sections of the chapter look outside the dance studio. They consider how independent as well as state-funded performances presented works that allegorically critiqued state violence, particularly during the waning, less repressive years of the dictatorship. The successful Danza Abierta (Open Dance) festival followed the path forged by the well-known Teatro Abierto (Open Theater, 1981–85) movement, staging community and publicly celebrating the vitality of dance practice across the city. At the San Martín Theater, home to the newly instituted Grupo de Danza Contemporánea (Contemporary Dance Group), concert works by Renate Schottelius and Alejandro Cervera addressed the military dictatorship's grip on bodily movement that *Gente*'s image so effectively rendered. To reconstruct the numerous forms of moving otherwise considered in this chapter, I draw on a breadth of personal and published interviews, archival materials, and movement analysis.

In all the cases considered here, moving otherwise hinged on dance's continued marginality within the arts generally, and politically committed art specifically. Where the first and second chapters of this book document how contemporary dance functioned as a site of political engagement under earlier periods of dictatorship at the same time that dancers fought to gain greater visibility within the broader Buenos Aires art scene, this chapter demonstrates how dance located possibility in what literary scholar Francine Masiello calls the "advantage of marginal space."[8] Writing about how both elite and popular culture went "underground" during the last military dictatorship, she argues that the margins offered "a safe refuge for spontaneous as well as planned oppositions" aimed at in-the-know audiences.[9] The government identified the cultural forms that Masiello considers (fiction, music, and humor) and other arts (theater and the visual arts) as hotbeds of subversion. Artists associated with these practices experienced explicit forms of censure and blacklisting that, for the most part, did not extend to contemporary dance.[10] While other forms of cultural production adapted to the margin, contemporary dance continued in an established tradition of tactical survival—both of the form and the dancing bodies themselves.

It is critical to note, however, that contemporary dance spaces were by no means fully out of the reach of the dictatorship's watchful eye. They were also not free of the practices of self-censorship and suspicion of "subversion" ingrained in citizens' bodies that actively sustained and perpetuated military violence and control. This chapter takes these limitations and complicities into account as it highlights the numerous ways that contemporary dance took advantage of dance's relative marginality. As choreographer Susana Tambutti lightheartedly phrased it while referring to the (relative) sense of security her group experienced in their rehearsals during the dictatorship years, "Who is going to come after three choreographers that want to dance in a room?"[11]

MOVING IN THE MARGINS

In personal as well as published interviews, dancers who were active during the last military dictatorship repeatedly testified that contemporary dance studios provided protected spaces for moving otherwise—even if the realities of the dictatorship were not always addressed explicitly. From amateur practice to professional company rehearsals, a range of dance spaces created, as Tambutti put it, a "refuge." Discussing her experience forming the influential Nucleodanza company with Margarita Bali and Ana Deutsch in 1974, Tambutti succinctly articulates how dance spaces became sites of survival:

> The political intensity that accompanied our generation would transform into an asphyxiating military dictatorship that held us in suspense, and the presence of that blend of perplexity, incredulity, and terror made it necessary for those of us who had not participated in the political fight to find meaning and purpose. What happened in those years had a dark backdrop. We started to look for a sense of purpose in this, our small story as an independent dance group . . . . In small theaters like the Payró, Planeta, and others like them, we went about creating a refuge from the horror.[12]

As the dictatorship settled in, with its "mix of perplexity, incredulity, and terror," dance provided a sense of meaning within a climate where direct opposition now meant nearly certain death. Tambutti underscores that, unlike the dancer-militants considered in the previous chapter, she and the majority of the contemporary dance community did not militate with the organized leftist groups that continued to confront state power through the early years of the dictatorship. However, her description posits dance as a world-making practice that, protected by its marginality, offered a way of surviving the military's infiltration of the body.

Ana Kamien's studio, where Tambutti and Bali's early collaborations took place, served as one such refuge. In 1969, Kamien and her husband, Leone Sonnino, opened the multipurpose space in the San Telmo neighborhood of Buenos Aires.[13] Kamien taught contemporary technique and composition classes while Sonnino used the remaining space as a photography studio. In an interview with dance historian Marcelo Isse Moyano, Kamien recalled that during the last military dictatorship:

> The dance studios were relatively safe places. I think they were safer than theaters, where the word is used and things are said. They were gathering places. The studios were filled with people. Even though it seems odd, they were filled with men; the men felt safe, it was a place where they felt accepted in form and condition. The students felt they could express themselves, that they could be, that they could express themselves in all possible forms. They were, I believe, cultural and expressive asylums. It was a great boom.[14]

Kamien identifies the dance studio as a "safe place" and a "cultural and expressive asylum" that allowed the possibility to simply "be." She suggests that a common misconception about dance—how can it make meaning if there are no words?—in fact allowed the form to escape the policing and censorship directed at theaters.[15] Presumed innocent, the studio took advantage of dance's marginality, enacting "spontaneous oppositions" through physical expression outside of the dictatorship's sanctioned choreographies.[16]

Kamien also reports that male practitioners, often discouraged from pursuing concert dance, flocked to her studio in record numbers.[17] Kamien's comment affirms Judith Hamera's notion that the dance studio provides a context for negotiating "dominant, totalizing fictions of masculinity"—in this case, the specifically gendered aspects of the dictatorship's national project.[18] In *Disappearing Acts*, Taylor argues that the military framed the National Reorganization Process as a "masculine" struggle played out across the feminized body of the endangered patria, or homeland.[19] While the military set out to rescue the patria, it depicted the subversive enemy as the wayward and disobedient woman in need of discipline. The feminization of alleged subversives included their construction as "inverted homosexuals."[20] Clandestine torture practices operationalized national sexual economies, inflicting penetrative acts (often literally with the insertion of torture instruments into the anus and genitals) that constituted not only disciplinary action against the individual body, but also "a reorganization of the social and political 'body' into active (male) and passive (feminine/effeminate) positions."[21] The military demanded that citizens embody heteronormative gender roles as clandestine torture practices disciplined "deviant" bodies. Kamien's observation, then, that her studio served as a haven for men's physical expression implies that it offered the opportunity to explore ways of moving that the dictatorship's scripts for "proper" masculinity forbade in daily life. Her comment also hints at the studio as a space for expressing nonnormative sexuality. While Kamien does not explicitly address and/or presume the sexual orientation of male participants, the notion that her studio fostered an environment where all students could simply "be" invokes an ethics of acceptance and inclusion that dictatorship surveillance also foreclosed.

While Kamien's testimony addresses her privately owned studio, choreographer Alicia Muñoz recalled how the public dance school that she directed likewise offered the opportunity to "breathe a bit."[22] During the last military dictatorship, Muñoz directed the Jorge Donn Dance School No. 2, a public secondary school founded in 1974. Located in a quiet neighborhood on the west side of the city, the school offers training in ballet, tango, contemporary, and folkloric dance. During our interview, it became clear that Muñoz's role at the school during this period was as much about the tactical negotiation of a vigilant military state as it was overseeing the training of young dancers. Muñoz actively worked to both protect the teachers and students in her school, and to find opportunities to signal dissent within her day-to-day work there. For example, during a gathering on May Revolution Day (the holiday that marks Argentina's first steps toward independence), Muñoz boldly declared "we [Argentines] have still not achieved revolution. We still have not achieved freedom."[23] A clear reference to the oppression of the dictatorship, Muñoz's statement also echoed how 1970s leftist militant groups conceived of their fight as continuous with the revolutionary struggles of the independence era, a connection considered in the previous chapter. She recalled that during this period, "the teachers said my school was an oasis."[24]

During our conversation, Muñoz also recounted a telephone call she received from the authorities after several teachers took part in a strike during the later years of the regime. Her retelling demonstrates the improvisational response required to maintain the school as an "oasis":

> One day they called me on the phone and asked for the names of the teachers who had organized a strike. So I told them, "Sir, it is no inconvenience at all to give you the names. But, I believe that you'll understand me when I say that over the phone I can't be sure that you are who you say you are. I'd love to, I have no problem at all, I am going to give you the names, but why don't you come to the school in person?"[25]

No one ever did come to the school. Muñoz's quotidian act of resistance mobilized the military's own tactic of encouraging of vigilant suspicion of other citizens. She improvised on the state's mandate that no one should be trusted—using the idea to simultaneously convince the caller of her obedience to the military government *and* protect the school's instructors from potential detention. By requesting that the caller come to the school and identify himself, Muñoz invoked the common military practice of demanding to see citizens' identification documents when encountered on the street. She adds that, "in this sense you negotiated things, but I'll tell you, truly, every time I left the school I checked to see if there wasn't some [Ford] Falcon parked outside."[26] Ford Falcons were synonymous with military power. These vehicles were frequently used for surveillance and to execute forced disappearances. Practicing countersurveillance, Muñoz performed vigilance against subversion for potential military personal while also attempting to ascertain if the school was being monitored.

Muñoz's actions adapted principles of dance training for everyday survival. A quotidian "dancerly strategy," as Ramón Rivera-Servera defines it, "pays attention to the nuances of moving from one place to another," or, in this case, to simply surviving in a city gripped by state terror.[27] Muñoz's ability to improvise on the spot and tactically replicate verbal discourses and physical repertories of proper citizenship suggest the mobilization of dance training within acts of resistance—however small and quotidian. While Muñoz's protection of the dance school had its limitations, her actions instantiate how sustaining dance spaces as "oases" required that dancers risk their safety to subvert and improvise on the dictatorship's disciplinary practices, in effect its "scores" for movement.

As Kamien's studio and Muñoz's school provided relatively protected spaces for bodily expression, professional companies' regular rehearsal and creative activities also preserved the possibility of moving otherwise. In the midst of the last military dictatorship's most violent years, Kive Staiff, then director of the San Martín Theater, negotiated funding for the Grupo de Danza Contemporánea (Contemporary Dance Group, later renamed the Ballet Contemporáneo, or Contemporary Ballet) and established an associated conservatory-style training program, the Taller de Danza Contemporánea (Contemporary Dance Workshop) in 1977.[28] Argentine dance critics and historians widely consider the 1977 company a continuation of Oscar Araiz's Ballet del San Martín, which operated at the theater from 1968 to 1971. Given its association with a prestigious municipally-supported institution, the Grupo de Danza Contemporánea quickly became (and continues to be) the most visible stage for contemporary dance in Buenos Aires and the professional standard for its middle-class viewing public. The company's movement style has shifted with each new artistic director; however, an emphasis on technical virtuosity remains consistent.

In 1977, young choreographer Ana María Stekelman became the company's first director. Stekelman struggled, she stated, "to be a choreographer and to form the group because we are people brought up in fear."[29] Despite the climate of fear and their location within a municipal institution, dancers reported a sense of relative autonomy (figure 3.1). In original company member Mónica Fracchia's recollection, "the place was a kind of untouchable stronghold where we didn't have censorship, or they underestimated us, I don't know."[30] In our interview, Stekelman recalled how Staiff consistently reminded the heads of various departments that the San Martín Theater was an "island."[31] The theater, she continued, "was not the reality of what was happening outside. What they wanted to say was that we should be on alert."[32]

In interviews, Fracchia and another company member, Ana Deutsch, corroborated the notion that the theater was an "island" apart from the external reality of the dictatorship. They agreed that the intense labor of professional dance managed to shut out the terror occurring beyond the theater's walls and provided a physical release from the strain of adhering to the dictatorship's strict corporeal codes.[33] Reflecting on the intense hours spent training and rehearsing, Deutsch stated, "I believe that the activity was a refuge."[34] For her, constant work toward technical mastery provided an

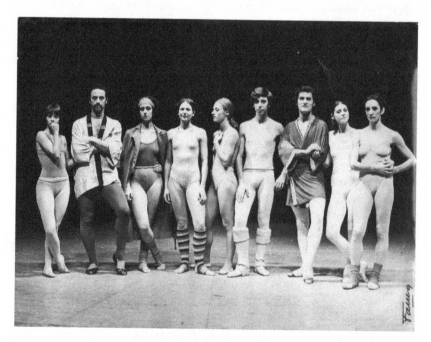

Figure 3.1 Grupo de Danza Contemporánea of the San Martín Theater, 1977. From left to right: Mónica Fracchia, Mauricio Wainrot, Lisu Brodsky, Margarita Bali, Liana Sujoy, Guillermo Arrigone, Carlos Zibell, Ana Deutsch, and Norma Binaghi. Photograph: Jorge Fama. Courtesy of Ana Deutsch.

outlet from the dictatorship's censure of bodily expression. In other words, the Grupo de Danza Contemporánea offered company members the ability to move otherwise through embracing the rigor of contemporary dance technique. It is worth recalling here that dance technique itself is a "system of command" that "implements, needs, produces, and reproduces whole systems of obedience" often predicted on horizontal power structures.[35] The Grupo de Danza Contemporánea dancers' experiences emphasize that moving otherwise does not necessarily imply a challenge to the power relations or disciplinary structures of creative practice itself, or even an explicitly oppositional stance to state power (as in Muñoz's statements on May Revolution Day). In this case, moving otherwise represents a situated practice of survival—a way of finding purpose and meaning under a dictatorial state.

For the dancers at the municipal-affiliated San Martín Theater, their "island" offered notably different political possibilities from those Rachmi Diyah Larasati attributes to Indonesian national troupe dancers in the wake of that country's violent campaign against leftist subversion (1965–66). While dancers were charged with presenting a harmonious image of national identity in the midst of H. Muhammad Suharto's ongoing dictatorship (1967–98), Larasati demonstrates that the offstage mobilities and socialities the dance troupe fostered became "a powerful form of resistance to dominant and dominating cultural and political narratives."[36] The Indonesian national troupe, unlike the Grupo de Danza Contemporánea, performed at state and diplomatic events, which meant the dancers' carried diplomatic passports and were officially designated as civil servants. While Indonesian national troupe dancers found tactical opportunities to challenge cultural and political narratives through the particular mobilities state affiliation afforded, for the Grupo de Danza Contemporánea dancers, government affiliation meant their movements otherwise were limited to the "island" of the San Martín Theater. As Stekelman pointed out, keeping the space secure demanded that staff and artists remain "alert" despite—or especially in light of—the theater's municipal affiliation. The island was maintained, it seems, so long as the Grupo de Danza Contemporánea confirmed contemporary dance's supposed marginality among the politically committed arts and fulfilled its function as a virtuosic company that catered toward a middle-class audience.

Throughout the last military dictatorship, a wide range of dance studios and schools functioned as spaces for practicing alternate forms of bodily expression. Tambutti, Kamien, and Muñoz's testimonies highlight the importance of studios as relatively safe and inclusive communal gathering spaces, while original members of the Grupo de Danza Contemporánea emphasize how a municipal theater—and the pursuit of technical excellence—likewise offered a refuge. In the following section, this chapter continues to document the importance of the dance studio as a marginal space during the period by examining *expresión corporal*—a practice linked to contemporary dance that was understood by its founder and its practitioners as uniquely situated to address the corporeal effects of living under dictatorship.

In closing, however, it is critical to note that maintaining these spaces as "cultural asylums," to invoke Kamien's phrasing again, at times involved policing and restricting access to them. One interlocutor—who requested that specific identifiers and details remain undisclosed—referenced the painful ways studio owners and theater directors turned dancers away precisely because of alleged ties to subversive activity. When this dancer most needed a refuge, it was outwardly denied. This excommunication, and others like it, actively reinforced the government's discursive construction of "subversives" as corrosive "diseases" (to recall Foreign Minister Guzzetti's phrase) that posed a threat to the health of the national body. Just as the military's grasp over public and private spaces was ultimately incomplete, then, dance spaces as inclusive asylums were likewise limited by the ways they enforced the practices of policing and exclusion that upheld military rule.

EXPRESIÓN CORPORAL: DANCING AS THE PRESERVATION OF LIFE

As dancing bodies found respite from the dictatorship's movement scores in studios across the city, a branch of contemporary dance known as *expresión corporal* also experienced a boom (to borrow Kamien's descriptor). *Expresión corporal's* popularity and institutional presence expanded so notably during this period that a 1982 *Clarín Revista* article enthusiastically declared, "Corporeal Expression, the New Fever of the Porteños."[37] Developed by Patricia Stokoe in the 1950s, *expresión corporal* aimed to put "dance within everyone's reach" through structured improvisation and creative exercises designed to explore the unique movement potential of practitioners' bodies.[38] Trained in classical ballet and modern dance, Stokoe drew inspiration from the theories of and approaches to movement espoused by Isadora Duncan, Moshé Feldenkrais, and Rudolf Von Laban.[39] *Expresión corporal* rejected techniques that emphasize aesthetics and uniformity among bodies, aiming instead to cultivate proprioception, wellness, and an awareness of the social and cultural aspects of embodied identity.[40] Although *expresión corporal* can resemble a number of movement practices globally, its development and application in Argentina is specific. As dancer and scholar Patricia Dorin notes, however, the practice itself varies widely and often reflects the interests and backgrounds of specific teachers and practitioners.[41]

Stokoe's earliest teaching took place at the Buenos Aires Collegium Musicum, and in 1968 she opened the Patricia Stokoe Studio and launched a teacher-certification program. By 1972 the curriculum of the National Dance School (Escuela Nacional de Danzas, now the Department of

Movement Arts of the National University of the Arts) incorporated the practice.[42] During the 1970s and 1980s, Stokoe and other teachers also focused on working with youth and advocating for the inclusion of *expresión corporal* in Argentine primary and secondary education. Furthermore, in an effort to develop the compositional potential of the practice, Stokoe founded Grupo Aluminé in 1974. She conceived of the group as both a performance troupe and a laboratory for developing *expresión corporal* methodologies.[43]

The growth of *expresión corporal* during the height of political violence actualized Stokoe's conception of the practice as one that "preserves life."[44] Stokoe trained and performed in London during World War II and witnessed the violent devastation of this period. This experience motivated her to create *expresión corporal* as "a proposal to address the need for new relational patterns between people and to help rediscover the joy of life through dance after so much death and destruction."[45] During our interview in the current Kalmar Stokoe Studio, Stokoe's daughter, and lifelong *expresión corporal* practitioner, Déborah Kalmar articulated how the practice responded again to violence during the last military dictatorship:

> It arose as a vital response to preserve life, that is, as the essential possibility of spreading life in relationship to earlier periods with different forms of violence than those of today, that is, those of the last military dictatorship and World War II. I mention this because of Patricia's history when, at eighteen years old, she went through the bombings in London. Me at eighteen, the last military dictatorship. That is, [*expresión corporal* came out of] the period of going out into the world, with the greatest vitality and with all this creative energy, but also with everything that repression implies . . . . For me, dance is always united with life, even if speaking of the greatest pain.[46]

Both Kalmar's and Stokoe's statements equate dance with life. They consider movement the literal condition of possibility for their survival within the transnational climates of violence that shaped their lives.[47] For them, *expresión corporal* "preserves" life by calling all bodies to movement, facilitating "new relational patterns" that undo self-censorship and suspicion of the other. In this sense, *expresión corporal* aims to dislodge political violence's hold over the body.

Recall here that one of Kalmar's insights inspired this book's notion of moving otherwise. Succinctly identifying the political stakes of movement under repressive political regimes, she stated: "It's as if someone else, not oneself, is moving. There is a reason why the most explicit, implicit, or covert forms of repression have to do with restraining the body."[48] In the context of the last military dictatorship, *expresión corporal*'s emphasis on movement as an ethics of life—transmitted through classes in private studios and public schools across the city—worked explicitly to empower bodies and offer countertechniques to the dictatorship's politics of death.

Expresión corporal, like the contemporary dance spaces considered in the previous section, largely enjoyed the advantage of marginal space. However, like Kamien's studio and the San Martín Theater's Grupo de Danza Contemporánea, *expresión corporal* spaces were likewise subject to the dictatorship's choreographies of fear and control even as they offered asylum. Musician Osvaldo Aguilar, who accompanied *expresión corporal* classes at private studios as well as the National Dance School during this period, recalled his strong (but unconfirmed) suspicion that undercover intelligence officers had been sent to classes to scout out "subversive" activity.[49] When I asked Aguilar to expand on his comment, he stated that he could sense, through the uninvested ways certain participants engaged with the movement exercises, that they were not there by their own choice.[50] Just as Muñoz improvised on the military's own codes of conduct to protect her school, Aguilar relied on his trained eye to detect "inauthentic" movement execution as a sign of potential surveillance. Whether or not there were government surveyors present, Aguilar's comment evidences the vigilance citizens practiced to survive during the dictatorship years.

The development of Grupo Aluminé's first work exemplifies how *expresión corporal* choreographed room for (safe) dissent in the midst of the last military dictatorship's surveillance culture. Titled *La línea (The Line)*, the group based their creation process on Beatriz Doumerc and Ayax Barnes's children's book, which was published in Buenos Aires in 1975. Stokoe felt the book's concept and images offered timely material that would translate well into movement exploration.[51] Through the story of the relationship between two human figures and a red line, the text and illustrations emphasize cooperation and underscore the ability of individuals to join together and effect change. In addition to the text's broadly left-leaning values, the redness of the line invokes the color's historical connection to socialism and workers' rights movements.

The final images of *La línea* are the text's most direct tie to the leftist imaginary; it ends with images of a tree that bears fruit for all, a peace dove calling for love and tolerance, and a sun representing an inclusive patria "where the new man lives."[52] The "new man" references Ernesto "Che" Guevara's enlightened political subject.[53] As discussed in chapter 1, Susana Zimmermann's Laboratorio de Danza drew on the language of the "new man" in the late 1960s to frame its sociopolitical investment, which attracted many of the militant dancers considered in chapter 2. Further strengthening *La línea*'s connection to revolutionary politics, the year of its publication it received a prize from the influential Cuban publishing house Casa de las Américas. Estela Maris's *Juana Azurduy*, also considered in chapter 2, was based on Andrés Lizárraga's Casa de las Américas prize-winning play *Santa Juana de América*. These repeated references to Guevarism and engagement with texts recognized by a cultural institution closely associated with leftist movements point to Argentine dance's continued connections to a broader Latin American leftist imaginary.

As Grupo Aluminé prepared to premiere their movement adaptation of the text in 1976, *La línea* appeared on the government's list of prohibited books. The risk associated with performing the piece publicly was too great; however, they did not abandon the work's principles (ideological or choreographic) in their studio practice. Rather, Grupo Aluminé continued to work with the concepts that came out of the text, a process that fundamentally shaped the refinement of their creation methods throughout the period of the last military dictatorship.[54] In this sense, *La línea* functioned similarly to Larasati's understanding of Indonesian women's covert transmission of folk dance techniques in villages and family compounds during the dictatorship. Under threat of punishment for practicing particular dance forms outside of official government channels, learning technique effected "a coded distribution of different types of narratives concerning history, power, and state order, narratives aimed at an eventual *coming to fruition* in the form of resistive practice."[55] The "coming to fruition," for Grupo Aluminé, took place when they finally premiered *La línea* in 1983, after the return to democracy. In Stokoe's words, the piece was "a mature choreography after so many years of learning."[56]

Video documentation of the piece features an ensemble cast of ten dancers clad in flesh-toned leotards and tights.[57] The movement vocabulary of the piece oscillates between defined, shape-driven gestures drawn from contemporary dance vocabulary (including leaps, arabesques, and floor work) and mimetic action that references the *La línea* text. The choreography blends ensemble movement with duets and trios, but avoids romanticized pairings between male and female dancers. Hand-painted banners displaying lines from the text appear multiple times. A literal line, in the form of a rope, materializes only once in the piece. Two dancers hold the rope taut as another dancer interacts with it. As in the illustrations in the book, the dancer playfully leans on, leaps over, and rolls under the rope/line (video clip 3.1 ▶).[58] In the book, exploration of the line represents individuals' agency over the course of history as well as the different "lines" of thought and ideology that cause conflict. As the opening text states, "Line: succession of points. History: Succession of facts. Points make a line. Men make history."[59]

A score featuring jazz and folk influences echoes the predominately light-hearted mood of the piece, which is interrupted by only one episode in which four menacing figures surround a group of dancers clumped together tightly. As the dancers dodge impending blows from these aggressors, the stage goes dark. When the lights come back up, the stage is strewn with motionless bodies, some piled on top of one another. The dancers remain still in this tableau for a lengthy one-minute hold before slowly and stoically rising to their feet (video clip 3.2 ▶).[60] This section corresponds to the moment in the book when the line becomes hostile; it restricts, hinders, and even kills the illustrated figures. Recovering from the violent turn, the text reminds the reader of "man's" relationship to history—he or she can march "against" it.[61] In Grupo Aluminé's work, the dancers recuperate from the devastation by moving into a series of gentle and tender weight sharing movements in pairs.[62]

Though the piece did not make it to the stage until the return to democracy, the group's continued work with its agential message—that change is indeed possible through the actions of committed bodies—quite literally danced hope within the relatively protected walls of the dance studio. When the work ultimately premiered following the return to democracy, as the extent of human rights violations were slowly beginning to come light, the fight and death scene created a space to reflect on the effects of violence on citizen bodies. The work both mourned the *desparecidos* and made visible the military government's clandestine violence. The lengthy stillness following the blackout literally held space for seeing and reflecting on the physical effects of political violence. Translating *expresión corporal*'s aim to preserve life into a concert work, the development of *La línea*'s ideas and choreography across the years of the dictatorship moved otherwise.

Where contemporary dance practices provided protected spaces for moving otherwise during the earlier and most repressive years of the last military dictatorship, public dissent began to explicitly push back against government repression in the later years of the regime. These movements joined the Madres de Plaza de Mayo, who first launched their well-documented activist performance in 1977. Carrying images of their disappeared children as they circled the plaza in front of the presidential palace on a weekly basis, these women demanded to know their children's whereabouts. Later joined by the Abuelas de Plaza de Mayo, these women-led organizations significantly increased national and international awareness of human rights violations.[63] Additionally, by the early 1980s changes in government leadership and a series of military and economic failures loosened the dictatorship's control. These shifts did not eliminate risk associated with resisting the government; however, a growing sense of national dissent provided momentum for increasingly visible social and cultural movements against state violence.

In the following sections, I turn to the dance community's role within this broader climate of building resistance, following dancers' steps from inside studios and schools out onto Buenos Aires's streets and stages. While contemporary dance still operated from the margins of cultural production and government surveillance, the cases I consider emphasize how contemporary dancers and audiences began to publicly move otherwise in the early 1980s.[64] I first consider how the Danza Abierta festival (1981–83) performed inclusion and community in the face of the regime's efforts to still and isolate bodies by generating movements otherwise on city streets as well as stages. The final section of this chapter analyzes two concert works presented by the Grupo de Danza Contemporánea that critiqued the offstage power dynamics and human rights violations of the dictatorship.

LINING UP AT THE THEATER: INCLUSION AND "HYBRID" SPECTATORSHIP AT DANZA ABIERTA

Danza Abierta emerged out of the Teatro Abierto (Open Theater, 1981–85) movement, which has been hailed as one of the most important Argentine theater movements of all time.[65] The theater community produced Teatro Abierto in protest of government measures that banned and censored plays, blacklisted playwrights, and removed theater history courses from secondary and higher education curriculums.[66] The popular festival sent a clear message to the government that Buenos Aires theater was alive and committed to its rich history of political critique.[67] Planning for Danza Abierta began with the assistance of Teatro Abierto director Alfredo Zemma.[68] Danza Abierta's three cycles took place in the Bambalinas (1981), Blanca Podestá (1982), and Catalinas (1983) Theaters, all of which donated their space and technical support.[69] Danza Abierta 1981, the focus of my analysis here, ran from November to December, presented the work of more than seventy choreographers, and featured more than five hundred dancers.[70] Danza Abierta 1982 took place from August to October, and grew to include around ninety choreographers, though the 1983 program was significantly smaller.[71] The festivals united an unprecedented number of choreographers working in contemporary dance, folklore, flamenco, tango, jazz, and classical ballet. Like Teatro Abierto, Danza Abierta aimed to keep ticket prices low to allow for broad attendance. While invited playwrights wrote specifically for Teatro Abierto with the theme of the festival in mind, following a series of debates, Danza Abierta organizers opted to open the program to anyone who wanted to participate, regardless of previous experience, dance genre, or thematic content of their contribution.

This inclusivity became the cornerstone of the Danza Abierta festival, and promotion materials emphasized the festival's populist ethics (figure 3.2). The 1981 flyer read:

What is it? Danza Abierta is a spontaneous, not-for-profit movement organized by artists that represent Argentine dance who are concerned with demonstrating the validity and vitality of dance in our country. Why? Because we need to make sure everyone knows that dance is not an elite art, but rather one of the most beautiful and popular expressions of the spirit. We want to make sure that it reaches our community—with very affordable ticket prices, high quality, and a large quantity of creators.[72]

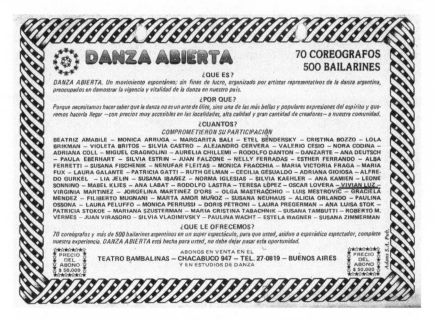

Figure 3.2 Danza Abierta Flyer, 1981. Courtesy of Vivian Luz.

While Danza Abierta's lack of selection criteria generated anxiety over artistic standards, my interviews with a number of participants suggest the festival's approach created much-needed space for validation and expression within a political environment literally defined by the excision of allegedly subversive bodies.[73] As Tambutti states, "someone who had just begun did their first three-minute piece, it was great, it was all good, and those of us who had a little bit of recognition . . . we were all there."[74] For Nucleodanza member Nora Codina, Danza Abierta's inclusivity fortified the contemporary dance community in particular: "it was tremendous . . . it was a moment that brought contemporary dance to its peak . . . everyone who wanted to dance, danced."[75] Even Muñoz, who expressed reservations about the lack of criteria, added, "There wasn't the least bit of screening: if you wanted to dance, no one asked if you had or hadn't danced before, and you danced. It was good, in the face of so much gagging and silence, in the face of so much lack of expression."[76] The flyer's call for Danza Abierta to demonstrate the "validity and vitality" of dance not only speaks to this need for physical expression, but also acknowledges the movements otherwise already occurring in studios and schools across the city. The overwhelming response to the open call demonstrated the sheer number of Buenos Aires dancers who had sustained and perhaps begun their practice during the most violent years of the dictatorship. Their numbers evidence, once again, the importance of dance as a strategy of survival from the margins.

In addition to uniting a growing community, Danza Abierta 1981 also made good on its aim to reach as many people as possible, reportedly attracting the largest audience attendance at a dance performance in recent history.[77] In a 1981 *Clarín Revista* article titled "Danza Abierta: Freedom's New Paths," Ana Kamien, Susana Zimmermann, and María Fux note that because tickets were sold in private dance studios as well as theaters, Danza Abierta produced an influx of people into studios as dancers simultaneously ventured out onto the Danza Abierta stage.[78] As Danza Abierta programming attempted to extend the refuge of the studio to the stage, ticket sales welcomed even more bodies into these "cultural and expressive asylums."[79] Codina observed that the demand for contemporary dance classes increased notably following the 1981 festival.[80]

The impressive audience attendance, of course, also defined the live event itself. In this book's introduction, I highlighted the image of Danza Abierta spectators waiting in a line that wrapped around a full city block in December 1981 as they waited to enter the Bambalinas Theater. Muñoz, Codina, Zimmermann, and Vivian Luz all recalled the lines wrapping around the block to enter the Bambalinas as the most impressive performance of Danza Abierta 1981.[81] For Muñoz, "This never, ever happened again save for Baryshnikov coming or something like that."[82] The lines of spectators performed solidarity with the festival's dancers—at the same time that the spectators' overt visibility directly challenged public space as the domain of the military regime. Though they gathered for ostensibly artistic rather than political reasons, spectators' willingness to take on public visibility—and vulnerability—to attend a dance festival staged against state violence and censorship boldly repatterned the highly policed circulation of bodies and their movements. Danza Abierta, before the performers even took the stage, generated new economies of corporeal circulation into dance studios as well as inside and outside of theaters, powerfully challenging the dictatorship's stagnating movement scores.

In addition to the inclusivity that marked the festival's programming and the defiant offstage choreographies of its viewing public, Danza Abierta also prompted strategically worded, public reflections on dance's ability to intervene in the dictatorship's management of citizens' bodies. While the 1981 flyer hints at the broader political context (the organizers are "concerned" with demonstrating dance's validity and vitality), the "Freedom's New Paths" article includes more direct references to political violence. Toward the end of the article, the unnamed author writes, "Kamien also accepts that in the last several years everyday men and women have been pushed to worry about their bodies, something that didn't happen before."[83] This veiled reference to forced disappearance appears unexpectedly and does not connect to the previous paragraph that discusses the Danza Abierta festival's unprecedented four-week length. Additionally, several of Fux's comments also suggest dance as a strategy for survival within contexts of bodily precarity. Echoing Kamien's reflections on the increased number of male students at her studio mentioned earlier in this chapter, Fux states, "In recent years, dance has received a large influx of people—notably many men who formerly had prejudices—and these people dance because they need to express themselves. Our bodies need to break out of solemnity and stereotypes. Ultimately, we look to free ourselves and dance is one way of finding that freedom."[84] For Fux, Danza Abierta extended the relative "freedom" of the dance studio to festival spectators: "We who love dance want the people to dance, dressed as they are, in the audience. With a suit on, but moving the body."[85]

Kamien and Fux's statements carefully articulated a public politics of moving otherwise through what Masiello, calling on the work of Mikhail Bakhtin, names "hybrid discourse."[86] Masiello notes that during the dictatorship cultural practices and the communities around them found ways of signifying that allowed them to express resistance while avoiding government accusations of subversion. These shrouded meanings were meant for "those who know to listen"—or to see, or move, otherwise.[87] While Kamien's statement is a coded recognition of government violence, in an interrogation it could have been justified as a reference to crime. Likewise, Fux's mention of dance as a form of "freedom" in the face of "stereotypes" and "solemnity" is general enough to have escaped charges of subversive language, even as it staked a claim for dance's political potential. While discourses around freedom in dance are common, Fux's formulation subtly called out the military's strict codes of corporeal comportment. Her desire to see the audience dance in their seats—note that they are wearing suits, invoking the military's image of the "proper," disciplined Argentine—is a radical call to action. For Fux, "freedom" is not the experience of a lack of constraints on one's movement. Rather, it is a dancer's ability and readiness to tactically negotiate normative movement patterns and ways of being (quotidian and theatrical) in a given time and place.[88]

My conversations with dancers about their experiences as Danza Abierta audience members also revealed how the featured works opened possibilities for "hybrid" spectatorship—an imaginative version of dancing in one's seat. Their memories and reflections evidence how the Danza Abierta program itself moved otherwise alongside the offstage choreographies and communities the festival convened. Although Danza Abierta works were not required to thematically address authoritarianism (and none explicitly claimed to do so), in interviews participants identified pieces that they remembered interpreting as symbolic commentaries on political violence. I found some consistency in the pieces invoked; for example, Tambutti and Kamien independently recalled the impact of Silvia Vladimivsky's *El día del campeón* (*The Day of the Champion*, 1981).[89] Vladimivsky's work explored the police chaos that ensued when two poverty-stricken children stole bread from a nearby bakery during a parade celebrating a boxing champion.[90] The police presence in the piece likely sparked resonances with the current political climate. Additionally, Patricia Dorin signaled Adriana Barenstein's *Bowling, o el orden establecido* (*Bowling, or the Established Order*, 1982).[91] In Barenstein's ten-minute work, several dancers embodied bowling pins that fellow performers repeatedly knocked down and set upright.[92] For Dorin, the manipulation of the human bowling pins made allegorical reference to the military's strict codes of physical comportment.[93] She recalls that the piece's impact on her was so great that it solidified her desire to pursue a career in dance.[94] On the Danza Abierta stage, Vladimivsky and Barenstein's works opened up possibilities for "hybrid" interpretations in Masiello's sense. Like Kamien's and Fux's statements in the "Freedom's New Paths" article, the works' themes were general enough to avoid reprisal. However, for Tambutti, Kamien, and Dorin, these pieces also created a space for reflection on and critique of political violence.

When I asked Vladimivsky and Barenstein if they conceived their works as critiques of dictatorship violence, the choreographers indicated that though not devised in that spirit, in retrospect they understood their colleagues' interpretations. In both instances, the choreographers reflected on what might have been their choreographic unconscious in creating these works for Danza Abierta. Vladimivsky expressed that *El día del campeón*, "was done almost unconsciously, I can't tell you that I wanted to do a work with social overtones."[95] In strikingly similar language, Barenstein explained that with *Bowling* "it is so unconscious . . . . That had symbolism, I didn't realize it in that moment, but it symbolized, if you like, the people they were killing."[96] The recollections of Tambutti, Kamien, and Dorin of the spectatorial impact of Vladimivsky's and Barenstein's works, as well as the choreographers' own retrospective commentaries regarding their hybrid significations (unconscious or otherwise), emphasize contemporary dance as a world-making practice then and there, as well as here and now. Vladimivsky and Barenstein's reflections—even thirty years later—on their works as potential social and political critiques transmit how contemporary dance, and Danza Abierta in particular, is part of a living narrative of cultural resistance to the last military dictatorship.

Mobilizing a politics of resistance in dancers, choreographers, and spectators alike through on- and offstage performances of community and critique, Danza Abierta moved bodies otherwise on an unprecedented scale. The independent dance community's show of solidarity against the dictatorship extended the "cultural asylum" of the studio into public space and demonstrated their impressive numbers. As *El día del campeón* and *Bowling* offered symbolic critiques of the dictatorship's disciplinary choreographies at the Danza Abierta festivals, two works that premiered at the San Martín Theater moved otherwise on the municipal stage. In the final section of this chapter, I offer close readings of how these two works moved otherwise in a markedly different production context from the grass-roots ethos of Danza Abierta.

DANCING ALLEGORY ON THE MUNICIPAL STAGE: *PAISAJE DE GRITOS* (1981) AND *DIRECCIÓN OBLIGATORIA* (1983)

While early works presented by the San Martín Theater's Grupo de Danza Contemporánea featured themes unlikely to raise the government's alarm— helping secure the theater's status as the "island" original company members remembered—pieces that premiered during the later dictatorship years clearly alluded to state violence.[97] Renate Schottelius's *Paisaje de gritos* (*Landscape of Screams*, 1981) and Alejandro Cervera's *Dirección obligatoria* (*One Way*, 1983) premiered alongside independent cultural movements, like Danza Abierta, that expressed a growing climate of dissent against the military government. Like *El día del campeón* and *Bowling, Paisaje* and *Dirección* did not explicitly cite the Argentine national context—*Dirección* came close, but *Paisaje* was outwardly about the Holocaust. As was the case with the works presented as part of Danza Abierta, the Grupo de Danza Contemporánea pieces extended contemporary dance as a practice of survival by offering critiques, through "hybrid" significations, of how the last military dictatorship choreographed bodies in public and private space.

While Danza Abierta and the Grupo de Danza Contemporánea both created space for hybrid significations on the concert stage, the former's grass-roots production and populist ethics distinguishes it from the latter's state affiliation and emphasis on technical virtuosity. Notably, Cervera was one of the few Grupo de Danza Contemporánea-affiliated dancers who elected to participate in Danza Abierta. He considers the work he presented on the 1981 program, *Ilusiones de grandeza* (*Illusions of Grandeur*), a precursor to *Dirección obligatoria*.[98] Furthermore, the stakes of attending the San Martín Theater were different from those of attending Danza Abierta. While the very act of attending the Danza Abierta and Teatro Abierto festivals moved otherwise to the dictatorship's scripts for occupying public space, going to the San Martín Theater fit within government-sanctioned modes of middle-class cultural consumption. Here we might recall that Kive Staiff, the theater's director, negotiated funding for the Grupo de Danza Contemporánea in 1977 at the height of repression. While going to the San Martín did not constitute a form of moving otherwise in and of itself, for company members, dance practice and performance at the theater opened up possibilities for bodily autonomy. As considered earlier in the chapter, Grupo de Danza Contemporánea dancers testified to the sense of purpose that the labor of dance afforded in the earlier and most repressive years of the dictatorship. During the regime's later years, Schottelius's *Paisaje* and Cervera's *Dirección* began to process the physical toll of life under dictatorship and challenged the San Martín Theater's public to confront the violence of their recent past.

Schottelius's *Paisaje* premiered in March 1981, several months ahead of the opening of the Danza Abierta festival. Schottelius created *Paisaje* toward the end of her distinguished performing and teaching career, which began in Buenos Aires in the 1940s and shaped the development of many influential dancers and choreographers. She choreographed the piece following her return to Buenos Aires after over a decade teaching and presenting work in the United States and Europe. Schottelius came back to Argentina when Ana María Stekelman—her former student and then Grupo de Danza Contemporánea director—invited her to lead composition and technique classes, and set a piece on the company.[99]

Schottelius choreographed *Paisaje* through the prism of her personal history as a German refugee. Due to her mother's Jewish heritage and the rise of the Nazi state in Germany, Schottelius immigrated to Buenos Aires in 1936. She made the journey alone at the age of fourteen after an uncle living in Argentina wrote that he was able to receive one family member.[100] Several years later her parents immigrated to Colombia; however, Schottelius's father passed away from illness before the family was able to reunite in Argentina.[101] *Paisaje* invoked the pain of the Holocaust through the archive that it drew on. The piece is titled after the Nelly Sachs poem "Landschaft aus Schreien" (1957), which depicts the horror of concentration camps, and the score featured Maurice Karkoff's musical interpretation of the poem. The piece further explored the archive of Holocaust memory by including a program note from *The Diary of Anne Frank*: "I feel the suffering of millions; and yet, when I look up at the sky, I somehow feel that everything will change for the better . . . because I still believe in the innate goodness of man."[102] This quote both invokes the horror of Holocaust violence and articulates hope in the face of mass devastation. Despite these direct references, in a 1981 *Clarín* article previewing *Paisaje*'s premiere, Schottelius's description of the work distances it from association with any specific context: "It doesn't deal with a story, but rather with . . . human ties and relationships."[103] Schottelius's broad statement previewed the general, yet evocative, language Fux and Kamien used only a few months later in the "Freedom's New Paths" article that promoted Danza Abierta. Like their subtle statements about dance as a form of freedom in the face of physical restriction, Schottelius's statement also invited reflection on the current political climate's rupture of human ties while stopping short of naming the practice of forced disappearance.

The piece, which lives on in video documentation, explored "human ties and relationships" through two duplicated casts (figure 3.3). The casts are composed of five archetypal characters: the mother, the young woman, the woman, and two men.[104] The costuming is simple. The mothers wear a flowing dress and headscarf, and the other women wear plain midlength dresses. The men wear pants, with two dancers clad in a tank top and the others in an open, short-sleeved shirt tied at the navel. Throughout the piece, one cast performs downstage while the other dances upstage. The upstage cast comes into and out of visibility behind a stage-width scrim. At several points, the two casts join together in the downstage space.[105] Throughout, the use of the doubled cast and scrim invites interpretations around the divisions between life and death, the past and present, and experiences of separation and exile relative to both the Holocaust and political violence in Argentina.

Choreographically, the piece combines a Graham-inspired sense of weight and line with an emotional intensity critics frequently associated with Schottelius's early contact with German expressionism.[106] In the 1981 *Clarín* article, Schottelius distinguishes her work from the younger choreographers with whom she shared the program—the program also included the premieres of Elena Orfila's *Las hadas* (*The Fairies*) and Mauricio Wainrot's *Fiesta* (*Celebration*). While she read their works as "searches" for new ways of moving, she saw her own work as rooted firmly within the modernist movement vocabulary that marked her career.[107] The highly technical choreography is not narrative; rather, movement dynamics match the haunting musical score. As Karkoff's score emits piercing notes alongside sung and spoken

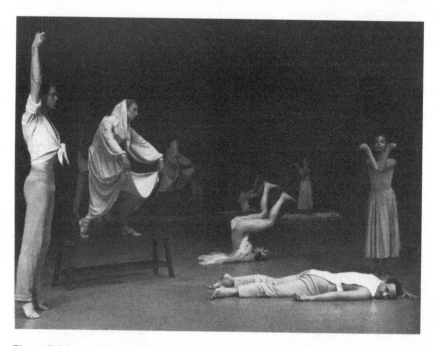

Figure 3.3 Grupo de Danza Contemporánea of the San Martín Theater in *Paisaje de gritos*, 1981. Photographer unknown.

fragments of Sachs's poem (in German), the dancers sharply twist, turn, leap, and contract (video clip 3.3 ▶). As the score takes on a more mournful quality, so do the dancer's movements—sustained leg extensions and slow floor work signify pain and suffering. The musical score also features the third choral prelude from Bach's *Orgelbüchlein* (*Little Organ Book*), and in these moments the movement takes on a faster-paced and more hopeful quality. In the ending image of the piece, both casts join together in front of the scrim. Led by the mother characters, the dancers reach their hands toward the audience in a gesture of pleading that could also be read as an invitation for connection. Simultaneously, the male dancers lift the "young woman" characters onto their shoulders as the women reach their arms toward the sky.[108]

By invoking the Holocaust in the context of Argentine state violence, *Paisaje* echoes Susana Zimmermann's 1969 *Polymorphias* (discussed in chapter 1). In the midst of Juan Carlos Onganía's relatively less brutal military dictatorship, *Polymorphias* signaled a "state of alert" around national authoritarianism through the prism of a temporally and geographically distant trauma that is also very much a part of the personal histories of Jewish Argentines. *Paisaje* similarly functioned as an allegory that called attention to the violence that had been and was happening on Argentine soil, while creating enough thematic distance to avoid government reprisal. The piece invited spectators to see the pain suffered by the onstage characters as a reflection on the absences thousands of Argentine families were grieving.

However, *Paisaje*'s citation of the Holocaust also offered a transnational model for grieving itself. The piece's "scream" responded to the multiple traumas that crossed Schottelius's life—the Holocaust and the last military dictatorship—and choreographically questioned how to express grief and find a way forward together. As a range of artists and activists were beginning to struggle toward representing the inconceivable violence of the dictatorship, *Paisaje de gritos* literally cried out. Notably, the "mother" characters' headscarves in *Paisaje* echo the white cloth diapers the Madres de Plaza de Mayo wore as headscarves during their weekly marches, which at the time constituted one of the only examples of public grief. Onstage, *Paisaje* boldly placed grief at the forefront before a population still gripped by fear and with only partial knowledge of the extent of government human rights violations.

While the 1981 premiere of the piece maintained a safe distance from any direct reference to Argentine state violence, press coverage of the Grupo de Danza Contemporánea's 1993 restaging of the work acknowledged *Paisaje*'s clear analogue to the violence of the dictatorship. The piece was presented as part of the twenty-fifth-anniversary celebration of the founding of the company.[109] In her discussion of the piece in the text published to mark the anniversary, Schottelius explicitly describes the piece as an "antiwar" and "antifascist" work that premiered "in full military dictatorship."[110]

While Schottelius's *Paisaje* allegorized political violence "in full military dictatorship," Cervera's work took the stage two years later amid the government's decline and uncertainty about when democratic elections would be held.[111] *Dirección* premiered in May 1983, five months before the democratic elections in October that brought President Raúl Alfonsín into power. According to Cervera, movements like Danza Abierta inspired the work, as did the political "free fall" precipitated by the 1982 Malvinas conflict with the United Kingdom.[112] The Malvinas are a collection of British-controlled islands located off the coast of Argentina in the South Atlantic. By 1982, there had been over two centuries of conflict over the sovereignty of these islands. In an ill-fated nationalist exercise, the faltering military government invaded the islands, hoping to bolster public support. Large swaths of the Argentine public initially supported the operation, and Taylor has demonstrated how press coverage used the conflict as an opportunity to unite the nation around "feelings of communal struggle and identity."[113] However, British Prime Minister Margaret Thatcher deployed troops that effectively quashed the underprepared, underequipped, and overwhelmingly young Argentine conscripts, resulting in nearly one thousand deaths. The lost lives, collective sense of betrayal, and perceptions of ineptitude—all exacerbated by rising inflation and a failing economy—accelerated the military government's decline.

In the wake of these events, Cervera felt compelled to create a work embedded in the physical experience of life under dictatorship. Where Schottelius's work acknowledged dictatorship violence through the prism of the Holocaust, *Dirección* tried to make sense of how the dictatorship had exercised control over Argentine bodies. Cervera recalled the urgency behind this exploration during our conversations, stating that "when the San Martín asked me to make a piece, I said to Kive Staiff: I can't do any work but this one right now. I would love to make a work where everyone is dancing and happy, but I can't do that. It wouldn't be sincere."[114] Staiff, still serving as general director of theater at the time, agreed to support Cervera's vision. By 1983, Cervera had an ongoing relationship with the San Martín Theater's Taller de Danza Contemporánea and Grupo de Danza Contemporánea. Following the establishment of both in 1977, Cervera gave music classes for dancers and later joined the company as a performer. Cervera developed his choreographic voice through smaller, collaborative works across the late 1970s and early 1980s, but he considers *Dirección* his first major work.[115]

Cervera set *Dirección* to minimalist composer Steve Reich's instrumental *Music for 18 Musicians*. The central choreographic concept is the continual movement of dancers from the right to the left side of the stage (from the perspective of the viewer). With a few notable exceptions, the large ensemble cast enters and exits in continual waves of linear movement for the piece's twenty-minute duration. The choreography actualizes the title's mandate to move "one way," a reference to street signage that comments on the military dictatorship's tight scripts for movement and the severe consequences of movements otherwise. The lighting design of the piece creates the sense of a confined, "passage-like" space where, as Cervera described in an interview, "one cannot leave, where there is the obligation to keep moving toward the same place."[116] Linking this scenic space and the obligatory current of movement to everyday life under dictatorship, Cervera stated, "I believe that this was what happened to people, there was no way to change."[117]

While Cervera understood the dictatorship's obligatory choreographies as a collective experience for Argentines, the piece carefully explored the specificities of how the dictatorship's movement scores animated differently situated bodies. As evidenced in video documentation of the work, successive "waves" of left-to-right movement cite different social identities through stylization of the everyday movement repertoires associated with middle-class professionals, military and police officers, and political activists (video clip 3.4 ▶). The episodic piece moves through scenes that explore each of these identities. In one early episode, dancers carrying orange suitcases sweep across the stage (figure 3.4). Their movements depict an urban, middle-class morning commute to work. Some dancers run and swing their suitcases, others pump their heels and raise grasped fists toward the sky as if standing while riding the bus, still others shuffle along briskly or read the newspaper. Two dancers reminiscent of police officers survey the scene and hold up scroll-like signs, ensuring the flow of movement continues. They quite literally personify André Lepecki's notion of choreopolicing, or the social processes that enforce "a forced ontological fitting between pre-given movements, bodies in conformity, and pre-assigned spaces for circulation."[118] They make certain that dancers who linger too long reading the paper continue on to their destination in a timely fashion, and on the prescribed path.[119]

As dance scholar Juan Ignacio Vallejos demonstrates in his analysis of Cervera's *Dirección,* these references to middle-class professional life— particularly the morning commute to the office—were especially significant given the San Martín Theater's bourgeois audience.[120] Large portions of the urban middle classes initially supported the military junta as a welcome corrective to the instability that successive government changes and political movements precipitated in the 1960s and early 1970s. Cervera's piece makes direct reference to middle-class professionals who were not directly involved in politics or political mobilization—the group historian Sebastián Carassai refers to as the Argentine "silent majority"—whose own daily choreographies matched up with the government's emphasis on order, and who likely made up members of its audience.[121]

The morning commute gives way to an exploration of military choreographies. A male dancer dressed in a military-style hat and black boots

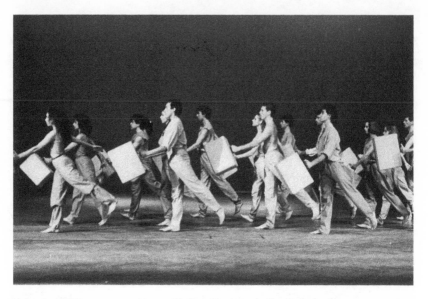

Figure 3.4 Ballet Contemporáneo (previously Grupo de Danza Contemporánea) of the San Martín Theater in *Dirección obligatoria*, 1993. Photographer: Carlos Flynn. Courtesy of Alejandro Cervera.

appears first, followed by soldiers who move in precise unison across the stage. Additional soldiers appear carrying batons held as rifles. They move across the stage in slow, controlled lunges with their weapons poised to fire. As they march, two dancers fall to the ground as if shot, invoking the recent military deaths in the Malvinas. Following a series of romanticized duets between fallen soldiers and female dancers (presumably their widows), two dancers enter with large brooms and "sweep" the soldiers offstage. The soldiers perform a series of back-rolls as the dancers advance with the brooms. This encounter in particular calls attention to disposable life in military conflict as well as under dictatorial rule. In the first case, the affectless sweeping motion of the dancers suggests the military's disregard for the young soldiers' lives by sending them to war woefully underprepared. It also echoed the military government's merciless disposal of *desaparecidos* in mass graves. By 1983, the extent of the dictatorship's human rights violations was just coming to light— particularly the government's treatment of bodies it had insisted simply "disappeared." By opening these dual interpretive possibilities, as Vallejos points out, *Dirección* joined other contemporaneous cultural productions in which "the revelation of the horrors to which the military had subjected the young Argentine soldiers functioned as an alert for a large part of the population that was beginning to become aware of the scope of state terrorism over the past years."[122]

One episode of the piece highlights resistance and opens possibilities for moving otherwise within a climate that demands compliance. A group of dancers move across the stage holding posters and banners, collectively invoking choreographies of protest. Another dancer passes out flyers and makes one of the first attempts to move in the opposite direction, but a mass of suitcase-carrying dancers, as well as the two police figures from the morning commute, discipline the dancer back into the normative flow of movement.[123] This politicized group evokes the members of the working- and middle-classes that engaged in militant political activity during the late 1960s and early 1970s as well as the gatherings of working-class masses that defined political demonstration in the Peronist era.

The final moments of the piece, however, manage to break fully with the obligatory direction. In one evocative scene, dancers attempt to move toward the opposite side of the stage with their palms pressed forward as if against a wall. The incline of their bodies against an invisible force that pushes them in the normative direction makes palpable the struggle to—and physical risk of—moving otherwise. Shortly after a military figure in a wheelchair appears, offering a visual index of the military's literal degradation of the returning soldiers' bodies. In the ending image of the piece, the full ensemble appears onstage in dark trench coats and top hats. The dancers cluster together toward the side of the stage where they normally exit as one female dancer breaks from the group. She removes her coat and hat and slowly walks offstage in the opposite direction as the lights fade to black.

Dirección literalized the military's invisible yet insidious grip over citizens' movements across a spectrum of social identities, recalling the image in the *Gente* article of tiny, colorful soldiers occupying the body that opened this chapter. In a critical moment of political transition, the piece also explicitly placed potential in the power of moving otherwise, ultimately made literal in the dancer's final exit in the opposite direction. In the final months of the dictatorship, *Dirección* continued the tradition of contemporary dance as an embodied strategy of survival while also joining works like those featured in Danza Abierta that helped open an onstage choreographic conversation about the corporeal experience of life under dictatorship. Together with Schottelius's *Paisaje, Dirección* evidenced how the San Martín Theater's Grupo de Danza Contemporánea, from a position of institutional privilege and government affiliation, featured works that grappled with the climate of violence and control that characterized the previous decade. Schottelius's work, which mapped her personal connections to the Holocaust as well as the last military dictatorship, proposed movement as a modality for expressing grief. Cervera's *Dirección*, with its literal invocation of military figures and disposable life, demanded that spectators begin to come to terms with the scale and severity of human rights violations under the dictatorship.

ON EMBRACING THE FUTURE WHILE GRAPPLING
WITH THE PAST

This chapter has demonstrated how a broad range of dance practices—in studios and on stages—moved otherwise to the last military dictatorship's stifling grip on corporeality, often through the "advantage of marginal space."[124] Across this period, contemporary dance practices provided strategies for survival in the form of artistic projects and communities that gave life purpose, offered possibilities for strategic critique, and allowed for the imagination of alternate futures. The first half of the chapter considered how studios, schools, and professional companies served as relatively secure spaces for expression. Dancers' testimonies suggested that a range of practices—from those emphasizing technical virtuosity to *expresión corporal's* valorization of accessibility—all nurtured the body within a political project predicated on physical censure. In the case of Grupo Aluminé's *La línea*, this choreography kept alive the revolutionary dreams of the 1960s and early 1970s and allowed the group to transmit a different historical narrative from the one propagated by the military government. At the same time, it is also critical to recall that keeping studios and companies safe sometimes meant replicating the military's own practices of exclusion.

The second half of the chapter turned to contemporary dance's emergence from the studio and onto the stage in the relatively less repressive years between 1981 and 1983. The 1981 Danza Abierta festival demonstrated the vitality and size of the dance community as its enthusiastic audience reconfigured sanctioned forms of circulation in public space and read resistance in works featured on the program. Finally, Schottelius's *Paisaje de gritos* and Cervera's *Dirección obligatoria* moved otherwise to dictatorship choreographies as they centered performances of grief, resistance, and complicity on contemporary dance's most visible stage. While dance's relative marginality among the arts in fact facilitated many of the forms of moving otherwise considered in this chapter, taken together, these practices make contemporary dance seem anything but marginal.

The return to democracy in 1983 ushered in a period of broad cultural expansion throughout the late 1980s and early 1990s, and the contemporary dance community was no exception. A plethora of independent artists and companies in Buenos Aires grew with new cultural institutions. The Recoleta Cultural Center (Centro Cultural Recoleta) and the University of Buenos Aires-affiliated Ricardo Rojas Cultural Center (Centro Cultural Ricardo Rojas) were particularly important centers of production. Adriana Barenstein, whose work *Bowling, o el orden establecido* formed part of the 1982 Danza Abierta festival, was appointed coordinator of the Rojas's dance program in 1983, and is where she based her own performing group until 1994.[125] In 1984, Susana Zimmermann accepted a position as dance advisor to the national

secretary of culture. As part of this position, she directed the dance programming at the federally supported Cervantes National Theater (Teatro Nacional
Cervantes)—a position she held until the late 1980s. Nucleodanza's national
and international recognition continued to grow throughout the 1990s, as did
that of newer groups including Stekelman's Tangokinesis, El Descueve, and
many others.[126] The late 1980s also marked important developments in public
dance education at the primary and secondary levels, and advances toward
higher degree programs in contemporary dance at what is now the National
University of the Arts.[127]

As the Buenos Aires contemporary dance scene grew, the Argentine nation
faced the enormous task of bringing to light—and coming to terms with—
the period of the last military dictatorship. The following chapter examines
how contemporary dance engaged the personal and collective trauma wrought
by the dictatorship generally, and forced disappearance specifically. Like the
final section of this chapter, it is dedicated primarily to close analysis of
concert dance works. It demonstrates how postdictatorship works by three
choreographers who have already crossed *Moving Otherwise*'s pages—Susana
Tambutti, Silvia Hodgers, and Silvia Vladimivsky—invoke tango as a means of
dwelling in and making sense of the violent past.

CHAPTER 4
Moving Trauma

In the wake of the last military dictatorship (1976–83), Argentina faced the tremendous task of publicly reckoning with state violence and rebuilding the democratic processes that had been suspended under military rule. Following his democratic election in 1983, President Raúl Alfonsín appointed the National Commission on the Disappearance of Persons, which produced the 1984 *Nunca Más* (*Never Again*) report. This report made a first attempt to count and identify disappeared persons, detail the methods of abduction and torture used by the military and police, identify clandestine detention centers, and outline preliminary recommendations for juridical action.[1] A subsequent 1985 civilian trial found leaders guilty of human rights violations.[2] However, the climate of accountability that accompanied these early actions quickly shifted. Responding to pressure from the still-influential military, laws in 1986 and 1987 prevented further trials, and government rhetoric began to encourage the nation to move on and forget the violent past.[3] Shortly after assuming the presidency in 1989, Carlos Menem pardoned military officers awaiting trial.[4] In December 1990 Menem also pardoned former junta leaders Jorge Rafael Videla and Emilio Massera, releasing them from their life sentences. Menem justified the pardons—which were bitterly opposed by survivors and family members—as part of his administration's emphasis on looking toward the future and letting go of the past.[5]

In the years immediately following the return to democracy, some contemporary dance works first moved with the government's initial efforts to understand the dictatorship's legacies of violence. However, following the 1986 and 1987 laws and later pardons, a broader range of contemporary dance works boldly moved otherwise to the national mandate to move on. In the immediate and extended postdictatorship period, cultural production and activism played critical roles in reconstructing the past, provided spaces for mourning, and advocated for accountability on national and international scales. Dance's foundation in bodily movement offered a method of grappling with a history of violence experienced at the level of the body and its movements. Policing bodies' presentation and circulation in public space was central to the military's authoritarian strategy, and moving otherwise often resulted in shattering experiences of loss, exile, torture, and even forced disappearance. Following the dictatorship, dancing bodies in motion fleshed out corporeal experiences of state violence and worked to find ways to remember, honor, and mourn the disappeared.

As the democratically elected governments worked to remember and then forget, contemporary dance choreographers turned toward the tango, the most (in)famous of Argentine dance genres. This chapter examines how and why choreographers integrated tango themes in contemporary dance works that engaged the physical and psychic trauma of the last military dictatorship.[6] Contemporary dance choreographers saw tango—which initially emerged as a partnered social form in Buenos Aires at the turn of the twentieth century—as rich territory to explore the recent past. A number of pieces created in the years immediately following the country's return to democracy and stretching into the early 2000s engage tango's movement vocabulary, music, cultural lore, and lyrical themes. The move to blend tango culture with contemporary dance vocabularies and creation processes was not a new or uniquely postdictatorship phenomenon.[7] However, in the wake of the dictatorship, choreographers repeatedly invoked tango as an embodied paradigm for approaching the trauma of political violence, both collective and individual.[8]

This chapter charts two principal ways that postdictatorship contemporary dance works mobilized tango to engage with trauma. On the one hand, choreographers drew on tango's own history of moving otherwise to early-twentieth-century marginalization, specifically the discrimination, poverty, and dislocation experienced by the immigrants associated with the dance's emergence. For these choreographers, summoning this history became a way to situate their lived experience of dictatorship violence within a broader historical continuum of social exclusion and resistance in Argentina. Tango culture and movement functioned as palimpsests of embodied responses to collective trauma across the twentieth century and combined with contemporary dance vocabulary and creation processes to offer a way of dwelling in the more recent past. In this sense, tango's presence emphasizes the collective experience of dictatorship trauma and dance's role in the construction and transmission of its memory.[9] On the other hand, socially danced tango's improvisational, leader-follower movement structure offered choreographers steps to explore deeply personal experiences of trauma, particularly the violent, sexualized power dynamics that marked practices of imprisonment and torture as well as the loss of loved ones to forced disappearance. While the leader (traditionally danced by a man) generally prompts the steps of the follower (traditionally danced by a woman) through subtle physical cues, the follower has agency over the interpretation of the movement prompt, and can thus influence how a dance develops. As a meditation on personal trauma, this approach theorizes dance as a site for recuperating agency and performing mourning; that is, as a way of continually processing the past.

This chapter argues that both these collective and individual approaches—and particularly the crossings between them—constitute strategies of "moving trauma." In the concert works I consider, moving trauma names the process of both revisiting movement linked to offstage experiences of violence and using codified (social and concert dance) movement as modalities for entering into, dwelling in, and sifting through the pieces of traumatic pasts.[10] Through moving trauma, dancers interrupted the logic of Menem's pardons and laws preventing trials that literally worked to still trauma's ongoing effects in the present by locking it motionless in the past. It thus echoes trauma theory's assertion that trauma is experienced in the form of returns and repeats and suggests that this structure itself is kinetic. In her foundational trauma studies text *Unclaimed Experience: Trauma, Narrative, and History*, Cathy Caruth draws on Sigmund Freud's work to suggest that "trauma is not locatable in the simple violent or original event in any individual's past, but rather in the way that its very unassimilated nature—the way it was precisely not known in the first instance—returns to haunt the survivor later on."[11] These returns, however, are fragmentary in ways that escape everyday modes of comprehension and representation. As Caruth and others have pointed out, artistic genres offer possibilities for invoking aspects of trauma even as it defies complete understanding.

Diana Taylor has demonstrated how both staged and protest performances' efforts to recuperate dictatorship memory in Argentina—in the sense of coming to terms with the psychic-somatic effects of traumatic experience as well as calling attention to government impunity—encompass and expand what she considers the "individual" focus of trauma studies.[12] Taylor extends Caruth's argument to postdictatorship performance, noting that performance's basis in repetition assists survivors in coping with trauma's repeats as it not only represents the incommensurability of individual experience, but also publicly interpolates witnesses and grounds political mobilization in collective experience.[13] This chapter shows how "moving trauma" in contemporary dance works names a way to host trauma's returns (in Caruth's sense), amasses a convocation of witness in the service of political change (in Taylor's sense)—and illuminates the centrality of movement in experiences of trauma and healing.

I closely analyze three tango-inflected choreographic projects that exemplify how postdictatorship dance moved trauma. While these are not the only contemporary dance works that link tango to histories of political violence, their span from the immediate postdictatorship period into the early 2000s shows the ongoing nature of choreographers' engagement with tango and legacies of state terror.[14] Choreographically, the three works all intersect with dance theater broadly defined and invest heavily in the use of props (most notably shoes). I begin with Susana Tambutti's *La puñalada* (*The Stab*, 1985), a solo work that cites tango culture as a way of understanding military violence within a broader scope of twentieth-century Argentine history. I then consider Silvia Hodgers's *María Mar* (1998), an ensemble work that enlists tango's movement vocabulary to confront Hodgers's experience as a political prisoner in the early 1970s, the loss of her partner to forced disappearance, and her exile in Geneva, where she continues to live today. Tambutti's and Hodgers's works do not explicitly stage partnered tango dancing, but rather reimagine tango movements and culture through contemporary dance vocabularies. Finally, I examine Silvia Vladimivsky's *El nombre, otros tangos* (*The Name, Other Tangos*, 2006), a work that calls on tango's historical roots to speak to collective experiences of national trauma as well as the form's movement structure to help articulate Vladimivsky's personal loss of a loved one. Vladimivsky's choreography moves between staging partnered tango and contemporary dance-based movement. Both movement genres combine to depict the experience of loss and represent the violence of the last military dictatorship. In my discussion of all three dances, I draw on video documentation and interviews, and in the case of Hodgers's and Vladimivsky's works, on documentary films based on these choreographers' experiences of the dictatorship that offer rich insight into the creation processes behind *María Mar* and *El nombre, otros tangos*.

Tango, of course, frequently summons exoticized and eroticized images in the global imaginary. During the twentieth century, tango became synonymous with Argentine—and more broadly "hot" and "passionate"—Latin dance. An impressive Spanish- and English-language literature has documented and analyzed the genre's transnational past and present as a social and, more recently, theatrical form.[15] Most notably, dance scholar Marta Savigliano's influential *Tango and the Political Economy of Passion* compellingly traces how a dance that grew out of the experiences of marginalized bodies in Argentina became central to the global exotification of Latin American dancing bodies as well as a symbol of national identity. The political economy of passion names the market for and consumption of the "exotic" other within a global cultural economy that replicates and perpetuates colonial frameworks. A number of scholars credit the emergence of commercial theatrical productions such as *Tango Argentino* (premiered in Paris, 1983)—the choreographed scenes of which heavily marketed macho tango men and seductive tango women—with reinvigorating national and international interest in the form during the postdictatorship period.[16] Folklorist Ana Cara refers to this tango, which aims to profit from global consumption of the exotic, as the "export" tango.[17] Choreographies about the violence of the last military dictatorship, however, appeal overwhelmingly to what she designates the "home" tango. For Cara, "home" names the improvisational tango danced among Argentines themselves that articulates "local values, memories, and performative styles of home, regardless of their geographical location."[18]

As it engages explorations of "home" tango in works by Tambutti, Hodgers, and Vladimivsky, this chapter resists a reading that reduces these choreographers' turn to tango as the search for something "authentically" Argentine in the wake of a national trauma. As Savigliano and others have argued, fetishizing the "authenticity" of global-south cultural practices is central to their value and circulation in the global cultural economy. The creative processes, movement vocabularies, and choreographic structures of these works are rooted in contemporary dance—a movement genre that these works (and this book) suggest is just as "Argentine" as the tango, in the sense of its extended historical trajectory in Argentina as well as its role as a site of cultural expression and contestation. However, these choreographers' works—all three of which developed in dialogue with European and US audiences—are inevitably bound up in the machinations of the global political economy of passion and the "export" tango it privileges. As Cara notes, "home" and "export" practices of the tango are inevitably entangled, with audiences and motivations that at times overlap and intersect. Nucleodanza toured *La puñalada* extensively throughout the United States and Europe; Vladimivsky developed her work partly in Italy; and as a political exile in Geneva, Hodgers premiered her work before a Swiss audience. My analysis considers how all three resisted the pressure from the international scene to sell exoticized Latin passion, even as they benefited from the air of authenticity that their inclusion of tango lent on the global stage.

The tango-inflected dance works highlighted in this chapter contributed to the energy generated by a breadth of activist groups and artistic projects that utilized performance tactics to both remember dictatorship violence and call for justice in the postdictatorship period. The Madres de Plaza de Mayo, who had demanded to know the whereabouts of their disappeared children since 1977, continued to march.[19] The 1983 *Siluetazo* project, conceived by artists Rodolfo Aguerreberry, Julio Flores, and Guillermo Kexel, proliferated depictions of outlines of bodies throughout Buenos Aires. These outlines often included the names and dates of disappearance of *desaparecidos* or the word *presente* (present), making visible the violence of the recent past by physicalizing absent bodies.[20] Beginning in 1995, the organization H.I.J.O.S. (the acronym for the organization Hijos e Hijas por la Identidad y la Justicia contra el Olvido y el Silencio [Sons and Daughters for Identity and Justice Against Forgetting and Silence]; *hijos* means "children" in Spanish) began to stage *escraches*, or public shaming acts. *Escraches* called attention to government impunity by staging demonstrations outside the residences of known torturers and former clandestine torture centers.[21] The Argentine theatrical community continued its rich tradition of critique and resistance. Beginning in 2000, the Abuelas de Plaza de Mayo partnered with playwrights, actors, and directors on the Teatro por la Identidad (Theater for Identity) festival, which featured productions largely (but not exclusively) related to kidnappings that occurred during the dictatorship.[22]

As these prominent examples suggest, Argentine human rights movements have centered normative ideals of family and filial and/or spousal connections to *desaparecidos* as paradigms for approaching dictatorship violence. A burgeoning body of scholarship has begun to deconstruct the heteronormativity of Argentine memory practices—and subsequent academic studies— and advance alternate concepts of kinship relative to collective trauma.[23] While the dance works featured in this chapter often reinforce the heteronormative frameworks that mark memory practices (as well as the tango itself), in some instances they also create space for alternate histories and narratives.

Unlike the more visible and systematically documented memory practices noted above, dance's contributions to postdictatorship efforts to create collective spaces for interrogating the past's presence remain largely unexamined.[24] Works that engage tango culture—a form with its own history of dissent— evidence how contemporary dance practices moved with efforts to remember as well as how they moved otherwise to national imperatives to move on. In its analysis of projects created by Tambutti, Hodgers, and Vladimivsky, this chapter hopes to invite a broader conversation on moving trauma in Argentina and beyond.

A DANCE OF MANY BODIES: *LA PUÑALADA* (1985)

In a dance filled with arresting images, the closing episode of Susana Tambutti's *La puñalada* is one of the most impactful (figure 4.1, video clip 4.1 ▶). A solo female dancer sits on a chair, clad in a leotard and corset. Her costuming suggests she is a performer—perhaps a vaudeville or even ballet dancer. One arm animates the sleeve of a gray trench coat suspended on the chair; a white scarf draped above the coat collar and a black fedora give the impression of a head. The coat-covered arm grips a knife, poised to strike. The trench coat, white scarf, and fedora invoke the image of the *compadrito*, the mythic man who first practiced tango in turn-of-the-century Buenos Aires. One dancer animates two bodies as the male figure brutally stabs the female figure to death, leaving the spectator with the image of a lifeless body as the lights fade.[25]

The eponymous stab that concludes the piece, however, is but one episode in Tambutti's twenty-six-minute dance. Skillfully manipulating props, costumes, and movement genres, the dancer continually crosses gender, dressing as a *compadrito* and comically exaggerating tango and vaudeville-style movements throughout the first portion of the piece. The second half of the piece includes

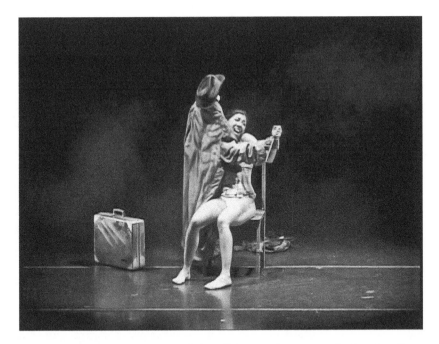

Figure 4.1 Luciana Acuña in *La puñalada*. Still from performance at the American Dance Festival, Duke University Reynolds Theater, Durham, North Carolina, July 2007. Courtesy of Susana Tambutti.

two episodes in which the dancer transforms herself into the female performer and male aggressor characters at the same time. The choreography of these two moments, which are separated by a parody of a military march, takes a serious turn in its depiction of sexualized violent encounters. I argue that the piece's shifts between movement repertoires and character transformations transmit traumatic cultural memory. I propose that *La puñalada* tells an evolutionary tale of the gendered production of bodies by the Argentine nation state from the nation-building projects of the early twentieth century through the moment of the work's premiere in the shadow of the dictatorship.[26] One of the first concert works to link tango with the violence of this period, *La puñalada* exemplifies how contemporary dance calls on tango's history to situate the dictatorship within a broader historical scope of social exclusion.

The Buenos Aires-based Nucleodanza company premiered *La puñalada* two years following the return to democracy. Tambutti and Margarita Bali's critically acclaimed company formed in 1974 and began their work at the height of dictatorship violence.[27] Tambutti and Bali first collaborated as students at Ana Kamien's San Telmo studio; chapter 3 demonstrated how this space, and others like it, provided a respite from the corporeal effects of authoritarianism in day-to-day life. Nucleodanza's works, in particular Tambutti's contributions, marked a reinvigorated interest in dance theater.[28]

Influenced by transnational developments in the field, particularly the work of German choreographer Pina Bausch and Chilean-born choreographer Ana Itelman (who developed her career in Argentina), Tambutti and Bali's choreography blended modern dance techniques with theater conventions; pedestrian gesture; humor and parody; and strategic citations of Argentine theatrical traditions, political figures, and other elements of the cultural imaginary.[29] Recall the discussion of Tambutti's *Patagonia trío* that figures in the book's introduction. This work, like *La puñalada*, exemplifies her repertoire's tradition of cutting cultural critique. At the same time that Tambutti was developing *La puñalada*, the company appeared in Fernando Solanas's well-known 1985 anti-dictatorship film *Tangos: El exilio de Gardel* (*Tangos: The Exile of Gardel*). The film depicts a group of Paris-dwelling Argentine exiles who decide to stage a *tanguedia* (tango + *tragedia* [tragedy] + *comedia* [comedy]) performance that combines dance, theater, and music. The film—like the contemporary dance works considered in this chapter—proposes tango as a privileged mode for processing the individual and collective trauma of political violence and exile.[30]

La puñalada begins as the lights gradually come up and the dancer comes into partial view, shadowed by dim lighting and smoke. She approaches the chair, the back of which faces downstage, wearing only a leotard and corset. A suitcase stands upright next to the chair. A gray trench coat is draped over the back of the chair, and the fedora and white scarf rest on a pole extending from the back of the chair. The trench coat, hat, and scarf signify a distinctively male body. Still for a moment, the performer rises to stand on the chair. She picks up a garter from the arm of the chair and puts it on her leg. The dancer then removes the white scarf from the pole and ties it around her neck. For the first time, she transforms herself into the figure of the *compadrito*. The dancer puts on the fedora, a fake mustache, a pair of sunglasses, and trousers to complete the transition as the music emits shrieks and gurgles—a sample from composer György Ligeti's composition *Aventures* (1962). As the tango song "La puñalada" begins to play, she briefly tangos solo and in caricatured movement falls to the ground to get back up again, looking to the audience for laughter. Intermittent hyperbolic citations of other movement vocabularies, including ballet, disco, and acrobatics litter the developing choreographic landscape.[31]

The series of embodiments that open *La puñalada* enact what queer theorist Elizabeth Freeman considers "temporal drag," in both the sense of drag as a "retrogression, delay, and the pull of the past upon the present" and as gender crossing.[32] The tango citations and *compadrito* body "pull" on the present as they invoke the complexity of tango's past, particularly its own history of moving otherwise. Tango first developed in Argentina amid the modernization projects that marked the late nineteenth and early twentieth centuries. As the introduction outlines, beginning in the post-independence period nation-building projects aimed to modernize (and Europeanize) Buenos Aires and populate its vast pampas (plains) with northern Europeans. As industrialization and large-scale agriculture changed the nature of the European economy at the turn of the twentieth century, Argentine private and national incentives aimed to attract agricultural labor and these "desirable" European immigrants. Immigration to Argentina boomed; however, the newly arrived population was largely Southern Italian, poor, male, and concentrated in the capital city.

Poor migrants—from abroad as well as rural Argentina—lived in *conventillos* (tenement houses) and gathered in bars now remembered as the birthplaces of the tango. Tango's musical and movement influences are diverse, and include the habanera (which traveled from Cuba to Spain and Argentina), the Andalusian tango, and the milonga, an Afro-Argentine form of popular dance related to Uruguayan candombe.[33] The oligarchical ruling class racialized the immigrant bodies most closely associated with early tango practice in opposition to the desired, whiter northern Europeans and constructed immigrants as "sexual inverts."[34] In these early years, tango became swept up in a national panic over mass immigration, race, class, and gender as its movement and lyrics captured experiences of marginalization, failed romance, broken families, and nostalgia for distant homelands.[35] Savigliano reads these tensions in the evolution of tango movement, particularly in the tightening of the embrace and shifts in footwork over time. She demonstrates how tango's steps are quite literally imbued with struggles of the past.[36] For scholar María Rosa Olivera-Williams, early tango music is likewise an aural ruin whose diverse musical influences and lyrics allow us to hear, in our listening in the present, the violence executed in the making of the modern Argentine nation.[37] She understands tango "as a nostalgic invention that is always fragmentary and inconclusive," much like Caruth's conception of trauma.[38] Through the figure of the *compadrito*, the dancer embodies the narratives of racialization and marginalization that excluded immigrant bodies from the desired national body and that live, materially, in the repertoire of tango.

In *La puñalada*, the *compadrito* body functions as Freeman's temporal drag not only in the sense of pulling a fraught past into the present, but also in the way it invokes the early-twentieth-century practice of female tango singers, or *cancionistas*, who would dress in drag to access the traditionally male role. Largely excluded from standard tango histories, according to scholar Sirena Pellarolo, *cancionistas'* "bold exposure of their femininity on stages . . . and occasional use of drag introduced the negotiation of alternative corporeal female styles in turn-of-the-century Argentina."[39] In his work on discourses of sexuality in turn-of-the-century Buenos Aires, Jorge Salessi highlights how prominent intellectuals read tango culture as a site for "masculine" women (female brothel owners and also *cancionistas*) and "feminine" men (*compadritos*).[40] These writings anxiously linked female brothel owners and the *compadrito's* attention to self-presentation and styling to same-sex desire.[41] The practice of men dancing tango together, ostensibly for practice, compounded this panic. In *La puñalada*, the temporal drag of the *compadrito/cancionista* body not only invokes the violence of modernization and embodied resistance to it, but also makes present a memory of nonnormative gender expression later overshadowed by the form's travels through the heteronormative political economy of passion.

The comedic, slapstick nature of the tango's invocation in these opening moments also draws on an Argentine theatrical genre that likewise grappled with the experience of modernization at the margins and became linked with tango in the early twentieth century: the *grotesco criollo* (creole grotesque). Tambutti has described *La puñalada* as "a small *grotesco criollo*."[42] Similar to the European grotesque, the *grotesco criollo* is characterized by the ironic mixing of the comic with the horrific to effect social critique. The genre's development was born out of the crash of middle-class aspirations post-immigration and is closely associated with the work of Argentine playwright Armando Discépolo, whose plays often took up themes of immigrant disenfranchisement.[43] Discépolo often collaborated with his brother, Enrique Santos Discépolo, a well-known tango lyricist.

For anthropologist Julie Taylor, the tango and *grotesco criollo* not only attest to the violence and trauma of modernization, they also embody resistance to the social exclusions it produced:

> As aesthetic creations, the social gatherings of milongas [tango social dances], like grotesque artistic genres in Argentina and other cultures, enact incongruities that give them the potential for elaborating the inherently dissonant experience of violence or trauma. Precisely because traumatic violence is outside the realm of socially validated reality, those who experience violence feel it to be profoundly incongruent with their everyday reality and often cannot speak about it . . . . The traditional worlds of the grotesque theater and of the tango protested modernization and the projects of capitalism with their harmoniously streamlined aesthetics. They asserted the importance of the body and pleasure, excoriated theory, exalted failure. Further, these worlds refused work ethics, indulged in excess, and reversed hierarchies of class and taste.[44]

Early tango and the *grotesco criollo*, then, might be read as strategies for moving otherwise, both in their rejection of the "hierarchies of class and taste" that accompanied modernization as well as in the space they afforded for expressing traumatic experiences that escaped everyday modes of representation and expression. In the opening of *La puñalada*, hyperbolic, kitschy citation of tango culture alongside clownish citations of other genres (ballet, disco, acrobatics) makes present the violence of modernization and points to tango's active resistance to its "streamlined aesthetics."[45]

By deploying elements of the tango and *grotesco criollo, La puñalada* exemplified the privileged role both genres played in processing the violence of the last military dictatorship. Julie Taylor, Savigliano, and others have noted that the social practice of tango became a way for Argentines at home and in exile abroad to express the experience of political terror.[46] Taylor notes that the economic violence "that formed the context of the invention of the dance . . . has been linked again and again in the minds of its victims with the political violence that has caused repeated exiles from Argentina."[47] While Taylor refers here to the social practice of tango, her passage captures the two primary ways contemporary dance works mobilize tango on the postdictatorship concert stage: as a mode of understanding the dictatorship within a continuum of social exclusion produced in the name of nation making, and as a way of confronting intimate experiences of "human ties destroyed," particularly the forced disappearance of loved ones and/or exile.[48] Just as the tango took on the weight of dictatorship trauma, around the time of the last military dictatorship the *grotesco criollo* also resurfaced as a way of ridiculing the excessive violence of this period—and, in so doing, ameliorating the pain it inflicted. Playwright Griselda Gambaro's work is closely associated with this turn, and she has gone so far as to claim that the *grotesco criollo* is a metaphor for Argentina itself.[49]

The tragicomedy of *La puñalada*'s opening sequences, rich in their invocation of multiple Argentine performance traditions linked to social critique, eventually gives way to a series of character transformations that feature explicit physical violence. In one such episode, the dancer places a sequined pointe shoe on her foot. Sporting an exaggerated smile, she mocks the kitsch of both revue-style dance and ballet as she bourrées across the floor, hands rested on bouncing hips. Wearing the leotard, corset, fedora, and glasses, she arrives at the trench coat—this time revealing its red and gold lining. She puts the coat on one side of her body, placing an arm in one of the sleeves and a leg in the other to create the image of a suit, reinvoking the figure of the *compadrito*. Here, the light, quick movements halt into abrupt stillness. The music changes briefly to Italian singer Carlo Buti's "La Romanina." The dancer puts a men's dress shoe on the foot of the trench-coated half of her body. Wrapping the white scarf around her head, she renders the body faceless (figure 4.2). Placing the hat on the head and putting on a white glove, the dancer sits on the chair, stomping what reads as a male leg in time with the beat. Extending and bending the bare, pointe-shoed leg in slow, sustained gestures as she fans her/his body with an ornate fan, the feminine leg crosses the masculine one. The gloved male hand tosses the bare leg off of his in rough rejection. Despite this cruel gesture, the leg rewraps around the male's, this time accompanied by the female arm. As the male figure compulsively stomps his foot on the ground and slaps his hand on his thigh, the sense of violence thickens when he raises the bodies from the chair. Seated once more, the male

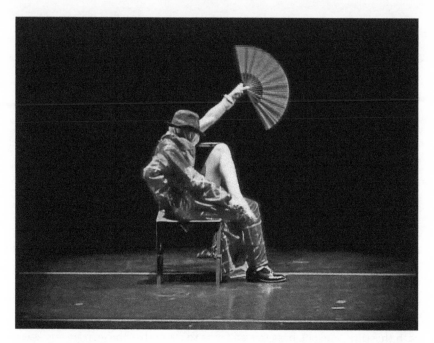

Figure 4.2 Luciana Acuña in *La puñalada*. Still from performance at the American Dance Festival, Duke University Reynolds Theater, Durham, North Carolina, July 2007. Courtesy of Susana Tambutti.

hand slowly reaches down to the floor to grasp the knife that is waiting beside the chair and stabs the female side of the body. He wipes the blade on the bare leg as if to clean it.[50]

Where the opening of *La puñalada* invoked the violence of turn-of-the-century modernization projects, the pedestrian movement in this episode summons the gendered and sexualized valences of the last military dictatorship's discourses and disciplinary practices. As outlined in the previous chapter, Diana Taylor has demonstrated how the military justified its actions as a masculinist struggle to save the endangered, feminized national body. In turn, military rhetoric depicted the "subversive enemy" as the wayward and disobedient woman in need of discipline.[51] Torture practices operationalized the military's "reorganization of the social and political 'body' into active (male) and passive (feminine/effeminate) positions."[52] In this episode, *La puñalada* denaturalizes the military's gendering of the national body by literalizing the construction of its two principal coordinates on one dancing body. As the upstage character, the feminized leg plays on tropes of femininity as undisciplined and sexually excessive—and is superseded by the cerebral order of masculinity. Perhaps most critically, the presence of the *compadrito* body juxtaposes the exclusions that modernization produced with the trauma of late-twentieth-century state terror. Although far more extreme in the scale of physical violence levied against citizen bodies, the military's construction of "subversives" as feminized, diseased agents infiltrating the nation and threatening its health and hygiene echoes the earlier panic over immigrant bodies made present through the tango citations. In this temporal juxtaposition, *La puñalada* visualizes how collective experiences of trauma accrue in the body and are transmitted through performance. Where the *compadrito* summons the cultural memory embedded in the tango, the contemporary dance-based strategies employed in this scene move otherwise to the dictatorship's gendered construction of the national body.

Shortly following the dually gendered body episode, the dancer performs another transformation that invokes the choreography of authoritarianism. Here, the performer once again wraps the scarf around her head and places the sunglasses over it, and wearing only the trench coat with the gray side turned outward, kneels on the stage so the coat is flush against it. Pulling her arms into the body of the coat and adjusting it to cover her neck, no flesh is visible. She exposes one hand and crosses it over her stomach, counting off by extending one finger at a time from a clenched fist as a discordant military march plays. The dancer then marches across the stage, coat sleeves waving as if orchestrating the music, in parody of a military parade. In tragicomic *grotesco criollo* fashion, the humor of the military march ceases and gives way to imminent violence as knives appear out of the cuffs.[53] In this episode, the faceless, body-less, trench coat could stand both for the estimated thirty thousand *desaparecidos* or the equally identity-less lower-level military figures responsible for their disappearance and torture. By parodically juxtaposing the consensus-building pomp of the military parade with a symbol of violence (the knives), this episode hauntingly summons violence executed in the name of national order. Once again, the embodiment of a collective trauma is concentrated in one moving body that serves as a conduit for transmitting the painful memory of dictatorship violence and as a site for estranging its disciplinary logic.

After completing the military parody, the performer transitions into the closing episode of the piece. As "La puñalada" plays, the dancer adjusts the gray trench coat on the back of the chair. Dancing with an empty coat arm, she moves it as if shaking a hand, before re-citing the movements that opened *La puñalada*—she tangos solo for a moment, comically slips and falls, and provocatively shimmies. Taking the glove out of the suitcase, she puts it on one hand prior to slipping the same arm into one of the sleeves of the trench coat. Now animated, the male arm slowly strokes the dancer's face. Beginning to sense impending violence, the performer frantically dances with the arm in an attempt to placate the masculine aggressor. As in the opening image of the piece, the dancer ties the white scarf around the pole extending from the chair. As the dancer begins to make her way around the chair, the trench-coated arm grabs her neck, bouncing her body on the chair. She moves to escape, but the man/military figure/*compadrito* covers her face with his hand, stopping her movement as she struggles and gasps. He reaches down to fondle her breast and grabs her between her legs as they shoot out in pain—face cringing, mouth open in a silent scream. The dancer reaches down toward the floor for the knife. As she lifts it, the male arm steals it from her hand and quickly and efficiently stabs her. Placing his hand over her expressionless face, he pats her motionless body as the lights fade out.

The most striking part of this episode is not the stabbing gesture in which the dancer enacts both aggressor and victim. Instead, it is the dancer's detailed process of constructing the scene itself, exposing again the centrality of violence to state power. What dies, then, in this final moment of the piece is not so much the "woman" herself. Rather, it is the persistent disciplinary logics that aligned feminized bodies with the subversive. The sexualized brutality and final stab make palpable the physical violence executed against bodies, particularly during the last military dictatorship. However, in the same instant, these movements also implicate the gendered and racialized power dynamics of the turn of the twentieth century that were made present earlier in the dance through tango music, movement, and historical figures. In *La puñalada*, the citations of tango culture, tragicomedy, and military figures together "moved" trauma. They destabilized the naturalized logics of violent nation-making projects and opened a space for remembering collective experiences of political violence during the early years after the return to democracy.

While I read Tambutti's work as exemplary of the move to invoke tango as a link between twentieth-century histories of national violence, in closing I want to reflect on the politics of representing violence and invoking tango on the global stage. Across our many conversations about the piece, Tambutti consistently pushed me to think critically about what gets lost if her piece is always, and only, about dictatorship violence. Tambutti's reluctance to consider her work in strict relationship to the dictatorship stemmed, in part, from Nucleodanza's experiences touring internationally. As the bearers of "Latin" contemporary dance, Nucleodanza experienced what Argentine writer María Negroni identifies as the expectation not only of the exotic and folkloric, but also the explicitly political.[54] In the wake of the 1970s dictatorships across Latin America, dramatic instability and political violence joined the exotic and folkloric as categories sutured to the region in the global imagination. US reviews of the company's 1989 American Dance Festival performance, which featured *La puñalada*, manifested this association. Two prominent newspaper reviews, Anna Kisselgoff's "Works That Cry for Argentina" and Jonathan Probber's "Latin Lovers, Lethal Props," both cited heavily circulated stereotypes themselves steeped in performance as they read *La puñalada* as a political protest piece.[55] Kisselgoff referred to the well-known song from Andrew Lloyd Webber's *Evita* ("Don't Cry For Me, Argentina"), while Probber summoned tango's femme fatales and (violent) macho men. Like these other North American critics, I too was eager to read *La puñalada* as a critique of the dictatorship's disciplinary practices—and I still do. At the same time, I am deeply indebted to Tambutti for pushing me to engage with the nuance embedded in the less explicitly violent moments of the piece, particularly those that feature references to early tango culture. Attention to these aspects of the piece not only produced a more expansive reading of how the work critiqued and remembered histories of violence, but also gave me a way to understand how tango functioned in a broad range of postdictatorship works.

In the following section, I turn to Silvia Hodgers's engagement with tango in her concert work *María Mar*, the rehearsal process of which is featured in the Swiss documentary film *Juntos: Un Retour en Argentine* (*Together: A Return to Argentina*). While *La puñalada* emphasizes how tango's historical relationship to exclusion lends itself to understanding the dictatorship within a broader continuum of collective cultural memory, in *Juntos* and *María Mar* the leader-follower structure of the dance form itself creates a space to reflect on Hodgers's personal experiences of trauma—particularly torture, the disappearance of a loved one, and exile.

AN ARGENTINE RETURN: *MARÍA MAR* (1998)

Chapter 2 explored how Silvia Hodgers's contemporary dance training and performance career informed her 1970s political militancy in unexpected ways. Recall that Hodgers was a member of the People's Revolutionary Army (ERP), the armed branch of the Marxist-Leninist Workers' Revolutionary Party (PRT), and she was arrested by federal police in 1971. Military officials tortured Hodgers and other political prisoners during this period, a practice that anticipated the intensification of state violence in the late 1970s. Between 1971and 1973, she remained incarcerated at the Villa Devoto and Rawson Penitentiaries, located in Buenos Aires and near the southern city of Trelew, respectively. At Rawson, Hodgers took part in the attempted prison escape that resulted in the military's execution of sixteen political prisoners on August 22, 1972. She used her dance training to help prepare prisoners in her unit for the escape. Following her release in 1973, Hodgers continued to work with the PRT-ERP until she fled Argentina with her son following the May 1976 disappearance of her partner Héctor Fernández Baños, a University of Buenos Aires law professor and PRT-ERP member.[56]

Hodgers continued to teach and performed briefly in Buenos Aires under an assumed name following her release from prison; however, she did not resume full-time work in the dance field until her arrival in Geneva as a political refugee in the early 1980s. Hodgers reinitiated her dance career as a professor at the University of Geneva and director of L'Atelier de l'Antichambre (The

Antechamber Workshop), the dance company with whom she created *María Mar*. Developed in 1998, *María Mar* explores Hodgers's memories of her periods of incarceration and the experience of exile.[57] The work was performed broadly in Switzerland—in theaters and schools as well as under the auspices of international human rights organizations.[58] Where *La puñalada* exemplifies how citations of tango can summon collective histories of social exclusion, *María Mar* weaves tango into its choreographic project to elaborate personal trauma and recuperate bodily agency through movement. *María Mar* also highlighted, in an international context, experiences the Argentine government insisted were best forgotten at the time of the work's 1998 premiere; in that sense, in exile, Hodgers was moving otherwise to compulsory forgetting.

Full-length footage of *María Mar* has been lost, so I base my movement analysis primarily on clips of the piece that are featured in the 2001 documentary *Juntos: Un Retour en Argentine* by Raphaëlle Aellig Régnier and Norbert Wiedmer as well as Hodgers's descriptions of additional scenes.[59] *María Mar*'s successful run in Geneva inspired Swiss filmmaker Aellig Régnier to propose a documentary project featuring rehearsals and performance of the piece alongside footage of Hodgers's trip to Buenos Aires in 2000, her first since leaving the country. A small, independent company produced *Juntos*, and the documentary circulated through film festivals in Switzerland and France following its 2001 release.[60] Although Hodgers does not maintain firm ties to the Buenos Aires contemporary dance community, press coverage of her 2010 visit to Buenos Aires detailed *Juntos* and her concert works that explore her experiences with state violence.[61] The documentary, like *María Mar*, centers on Hodgers's narrative as a torture survivor and traces the intersections between her political and artistic careers. *Juntos* follows Hodgers as she speaks with ex-PRT-ERP members about their unrealized political project and her decision to travel to Buenos Aires. She visits notable memory sites in the city and speaks with Estela de Carlotto, the president of the Abuelas de Plaza de Mayo. It also explores the loss of her partner to forced disappearance. Viewers witness heart-wrenching footage in which Hodgers learns her partner most likely died in a death flight, a method of killing wherein officials threw detainees (often drugged but still alive) from planes into the Río de la Plata that borders Buenos Aires and empties into the Atlantic Ocean. The documentary dedicates equal time to footage of Hodgers rehearsing *María Mar* in Geneva and narrating clips of a performance of the work.[62] In my reading of *María Mar*, I follow the invitation that *Juntos* extends to consider Hodgers's physical return to Buenos Aires alongside *María Mar*'s movement-based journey into the past.

The piece features six female performers. Five wear light-blue pants and tops reminiscent of prisoners' garb, and Hodgers understands two of these dancers as embodiments of the same character, María (one real, and one imagined); their doubling suggests both the fragmentation of self and the repetitions that characterize trauma's ongoing effects in the present.[63] It also signals Hodgers's own use of pseudonyms during her time as a militant. Another dancer clad in a uniform represents a prison guard. Like *La puñalada*, the piece draws heavily on props, including a table, chairs, and a collection of worn shoes. While the chair in *La puñalada* serves in some instances to animate a violent aggressor's body, in *María Mar* the furniture represents a prison cell. The imprisoned dancers engage the table and chairs with the full lengths of their bodies and from every angle, wrapping, arching, sliding, and occasionally striking their torsos and limbs against the objects.[64] These movements make the force of the prison's disciplinary power palpable with each impact. In Hodgers's description of the shoes' role in the piece, one of the Marías pushes the shoes (women's and children's) off the surface of the table and scatters them around the stage.[65] While in *La puñalada* the pointe shoe, taken on and off, represents an identity transformation across the performer's body, here the scattered, mismatched shoes call attention to absence—to bodies that never will be recovered and to lives disrupted by exile.

While *La puñalada* explicitly foregrounds tango through music, movement, and citations of figures like the *compadrito* and *cancionista*, *María Mar* draws on the form more subtly. It blends seamlessly into Hodgers's contemporary vocabulary, which in *María Mar* emphasizes tightly controlled floor work. The specter of tango emerges twice: once as part of a series of scenes featuring the guard and one María, and once in a moment danced by the prisoners. In *Juntos*, a series of clips conclude with a close embrace reminiscent of tango upper-body positioning that comments on power relationships between guards and prisoners. In the first clip, the guard stands on top of a small platform wearing a pair of flamenco shoes. The dancer who performed this role happened to be a flamenco dancer, and Hodgers prompted her to perform flamenco's characteristic foot strikes as if she were giving orders to the prisoners.[66] A microphone positioned underneath the platform amplifies what Hodgers chillingly describes as gunshot-like sounds, an effect that leaves the dancers, and surely the audience, with "goosebumps."[67] In the next clip, one María repeatedly slams her knee against the table in a gesture of self-discipline as the guard looks on. In the final clip in the series, the guard moves into a lead dancer's arm positioning in a close embrace, one arm wrapped around an absent partner's back, and the other extended to meet an invisible hand. Eyes closed, the guard slowly shifts back and forth in a moment of private reverie before lowering herself to her knees in front of one María. She gropes María's thighs and buttocks before pulling her into an embrace. María's body goes limp in the guard's arms as the guard sways her body (figure 4.3).[68] Fondled and manipulated in the guard's arms, María's blank stare and limp posture signal the loss of agency over the body as it becomes the object of sexualized violence.

In our interview, Hodgers explained that this choreography stemmed from her memories of a female prison guard's repeated attempts at sexual assault.[69]

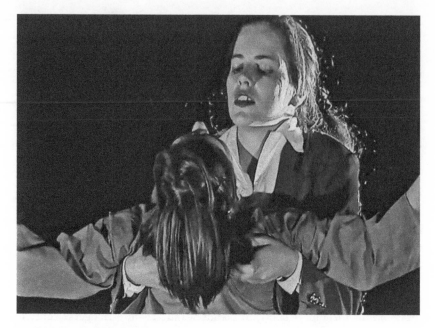

Figure 4.3 *María Mar* as featured in the documentary *Juntos: Un Retour en Argentine*, 2001. Courtesy of RaR Film and Biograph Film.

The flamenco foot strikes establish the guard's power over the prisoners, while the leader-follower structure of tango and its association with sexual encounters offers steps for denouncing the frequent inclusion of assault and rape within practices of torture and imprisonment. The guard's structured posture juxtaposed with María's motionless body exaggerates the leader's determination of how a dance would unfold, in turn mirroring the guard's position of power. Emanating from the leader position (traditionally danced by a man) the guard's movements comment on the military dictatorship's repeated masculinization of government power and feminization of "subversives" vis-à-vis torture, recalling *La puñalada's* critique of sexualized power dynamics through the construction of a dually gendered body.[70]

While the tango embrace employed in this scene alludes to uneven gendered and sexualized power dynamics, an additional episode cites tango elements to rechoreograph possibilities for self-determination and healing. In Hodgers's recollection, the scene begins when the guard leaves the two Marías and the additional prisoners with makeup and one high-heeled shoe each. They apply the makeup, and each puts on their one shoe. Mariano Mores's instrumental tango song "Taquito militar" ("Military Heel") begins to play. The title of Mores's song references early men's tango shoes, which derived from military boots. The heel provided a forward pitch that facilitated turning and the close embrace, and accented the foot strikes *milongueros* (male tango dancers) performed before asking a partner to dance.[71] Lying face down on the floor, the prisoners perform footwork (as best they can from such a physically limiting position) typically associated with a follower's steps in a tango pairing, particularly *ochos* (figure-eight steps).[72] As mentioned earlier, though the leader's movements generally prompt the follower in socially danced tango, followers have agency over the interpretation of the lead's signal and the option to add flourishes. These possibilities arise precisely from an intercorporeal awareness and responsiveness between leader and follower that is completely foreclosed in the guard scene. In her work on tango, theorist Erin Manning locates politics in this leader-follower negotiation. She writes, "Tango as a political gesture is the exhibition of the between: between my interpretation and your creation, between my lead and your response. Tango allows the mediality of experience to shine through, exposing the ethical dimension of that relation."[73] Manning's comments might be extended to encompass tango's mediation not only between two bodies, but also, as *La puñalada* so powerfully demonstrated, between experiences of the past and the present.[74]

Thus the steps performed while lying flat to the floor, or the "stomach tango," as Hodgers referred to it, play on tango's possibilities for improvisation and individual expression within a determinant structure.[75] In this case the "ethical dimensions" of the "medial" experience that Manning cites, however, do not index the particularities of the connection (or disconnection) between two dancers. Rather, they stage the possibility of reconnecting with one's own body and agency, a link that torture and imprisonment severed. By performing tango movements lying face down, in a position associated with a number of violent disciplinary acts (from arrest to rape), *María Mar* asks if tango might provide the literal steps for recovering the body's history and identity from a physical position often used to strip those elements away. It adapts tango movements and puts them to work in a context literally designed to discipline the body into stillness and silence. The makeup and the high-heeled shoes suggest both the mandate that female bodies make themselves desirable and the possible recuperation of a feminized sexuality muted by the threat of sexual assault. The "Taquito militar" musical reference makes present tango's historically heteronormative power dynamics (as well as those of the military) at the same time that *María Mar's* choreography evidences the space for tactical negotiation that tango's structure offers.

The internal focus of the stomach tango, directed as it is toward the floor immediately beneath the dancers' bodies, also powerfully resonates with dancer Nora Codina's description of how she turned to dance to survive her own clandestine detention. A member of the Nucleodanza company, Codina was detained in 1977 following the disappearance of her husband, a physician who provided medical care to impoverished neighborhoods, but had no ties to political organizations. She explains:

My husband, who was a doctor, disappears, and they take me as a hostage. I was there twenty days. What do I do to not think and to be able to survive? What was there to do there? I made choreography. I never put it on stage, but for me that was a resource at twenty-five years old, so I decided to isolate myself, to not listen, to not anything, and this helped me a lot.[76]

For Codina, choreographing served as both a shield against the sensorial on-slaught of the detention center as well as a way to connect with her body as it came under physical attack. In Codina's experience and *María Mar*'s chore-ography, choreographies serve as resources for sustaining and approaching, respectively, the trauma of detention. While she never publicly presented the specific choreography that she made during those twenty days, Codina ulti-mately did present works that, like *María Mar*, reflected the trauma of her husband's disappearance and her own experiences of torture and clandestine detention, including *Vivos* (*Alive,* 1984) and *Suicida* (*Suicide,* 1984).

In our interview, Hodgers used the verb "recuperate" to describe the rela-tionship between dance (contemporary and tango) and traumatic memory. Hodgers testified that dance generally and *María Mar* specifically served to "recuperate my body" following her experiences in the 1970s.[77] According to Hodgers, she "would not be who I am today" had it not been for "working with improvisation, getting the feelings out, expressiveness, and seeing that other dancers were also working with the political" after arriving in Switzerland.[78] Quite literally, the practice of dancing and choreographing moved trauma, allowing Hodgers to work through and live with experiences that can never be fully known. Her journey to Buenos Aires in *Juntos* emphasizes the ina-bility to assemble straightforward narratives of the past—conversations with ex-PRT-ERP members about shared experiences in particular reveal the insta-bility and mutability of memory across time. As mentioned earlier, she also comes face to face with the limited information available about her partner's death. Hodgers knows Fernández Baños most likely died in a death flight be-tween May and December 1976; however, his are not amongst the bones that have been recovered from the Río de la Plata.[79] The *mar*, or ocean, of the *María Mar* title suggests Fernández Baños's most probable final resting place. While Hodgers's experiences as a political prisoner motivated the creation of *María Mar*, the piece also mourns the absences left by forced disappearance. When describing a rolling motion during a rehearsal, Hodgers states, "It's as though one of the Marías wants to slip into the ocean, while the other holds her back a bit."[80] *María Mar* choreographically probes the sensations that bodies on death flights experienced and imagines, if only briefly, the macabre possibility of a re-encounter in the depths of the sea. In this sense, *María Mar* affirma-tively answers a question that Idelber Avelar poses about whether mourning, in the wake of military dictatorship, can be thought of as an act of productive doing as opposed to the Freudian negative process in which the object of loss must be released. He asks, "Can one mourn . . . as if learning *how to dance?*"[81]

Notably, just as the tango plays a subtle, yet constitutive, role in *María Mar*, the specter of tango also haunts Hodgers's literal return to Buenos Aires in *Juntos*. In the documentary, intermittent clips of Hodgers dancing and spending evenings at Buenos Aires milongas (tango social dances) frame her journey into the past.[82] Recalling that the documentary was created primarily for a European audience, the milongas indeed lend the film a marketable air of "authenticity" as they introduce the viewer to Buenos Aires through the eyes of Hodgers. That is, *Juntos* does not feature the flashy tourist tango of expensive dinner shows and La Boca street corners, but brings us to a traditional space where "real" *porteños* practice "home" tango, to recall Cara's formulation. At the same time, the milongas' persistent presence in the documentary, which pace the charged emotional scenes in which Hodgers directly confronts her past, also seem to visually underscore a statement that she makes early on: "You can never erase the past. I carry it with me every day, part of me is made of that past."[83] Hodgers makes only one direct comment about the milongas. In one of the final scenes, she recounts to a friend that a chance dance partner, a businessman, revealed that militants kidnapped him twice during the dictatorship. In that instant, the improvisatory space of the milonga brought together two experiences of the dictatorship otherwise unlikely to find a space for dialogue, let alone intimate physical proximity. As a framing device in the documentary and in the milonga encounter, the tango embrace creates "a space to reflect on power and terror," just as it does in *María Mar*.[84] For Hodgers, tango and contemporary dance provided the literal steps for mourning and moving otherwise to national narratives of erasure.

In the final section of this chapter, I examine Vladimivsky's *El nombre, otros tangos*, the creation of which is featured in the Italian-produced documentary *Alma doble (Double Soul)*. Vladimivsky's work combines *La puñalada* and *María Mar*'s approaches to weaving tango into choreographies about political violence. Emphasizing tango both as a way of transmitting Argentine cultural memory and as movement for mourning, Vladimivsky's work is also the most recent. She began showing versions of the work in Buenos Aires and Italy in the context of national political shifts that began to revise the official narratives of compulsory forgetting that marked the decades following the return to democracy. The left-wing Peronist administration of Néstor Kirchner (2003–7) reopened a federal conversation around memory of the last military dictatorship, including reinitiating trials of military officials. The next chapter goes into greater depth around government actions related to dictatorship memory in the early 2000s; however, it is important to mark here that, unlike *María Mar*, *El nombre, otros tangos* dovetailed with new attempts at government accountability. That said, Vladimivsky's work, like the others considered in this chapter, moved otherwise as part of ongoing activist and artistic efforts to call attention to—and mourn—the violent past.

DANCING TANGO'S REMAINS: *EL NOMBRE, OTROS TANGOS* (2006)

Like Tambutti and Hodgers, Vladimivsky's early career took place during the last military dictatorship. She studied technique and composition with prominent members of the Buenos Aires dance community, including Norma Binaghi, Ana María Stekelman, and Ana Itelman. Additionally, Vladimivsky studied acting and directing with Augusto Fernandes, and she locates her work at the intersection of contemporary dance and dance theater.[85] In 1981, Vladimivsky cofounded the dance theater troupe Teatro Fantástico de Buenos Aires (Fantastic Theater of Buenos Aires) with her late husband, actor Salo Pasik. That same year, she participated in both the Teatro Abierto and Danza Abierta festivals; the previous chapter considered how members of the Buenos Aires dance community recalled the political undertones of her work *El día del campeón* (*The Day of the Champion*).

While tango features in *La puñalada* and *María Mar*, in our conversations, Vladimivsky characterized *El nombre, otros tangos* as part of a broader artistic project, stretching across multiple works in her repertory, that "links dance theater with tango as [a form of] Argentine cultural expression."[86] Vladimivsky noted how this project frequently came into conflict with expectation of and demand for an exoticized version of the tango, especially during her years spent living and working in Italy between 1988 and 1993.[87] For her, succumbing to the political economy of passion (to use Savigliano's phrase again) risked "getting stuck" to what Cara designates the "export" tango.[88] To illustrate her point, Vladimivsky highlighted an instance in which she turned down a likely lucrative offer to co-direct a tango school and performance venue in Turin. She did so precisely because she felt the venture sold sexualized and racialized intrigue to its European clientele and limited tango's creative potential—a potential Vladimivsky felt she could best explore in dance theater works.[89]

Vladimivsky developed *El nombre, otros tangos* and agreed to document the work's creation in *Alma doble* precisely because the stage work and documentary film promised to offer international audiences an alternative perspective on the tango that attended to both the form's historical roots among socially excluded populations and its contemporary link to the exile and loss that dictatorship violence produced.[90] *Alma doble* also features prominent tango composer Gustavo Beytelmann's narrative of exile (he left for Paris in 1976) and follows the development of his score for a version of *El nombre, otros tangos* performed in Turin in 2006. Vladimivsky became involved in the project in

2005 through Patrizia Pollarolo, a tango performer and instructor based in Turin who proposed a collaboration between Vladimivsky and Beytelmann on the theme of memory of political violence. La Sarraz, a small Turin-based independent company specializing in documentaries and art films focused on social issues, produced the film. The project filmed in Buenos Aires and Turin as Vladimivsky developed a new version of *El nombre, otros tangos*, which she had started showing in Buenos Aires in the early 2000s.[91] The piece explores the trauma of political disappearance through the danced narrative of a heterosexual couple. A version of the work forms the basis of the documentary's culminating performance featuring Beytelmann, *El nombre, otros tangos* dancers Karina Filomena and Leonardo Cuello, and Pollarolo.

In this section, I begin by discussing *El nombre, otros tango*'s creation process as it is featured in the documentary, and then turn to the piece as a standalone stage work. As with the *Juntos* documentary, *Alma doble* provides rich context for understanding how tango functions in the featured concert work and constitutes an object of analysis in and of itself. I demonstrate how both the documentary and the stage work alternately mourn personal trauma and transmit collective cultural memory. Like *La puñalada*, Vladimivsky's work links the violence that marked the context of tango's invention in the early-twentieth-century with the violence of the last military dictatorship.

Alma doble begins with a site-specific *El nombre, otros tangos* rehearsal in an antique shop in Buenos Aires. In the opening scenes, clips of Pollarolo interviewing Vladimivsky among the antiques alternate with shots of Filomena improvising on the sidewalk outside the shop (figure 4.4). Vladimivsky has asked Filomena to generate movement based on the idea of recuperation, echoing Hodgers's assertion that dance allowed her to recuperate her body following torture and incarceration. In the improvisation, as Beytelmann's score plays, Filomena moves in relationship to a table and chair, invoking a milonga club, and manipulates a collection of worn, mismatched men's and women's shoes—props strikingly similar those used in *La puñalada* and *María Mar*. Her movement does not explicitly employ a tango vocabulary; rather, it draws on shapes associated with contemporary dance, including dramatic leg extensions, floor work, lunges, and back arches.[92]

In the interview clips, Vladimivsky explains the location of the rehearsal and the material that grounds Filomena's movement:

This is a very special neighborhood where the antiques in Buenos Aires end up, when they are apparently no longer useful. However, this shop is magical because it holds the story of people's lives. I'm working poetically to get at what we harbor inside ourselves. In Argentina, a country devastated by the dictatorship where so many young people died, it is very important to recuperate every last thing. Ultimately, tango is not something that you just dance for entertainment. Tango is also a way of being, in a word, metaphysics. It's mystical, where the past

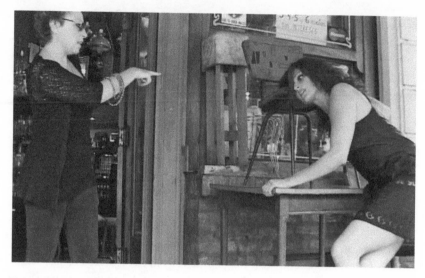

Figure 4.4 Silvia Vladimivsky directing Karina Filomena's improvisation on the sidewalk outside of the antique shop in the documentary *Alma doble* by Ivana Bosso and Francesca Gentile, 2007. Courtesy of La Sarraz Pictures srl-Italy.

is important . . . . She [the dancer] is looking for an answer in her innermost being. These are classic themes in the tango, but brought to a level of theatrical drama. She opens the coat and these men's and ladies' shoes fall out and she gets her memory back. Her hidden memories come out.[93]

Vladimivsky's commentary ends somberly with her recounting the story of her boyfriend's disappearance during the early years of the last military dictatorship. His name she notes, is missing from official records of disappeared persons, an absence reflected in the title of the stage work. As she pointed out in our interview, her cultural activities during the dictatorship also placed her at risk of disappearance.[94] Vladimivsky was active in theater, and as mentioned in the previous chapter, the military government closely monitored this community.[95]

By surrounding Vladimivsky and Filomena with objects from the past charged with the mystique of their own unknown stories, the setting gives allegorical form to Vladimivsky's mission to "recuperate every last thing." In Vladimivsky's usage, *recuperate* implies both collective and/or official reckonings with dictatorship violence (in the form of public commemoration and juridical trials of military officials) and performance's capacity to transmit the personal, embodied experience of trauma, itself fundamentally marked by absence and fragmentary knowing. As was the heartbreaking case for Hodgers's partner, Vladimivsky makes clear that she will never be able to recover her boyfriend's body or know how he died. Rather, *El nombre, otros tangos* comes from "a place of me [Vladimivsky] trying to poetically close a situation that isn't closed historically or legally."[96] Vladimivsky, then, does not purport to recover literal facts or complete narratives through dance, but instead invokes dancing as a site that allows pieces of the past to "flash up," to borrow Walter Benjamin's phrase.[97] Vladimivsky's notion that the dancer's movement in the antique shop improvisation recuperates "hidden" memories invokes Caruth's theorization of trauma's repeats. This "flashing up" also moves otherwise to ongoing juridical impunity for dictatorship-era human rights violations. As in *María Mar*, the collection of mismatched shoes, however, symbolizes the inevitable incompleteness of the past's returns. The repeated invocation of shoes, particularly "in the aggregate" in the *Alma doble* improvisation and *María Mar*, notably echo "one of the most common symbols of the devastation and loss of the Holocaust."[98] While none of the works considered in this chapter draw direct parallels between the last military dictatorship and the Holocaust, their use of shoes connects with a transnationally resonant representation of trauma. It also recalls earlier works like Susana Zimmermann's *Polymorphias* (1969) and Renate Schottelius's *Paisaje de Gritos* (1981), discussed in chapters 1 and 3 respectively, that explicitly placed Holocaust violence in conversation with Argentine political violence.

In Vladimivsky's theorization, contemporary dance combined with "classic" tango themes create a choreographic language for publicly hosting trauma's inassimilable returns. The antique shop scene develops this choreographic language vis-à-vis tango as a "way of being . . . where the past is important." Vladimivsky calls on the form to tell the story of her disappeared boyfriend, conceiving movement, as did Hodgers's work, as way of mourning his loss. By tapping into tango as a way of "being" in the past, Vladimivsky's choreography also follows in the tango's own palimpsestic tradition that Julie Taylor and María Rosa Olivera-Williams identify—it takes tango sounds and themes as occasions for dancing through trauma's returns. Where *La puñalada* performed a temporal drag that placed the context of tango's early-twentieth-century invention in conversation with the violence of the last military dictatorship, Vladimivsky's work inscribes the trauma of dictatorship violence into the tango as an aural and embodied ruin. *Alma doble* visually symbolizes this idea by literally surrounding Filomena and Vladimivsky with antiques. As *La puñalada* suggests, the periods share a basis in violence wrought by modernization projects different in scale and kind, but both forming part of Argentine collective cultural memory. Ultimately, the *Alma doble* antique shop improvisation invokes tango as an established repertoire for expressing the traumatic effects of national projects on the body. At the same time, the contemporary dance vocabulary and inclusion of theatrical elements like props and scenery (e.g., the shoes and the antique shop setting) allow Vladimivsky to choreograph absence and trauma beyond specific tango steps.

Another segment in the documentary imbues Vladimivsky's hybrid tango-dance theater vocabulary with the potential not only to host the repeats of dictatorship trauma, but also to dialogue with related histories of resistance against state violence. Following an interview scene in which Beytelmann identifies Teatro Abierto as "the most important demonstration of resistance against the dictatorship," the film cuts to members of Vladimivsky's Teatro Fantástico dancing in front of the downtown Picadero Theater.[99] The Picadero was the initial site of the 1981 Teatro Abierto festival; however, the theater experienced a devastating fire (under conditions some consider suspicious) prior to opening night.[100] In the scene, Vladimivsky leads the group in an improvisation meant to explore the "conspiracy of art" against power she feels Teatro Abierto represented.[101] A single male-female couple performs a slow, improvisational tango in close embrace; they maintain a tight kinesphere, as if dancing in a crowded club. As the couple dance, four additional dancers huddle against the doors of the theater. They transition into a tight clump, embracing one other and climbing over each others' bodies. The tangoing couple moves into the center of the group, and Vladimivsky instructs the crouched dancers to hold onto their legs and attempt to climb their bodies, "as if holding onto a tradition as well."[102] The "tradition" here might imply the preservation of a "home" tango rooted in national histories of exclusion that rejects the global political economy of passion. However, the scene also suggests that Vladimivsky asks the dancers, as they move in front of the Picadero's doors, to hold onto the memory of Teatro Abierto as evidence of a robust tradition of national resistance. The scene immediately cuts to a young Teatro Fantástico dancer who describes how, having not lived through the dictatorship, he only knows of the festival through theater history books. He reflects on the power of "being here," at the place where it all began. The documentary and Vladimivsky's choreography propose movement not only as a modality for making sense of individual experiences of the past, but also for viscerally transmitting collective histories of pain *and* resistance to younger generations.

Vladimivsky completed *El nombre, otros tangos* in 2006. She presented two versions of the work that year, one in Turin (presented under the title *¿Cómo te llamás?. . . Azul*, or *What is your name?. . . Blue*) and a second in Buenos Aires. Vladimivsky's continual return to and revision of the piece—recall that she developed the first versions in the early 2000s—itself embodies engagement with trauma as a process based in repetition.[103] Both 2006 versions are duets between a female dancer and a male dancer, and both incorporate tango music and partnered tango dance interludes alongside the contemporary dance vocabulary exemplified in Filomena's antique shop improvisation (video clip 4.2 ▶).[104] *El nombre, otros tangos* went on to appear on the 2007 Teatro por la Identidad program.

The Italian version features visual elements that literalize the conflation between tango, turn-of-the-twentieth-century economic violence, and political violence that the antique shop improvisation implied. Projections juxtapose images of archival tango photographs, impoverished immigrants standing outside a *conventillo*, images of the Argentine flag, and shots of the Madres de Plaza de Mayo. The inclusion of images of protest and activism echo the Picadero Theater improvisation from *Alma doble*, folding memories of resistance into the process of "recuperating" the past. The worn shoes employed in the *Alma doble* improvisation appear in the Buenos Aires version of the work, but in the Italian production they are replaced with suitcases, scattered clothing, and mannequin busts. In both versions, these various artifacts signal "a story inevitably in pieces."[105]

Like *La puñalada* and *María Mar*, the Italian production makes legacies of incarceration and torture present. While Tambutti and Hodgers's works stage acts of violation, *El nombre, otros tangos* presents only the violated body. In the opening moments of the piece, the male dancer appears alone on stage—naked, bound, gagged, and lying supine across the top of a metal bar that resembles a freestanding ballet barre. His pose is reminiscent of stress positions frequently incorporated into torture practices. The lighting design brings the intense image into and out of view as the projection design casts the montage of cultural and activist symbols (video clip 4.3 ▶). In juxtaposition to this archival footage, the dance offers a live, material body in pain. It quite literally brings the horror of clandestine torture practices, whose absence from public view allowed the military government to feign innocence, into the light. This act of making the invisible visible frames the choreography's subsequent journey into the history of the couple, making clear that the dramatic action unfolds as a result of devastating physical violence. It also acts as an enduring reminder of the past in the context of continued activist efforts to advance juridical recognition of human rights violations committed during the last military dictatorship.

Vladimivsky's *El nombre, otros tangos*, as it appears in the *Alma doble* documentary and on the concert stage, moves trauma as it invokes tango as both a practice of collective cultural memory and calls on the movement's ability to express deeply personal loss. In Vladimivsky's own construction, her work proposes a hybridized movement language for approaching the specificity of the Argentine experience—and claiming Argentine-ness—on its own terms. As it employs dance to help "close" (as Vladimivsky put it) a period that remains suspended juridically and historically, the piece theorizes movement as a method of mourning that acknowledges the necessary incompleteness of this task. *El nombre, otros tangos* powerfully posits movement as a site where the past might continually flash up in ways that honor the absences that mark the present.

MEMORY AS MOVEMENT

This chapter has demonstrated how contemporary dance works consistently explored the lasting effects of trauma through the body in motion in historical moments marked by early juridical strides, stunning government impunity, and renewed attempts to reopen the national conversation around dictatorship violence. For Tambutti, Hodgers, and Vladimivsky, contemporary dance in conversation with the tango provided the steps for moving through trauma's returns. Through its myriad character transformations, *La puñalada* rehearsed tango's, and the *grotesco criollo*'s, turn-of-the-century roots to situate tango music and movements as culturally specific palimpsests that activate and accrue collective absence and loss across time. While tango still inevitably marks the national in *Juntos* and *María Mar*, both the documentary and stage work posited the very act of dancing tango as a way of approaching personal trauma—in Buenos Aires milongas and on the concert stage. In the first instance in *Juntos*, the milonga facilitated a chance encounter between Hodgers and the businessman who had experienced kidnapping at the hands of militants. On stage, Hodgers's "stomach tango" questioned how these historically charged movements might aid in a conscious recovery of the body's agency in the wake of torture and sexual assault. *Alma doble* and *El nombre, otros tangos* drew on tango as a repository of collective cultural memory at the same time that tango themes provided a way to approach the loss of a loved one. In all three cases, tango functions as a privileged corporeal repertoire for moving into, dwelling in, and sifting through the pieces of the past—for moving trauma. These cases nuance a lively discussion on tango's many lives—on the concert stage and off. They also powerfully evidence contemporary dance's response to the individual and collective trauma of the last military dictatorship, and most critically, the possibilities of memory and mourning in motion.

As alluded to earlier, the works considered here are three among many projects that put contemporary dance to work as a site for representing and reflecting on the period of the last military dictatorship. The following chapter extends this focus on dance as a practice of collective memory, but with a specific focus on work—particularly the unification of memory politics with cooperative labor politics characteristic of multiple contemporary dance projects that emerged following Argentina's 2001 economic crisis. While the choreographers considered here came of age, built careers, and lost loved ones during the height of government repression, many of the dancers in *Moving Otherwise*'s final chapter were either young children or born following the return to democracy. Most have no direct relationship to disappeared persons. As they explored movement as a way of connecting to what they nevertheless saw as a shared past, these dancers simultaneously grappled with the material legacies of the dictatorship that shaped their lives in the present. The following chapter turns to dance projects that manifest the links and continuities between Argentina's history of dictatorial rule and the devastating economic crisis that gripped the country in the early 2000s.

CHAPTER 5

Common Goods

In December 2001, Argentina became engulfed in economic crisis. While liberalization measures first began during the dictatorships that marked the 1960s, 1970s, and early 1980s, the neoliberal policies advanced under the administration of President Carlos Menem (1989–99) formed the immediate context of the crisis. Under the direction of economy minister Domingo Cavallo, the government opened the country to free trade, increased flexibility in the labor markets, privatized state-run industries, and pegged the peso to the dollar to control inflation and provide security for foreign investors.[1] By the late 1990s, however, the economy began to buckle under the strain of unsustainable monetary policy and growing unemployment. Fernando de la Rúa assumed the presidency in 1999 and attempted to adhere to the International Monetary Fund's (IMF) structural readjustment demands in exchange for financial support. As a result, interest rates soared and pushed the domestic budget into deficit. Capital flight began in anticipation of peso devaluation—and, following the IMF's refusal of an emergency loan in 2001, banks lost 17 percent of their deposits. On December 1, the government capped bank withdrawals, inciting violent riots and mass protests.[2] Middle-class *cacerolazos*, in which participants banged pots and pans, and working-class *piqueteros*, where protestors occupied streets with bodies and blockades, took place across the nation.[3] Protestors unified under the cry *¡que se vayan todos!* (out with them all!), the unofficial slogan of movements calling for new political leadership.[4] De la Rúa resigned on December 20 as most of the population faced diminished standards of living and millions experienced poverty.

Throughout the immediate and extended post-crisis period, contemporary dance practices moved otherwise through practices of cooperative labor. In the days, months, and years following the events of December 2001, contemporary dancers as well as other artists, workers, and middle-class professionals embraced cooperative arrangements not only as a means of sustaining themselves, but also to contest neoliberal emphases on the market economy, individual achievement, and financial gain. As activist scholar Marina Sitrin points out, the concepts of *autogestión* (self-management) and *horizontalidad* (horizontality) became key to cooperative activism and art making alike. *Horizontalidad* "implies democratic communication on a level plane and involves—or at least intentionally strives towards—non-hierarchical and anti-authoritarian creation rather than reaction. It is a break with vertical ways of organizing and relating."[5] For example, the popular assembly movement, a form of direct democracy in which members discuss and vote on pressing issues, took root in neighborhoods and communities across Buenos Aires.[6] Artistically, groups including the Grupo de Arte Callejero (Street Art Group), the Taller Popular de Serigrafía (Popular Silkscreen Workshop), and Argentina Arde (Argentina Is Burning) strived to support worker movements by lending their production skills to the post-crisis struggle.[7] The Eloísa Cartonera publishing cooperative began to print literary works on reclaimed materials; *cartoneras/os* refer to recyclers who collect cardboard and other materials from refuse left for garbage collection.[8] Following the economic collapse, estimates placed the number of *cartoneros*—in Buenos Aires alone—in the tens of thousands.[9]

While a turn to cooperative labor marked a broad range of post-crisis dance practices, this chapter focuses specifically on dance initiatives where memory of the last military dictatorship figures prominently, both in how dancers conceptualize their missions as well as in the thematic content of their stage works.[10] While the previous chapter traced how a select set of stage works employed tango themes in their approaches to individual and collective trauma, the initiatives considered here explicitly link the last military dictatorship to the devastating effects of neoliberal crisis. Their work formed part of broader efforts to make the corporeal effects of the crisis legible within histories of national violence. In the post-crisis period, social movements identified a new generation of *desaparecidos*: the economic disappeared.[11] Bodies did not suffer the explicit censure—in the form of forced disappearance and torture—sustained during the last military dictatorship. However, as literary scholar Judith Filc points out, neoliberal precarity produced "elements of continuity with the diverse modes of social expulsion produced by state terror."[12] Sociologist Barbara Sutton adds, "human bodies disappear under the neoliberal logic, just as the last military dictatorship in Argentina disappeared the real, material bodies of many people who opposed precisely the purview of that kind of socioeconomic organization."[13] Economic disappearance, in other words, named the attritional, or "slow," violence of neoliberal capitalism.[14] This terminology also evidences how, as anthropologist Karen Ann Faulk demonstrates, injustices linked to the last military dictatorship indelibly marked the activist vocabularies and human rights discourses of the neoliberal era.[15] Furthermore, in the post-crisis period the state itself emerged as a prominent advocate for dictatorship memory. The left-wing Peronist Kirchner administrations (Néstor Kirchner 2003–7 and Cristina Fernández de Kirchner 2007–15) reinitiated juridical trials of military officials and fostered close relationships with groups like the Madres de Plaza de Mayo and Abuelas de Plaza de Mayo, reinforcing the link between dictatorship memory and advocacy for rights.[16]

This chapter begins with the 2007–8 labor dispute between the administration and members of the prestigious Ballet Contemporáneo of the San Martín Theater. A series of injuries and subsequent firings gave rise to the Bailarines Organizados (Organized Dancers) labor movement, which called attention to the dancers' short-term contracts that denied them access to benefits and job security. Bailarines Organizados linked their economic disappearance to political disappearance—from the images on their posters to their protest tactics, the group mobilized dictatorship symbols and broader memory discourses. In the wake of the labor movement, members of Bailarines Organizados formed the performing company Nuevos Rumbos (New Waves), later reincorporated under the auspices of the Secretary of Culture as the Compañía Nacional de Danza Contemporánea (CNDC, National Contemporary Dance Company, 2009–). The CNDC, in its initial years, was committed to a horizontal administrative structure and the production of work with a sociopolitical orientation, including a number of pieces that represent the last military dictatorship. In this chapter, I consider Daniel Payero Zaragoza's 2010 *Retazos pequeños de nuestra historia más reciente* (*Small Pieces of Our Recent History*). In my discussion of Bailarines Organizados as well as the CNDC, I draw on interviews with dancers, documentation of protests as well as stage works, and my own viewing of CNDC performances.

The chapter then turns to Bailarines Toda la Vida (Dancers for Life, 2002–), a community troupe I performed with for nearly a year. Focused on inclusive membership and collaborative creation, for fifteen years the group rehearsed weekly in a breadstick factory that was reopened by the labor cooperative La Nueva Esperanza (The New Hope) following the factory's closure during the 2001 crisis. The Grissinopoli factory (*grisines* are breadsticks in Argentine Spanish) is one of the longest-lasting worker cooperatives to emerge from the Movimiento Nacional de Fábricas Recuperadas (National Movement of Worker Recuperated Factories), a cornerstone of post-crisis labor mobilization.[17] Many factories, including Grissinopoli, reopened as hybrid cultural centers where manual and creative labor joined forces to support alternative management configurations—a phenomenon that gained international attention.[18] Like the CNDC, Bailarines Toda la Vida's repertory engages sociopolitical themes with a particular emphasis on dancing the memory of the last military dictatorship; here I consider . . . *Y el mar* (*. . . And the Sea*, 2011) and *La oscuridad* (*The Darkness*, 2006). In addition to engaging memory through their creative work, Bailarines Toda la Vida also frequently performs in cultural spaces associated with dictatorship memory, and the group consistently has worked to form alliances with prominent human rights organizations. My embodied experience as part of the group, Chillemi's writings on the project, interviews with group members, and materials documenting the group's choreographies collectively inform my analysis.

As post-2001 initiatives, Bailarines Organizados/CNDC and Bailarines Toda la Vida share explicit ties to labor movements that rejected neoliberal emphases on worker dispensability and hyperproductivity, working instead toward sustainable structures that support cooperative creative and administrative action. Both forged and maintain cooperative structures by linking economic disappearance to histories of political disappearance. This move contributes broadly to the transmission of the memory of the last military dictatorship at the same time that it contextualizes these groups' struggles within longer histories of national violence. It also "recuperates," to borrow the word used by the worker-run factory movement, the historical link between economic ideologies introduced during the last military dictatorship and the 2001 neoliberal crisis, and points to the continuities in physical violence that they share. In the worker-run factory context, use of the verb *recuperar* emphasizes the goal of returning the means of production to the working classes. It also, as the previous chapter demonstrated, resonates with discourses around the individual and collective trauma of the last military dictatorship. By "putting the body" in labor movements and day-to-day cultural work—*poner el cuerpo*, or the idea of fully committing the body to action, emerged as an overarching practice and ethics of political participation in the post-crisis period—these projects reckon with the past and present of neoliberal violence and evidence dance's ability to move new political subjectivities into being.[19]

LABOR MOVEMENT: BAILARINES ORGANIZADOS AND THE MOBILIZATION OF MEMORY

In 2008, I came upon a slightly faded—yet startlingly bold—black-and-white poster on my way through the halls of the prestigious Recoleta Cultural Center (figure 5.1). Pinned to the lower half of an announcement board, the poster read, "Look who is dancing . . .!!! In 9 months 7 accidents. In 6 months 12 fired (disappeared) dancers. In 10 months 6 performances. The Ballet of Terror."[20] The text framed an image of three dancers costumed in torso-skimming, full-length dresses, posed with legs extended to the side in grand battements. The faces of Kive Staiff, then director of the San Martín Theater; Mauricio Wainrot, then director of the San Martín's Ballet Contemporáneo; and finally, General Jorge Rafael Videla, were digitally fixed onto the dancers' heads. Videla, of course, has no association with the San Martín Theater, much less the Buenos Aires dance world. His is the highly recognizable face of the military

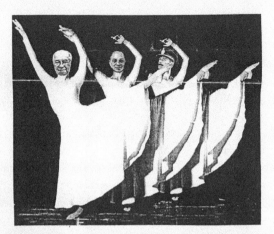

¡¡¡ MIRÁ QUIÉN BAILA...!!!

EN 9 MESES 7 ACCIDENTES

EN 6 MESES 12 BAILARINES DESPEDIDOS
(DESAPARECIDOS)

EN 10 MESES 6 FUNCIONES

EL BALLET DEL TERROR

Figure 5.1 Bailarines Organizados' "Ballet of Terror" poster, created with the support of the ATE, 2007–8. Courtesy of Bettina Quintá.

junta that orchestrated the political disappearances, here equated with the dancers' firings, which took place during the last military dictatorship. At the bottom corners of the page, the acronyms ATE (Asociación Trabajadores del Estado, Association of State Workers) and CTA (Central de Trabajadores de la Argentina, Argentine Workers Central Union)—two of Argentina's largest labor unions—were written in marker.[21]

As discussed in chapter 3, the Ballet Contemporáneo (then called the Grupo de Danza Contemporánea) was established in 1977 alongside a conservatory-style training program. It is the oldest and longest-running municipally supported contemporary dance company in Argentina, and it represents a standard of professionalization and technical rigor in the field. This poster, I discovered, was part of a 2007–8 labor dispute spurred by seven work-related accidents and the subsequent dismissal of twelve dancers from the troupe. None received worker's compensation or severance pay. The dismissed dancers first formed the Bailarines Organizados labor rights group, and eventually the CNDC performing company.[22] In this section, I consider how Bailarines Organizados conceptualized the events surrounding their dismissal as a question of labor rights, and identified themselves among the economic disappeared through the use of dictatorship symbols and language (as in the poster) that gave significant public weight to their cause. Their danced labor movement, I argue, critiqued the neoliberalization of dance practice and production in Buenos Aires through activist tactics imbued with the cooperative politics of 2001 mobilization.

Bailarines Organizados identified the Ballet Contemporáneo dancers among the economic disappeared as a result of both structural factors— namely the short-term contracts that formed the basis of company employment—as well as more insidious logics and practices that shaped artistic production at the theater and the professional dance field more broadly.[23] The former Ballet Contemporáneo dancers held *locación de servicio*, or sixth-month service agreements, that prevented dancers from procuring workers' compensation, health insurance plans (*obras sociales*), bonuses, or retirement funds granted to most government workers.[24] Many of the dancers who labored under these contracts had been with the company for nearly a decade as well-known soloists and award-winning performers. In fact, the year the labor dispute began, fired dancer Ernesto Chacón Oribe received the prestigious 2007 Clarín Award for notable figures in dance. In his widely viewed acceptance speech, broadcast as part of the televised awards ceremony, Chacón Oribe condemned what he characterized as the "discriminatory" nature of the dancers' contracts and the Ballet Contemporáneo's "artistic genocide" against the company's dancers.[25]

The San Martín contracts reflect wider patterns in the degradation of labor and retraction of state protections and services that accompanied the intensification of neoliberal reform in the post-dictatorship period. A San Martín Theater press release, reprinted in a 2008 article addressing the dismissals and ensuing labor dispute, articulated the firings as a simple matter of not signing new contracts:

> Given recent public demonstrations by ex-members of the San Martín Theater's Contemporary Ballet, the administration announces that these dancers were artistic personnel contracted under the regime "service agreement," which are contracts without benefits, honored only for a determined time, without a renewal clause, that meet the requirements of the Government of the City of Buenos Aires. As no new contracts were signed, with their expiration on 6/30/ 08 two of these contracts were automatically no longer valid.[26]

The dancers' short-term contracts embodied the logic whereby the disposability of laboring bodies, regardless of ability or consecutive years of dedication, maximizes profit and discourages labor organization. Production-wise, the Ballet Contemporáneo barely missed a beat. Emphasizing that the dismissed dancers were not scarce resources, the company moved forward with the planned season, mounted on the bodies of the many dancers waiting in the wings. The press release also reflects the increasingly corporate nature of government under neoliberalism. As choreographer Lucía Russo pointed out on the Bailarines Organizados blog, "Well, the San Martín is not a private business and the workers have the right to defend their contracts and labor rights."[27] By drawing a distinction between the responsibilities of the state versus private industry, Russo's comment calls attention to flexible labor's degradation of worker protections and valorizes collective resistance. It also evidences what Faulk identifies as a central tension of post-crisis activist vocabularies. Russo's comment—as well as Bailarines Organizados' own deployment of a rights-based vocabulary—ultimately articulates a liberal conception of individual rights through its appeal to the state.[28] As political theorist Wendy Brown has shown, rights-based discourses often legitimize the neoliberal state through their call for its protections.[29] Bailarines Organizados claim that as dancers "we have a right to rights!" undoubtedly affirms state power; however, the forms of collective social action that they took simultaneously contested neoliberal emphases on the individual and the market.[30]

In a personal interview, ex-San Martín dancer and Bailarines Organizados cofounder Bettina Quintá described the logics and practices that the group rejected in order to organize. As we sat in the small office off of the CNDC's rehearsal space in the National Center for Music and Dance, Quintá explained:

In Argentina, specifically, it's as if we are taught to dance, work, and be thankful that we can dance. . . . It's as if there are so few places to work and the moment you decide to be a dancer and live off of that, you have to take a good look at everything, or you leave the country and separate from your family and even then you can't be sure you'll find work abroad. So, what happens is that one holds onto the little work there is so tightly, it's as if everyone is afraid and no one expresses how they would really like things to be, or if there is something not right about the work, for fear of losing the job, you don't say anything. And the directors or those with administrative positions anticipate this and take advantage of it in most instances. Moreover, dancers come from a line of teaching with the structure of "The Director" so you can't speak, you have to be respectful. This is where individualism comes in also, like, it's better I stay quiet, protect my job, and if I advance in my career, even better. So, it's super difficult for dancers to join together so dance is respected, developed in more areas, and the dancer is respected as a worker.[31]

Quintá's observations characterize an individualized and precarity-driven—a neoliberalized—consciousness that tacitly discouraged organization among the dancers. As she articulated it above: "better I stay quiet, protect my job, and if I advance in my career, even better." During the last military dictatorship the permeating fear of forced disappearance often foreclosed collective mobilization, a condition that offers a figurative echo of dancers' fear of disappearing within unstable labor arrangements. So much so that many dancers played along with unfair practices, even if the conditions for extending employment by only six months at a time might mean an injury that could end their dance career. Where artistic production in general has proven to be amenable to the neoliberal push for "creative capital," dance, as a craft of the body, readily registers the corporeal effects of neoliberal management—in this case in the injured, displaced bodies of the premier contemporary dance company in Buenos Aires.[32]

The San Martín case takes on specific meaning within the Argentine national context; however, the theater's labor practices and the precarity that its dancers experienced is by no means unique within the global dance community. Quintá alludes to the persistent notion that dance does not constitute "real" labor, or if anything, consistent pay for a lucky few. Quintá also contextualizes her observations on individualism with broader commentary on the transnational corporeal tactics needed to succeed in a global dance market. Quintá, like many professional Argentine dancers, spent time abroad training and performing. She was a scholarship student at The Ailey School in New York City and a member of the Municipal Ballet of Santiago de Chile.[33] Quintá's time abroad also reflects her career's crossings between ballet and contemporary dance. Similarly, in Argentina she danced professionally with the Colón Theater Ballet as well as the Ballet Contemporáneo, the two most prestigious companies in the fields of classical ballet and contemporary dance, respectively. Quintá's career exemplifies the mandate for dancers in the neoliberal era to move smoothly between genres and across borders in the face of limited work opportunities, or what dance scholar Anusha Kedhar understands as the cultivation of "flexible bodies." Theorizing the various ways in which South Asian dancers are "flexible," Kedhar builds on concepts of flexible labor and citizenship:

> I understand flexibility here as a broad range of practices that includes, among other corporeal tactics, a dancer's physical ability to stretch her limbs or bend her spine backward to meet the demands of a particular work or choreographer, her ability to negotiate immigration regulations and restrictions in order to move more easily across national borders, and her ability to pick up multiple movement vocabularies and deploy them strategically to increase her marketability and broaden her employment prospects.[34]

The different kinds of flexibility Kedhar identifies not only account for Quintá's cross-border and cross-genre negotiations, but also speak to the demands for physical (over)extension that contributed to the Ballet Contemporáneo members' injuries and sparked the labor movement.

The Bailarines Organizados labor movement responded to local realities as well as professional dancers' broader strategies for managing market conditions. They did so through cooperative actions that mobilized post-2001 modes of moving otherwise while linking their plight to national histories of political injustice. The "Ballet of Terror" posters, hung throughout Buenos Aires cultural spaces and on the front doors of the San Martín Theater itself, visualized the corporeal continuities between political and economic disappearance in Argentina. In addition to the posters, the group also organized multiple protests. Like the "Ballet of Terror" posters, Bailarines Organizados' interventions recall the injustices of the last military dictatorship, in this case postdictatorship activist repertoires. In our conversation, Quintá referred to one of the group's protests—handing out pamphlets to theatergoers and government officials on the opening night of the company's first new season following the firings—as an *escrache*, or public shaming act.[35] As mentioned in the previous chapter, the H.I.J.O.S. activist group originally staged *escraches* in the 1990s in response to truncated trials of military leaders and government pardons. *Escraches* called attention to government impunity through their staging outside of the residences of known military officials and former clandestine torture centers. In the case that Quintá cites, Bailarines Organizados aimed to interrupt the smooth unfolding of the premiere by making sure attendees were aware of the theater's treatment of its former dancers. Quintá's designation of this intervention as an *escrache* follows a tradition of post-crisis social movements that also broadly referred to protest actions (particularly those staged inside and outside of banks) as *escraches*.[36]

Bailarines Organizados also organized demonstrations that involved dancing and chanting in the street in front of the San Martín Theater on days without performances, with representatives from labor unions standing alongside them in solidarity. These demonstrations did not involve the level of direct confrontation with theater and government officials that characterized the opening night intervention; however, their strategic location mobilized an *escrache*'s emphasis on the importance of addressing the physical site of injustice. The danced protests included a mix of gestures symbolizing defiance and unification—raised fists and clasped hands—alongside brief excerpts from the Ballet Contemporáneo's recent repertory (figure 5.2).[37] Shortly before the protests began, the company had performed Wainrot's neoclassical *El Mesías* (*The Messiah*, 1996) and was preparing, among other works, his version of *La consagración de la primavera* (*The Rite of Spring*, 1999) for the upcoming season.[38] Clad in jeans and T-shirts marking the thirtieth anniversary of the company, the dancers performed Wainrot's technically demanding choreography in the

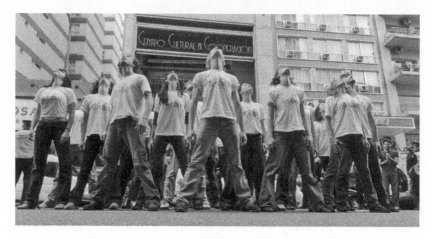

Figure 5.2 Bailarines Organizados' protest outside the San Martín Theater, 2008.
Photograph: Fernando Massobrio/*La Nación*. Courtesy of photographer.

middle of the street, performing soaring lifts, leaps, and movement into and
out of the floor, or in this case the pavement of bustling Corrientes Avenue.
Chanting, drumming, and speeches calling for dancers' rights provided the
sound score for the danced protest—these sounds replaced the repertory
works' classical music scores (set to Handel and Stravinsky, respectively).[39]
By performing selections of the repertory in the street alongside representatives from the unions, the protesters underscored their dancing as labor and
marked their displacement from the Buenos Aires theater, which was then
singularly associated with full time employment for contemporary dancers.

By imagining a labor movement that drew on dictatorship symbols
and adapted activist repertoires linked to human rights groups, Bailarines
Organizados engaged in a form of memory entrepreneurship. A concept developed by French historian Gérard Noiriel and Argentine sociologist Elizabeth
Jelin in their studies on collective cultural memory, the term memory entrepreneurship "implies elaborating memories in terms of, or in view of, a
project or endeavor."[40] Noiriel, building on work by Max Weber and Maurice
Halbwachs, argues that memory entrepreneurs emerge as protagonists
among a group of stakeholders in the formation of collective memory. As
entrepreneurs, they undertake the labor required to define, legitimize, and
make visible articulations of the past that support their communities and
identities within a particular political context, in the process accruing political capital as social actors. Memory entrepreneurs "choose which individual
experiences best represent their cause and then transform these into collective memory" through commemorative practices and other forms of memorialization.[41] In the Argentine context, Jelin identifies the Madres de Plaza

de Mayo and Abuelas de Plaza de Mayo as the first generation of memory entrepreneurs.[42]

Building on the work of Noiriel and Jelin, I expand memory entrepreneurship to include not only the production of collective memory, but also the process by which nonfilial groups deploy collective memories in view of *other* political projects—in this case, the ways in which Bailarines Organizados mobilized dictatorship memories in the service of post-2001 labor struggles. Within the post-2001 context, the concept offers a productive play on a term— entrepreneurship—firmly tied to neoliberal drives toward the accumulation of capital.[43] For Bailarines Organizados, however, memory entrepreneurship did not aim to advance dancers within the market conditions that literally left their bodies broken. Rather, the group's memory entrepreneurship accrued critical *political* currency that allowed them to call attention to the violence of neoliberalized artistic labor. The use of dictatorship symbols and protest strategies helped legitimize their labor movement by connecting their plight to memory politics, which by 2007 was driven by the federal government and activists alike. Bailarines Organizados' tactics illuminate how dictatorship memory provided the discursive ("economic disappeared"), visual (the "Ballet of Terror" posters), and physical (*escraches*) means for articulating a claim to rights and advancing a progressive political agenda.

Bailarines Organizados' memory entrepreneurship, in the form of the "Ballet of Terror" posters and San Martín Theater *escraches*, continues a tradition in which the deployment of the past is always already a politicized struggle for social recognition and political legitimacy in the present. By engaging in memory entrepreneurship, Bailarines Organizados not only contextualized their struggle within broader histories of injustice and connected their movement to prevailing legacies of activism, but also symbolically recuperated the historical link between economic and political disappearance. The group moved otherwise to the individualism that characterized their experiences of dance practice and production, as well as broader social structures. Contextualized by the post-2001 climate, the Bailarines Organizados movement embodied the fight for danced labor rights and placed demands on the responsibilities of a democratic state to its employees and citizens by making present the recent dictatorial past.

In the wake of Bailarines Organizados' efforts to call attention to precarious labor, the San Martín Theater granted dancers contracts that included health plans and pensions by city government order. None of the dancers fired in the midst of the labor dispute, however, were offered new contracts.[44] When I asked Wainrot if he might comment on the nature and outcome of the labor dispute during our 2011 interview, he declined.[45] As a new generation of Ballet Contemporáneo members rehearsed and performed as recognized city workers, the leaders of Bailarines Organizados carried on the legacy of their labor movement through their artistic work with the CNDC. With its inception, the company aimed to translate Bailarines Organizados' collective political action into a long-term creative project. In the following section, I narrate the company's formation and analyze Daniel Payero Zaragoza's 2010 *Retazos pequeños de nuestra historia más reciente*, one of the company's early works based on the last military dictatorship. Payero Zaragoza's work exemplifies how the company created a platform for choreographic work invested in exploring past and present social injustices. Then I consider the company's ongoing work to find an artistic and administrative structure that both supports the horizontal values that drove the group's foundation and functions within a vertical state structure.

THE COOPERATIVE COMPANY: LA COMPAÑÍA NACIONAL DE DANZA CONTEMPORÁNEA AND *RETAZOS PEQUEÑOS DE NUESTRA HISTORIA MÁS RECIENTE* (2010)

Nuevos Rumbos, a cooperatively managed independent dance company that engaged social justice issues, grew out of the energy that animated the Bailarines Organizados labor movement. During its brief period of activity, the company's repertoire extended the group's memory entrepreneurship onto the concert stage through an emphasis on the last military dictatorship.[46] In 2009, riding the wave of publicity gained from Bailarines Organizados actions, the Secretary of Culture reincorporated the company as the Compañía Nacional de Danza Contemporánea, making it the second "official" contemporary dance company in Argentina.[47] While CNDC dancers are eligible for the same benefits as other federal employees, the company continued to fight for an adjusted retirement age that realistically reflects the length of a professional performing career.[48] While the CNDC is based in Buenos Aires, the Ministry of Culture also facilitates company tours and workshops throughout Argentina's provinces. Though it has shifted management structure over the years, the company initially was run as a collective with members sharing artistic and administrative duties. Like Nuevos Rumbos, the CNDC's early repertory in particular emphasized social justice and human rights issues.[49]

The relatively rapid federal support granted to dancers that had been displaced by a municipal theater echoed the escalating conflict between the city government's socially and economically conservative head, businessman Mauricio Macri (2007–15, elected president in 2015), and President Cristina Fernández de Kirchner's federal government. Bailarines Organizados' labor struggle and the CNDC's investment in dictatorship-themed choreographies echoed the federal government's anti-neoliberal (and anti-city government) rhetoric as well as its official memory politics. Furthermore, it is likely that the residual cultural capital attached to these dancers vis-à-vis the prestige of the San Martín Theater helped secure them federal support while the vast majority of contemporary dancers in Buenos Aires continue to labor unevenly on a grant-by-grant basis, without the formal structure for receiving worker benefits or regular access to performance spaces that CNDC dancers enjoy.

While the ex-Ballet Contemporáneo dancers formed the original company, they soon held auditions for new dancers interested in building the CNDC's vision for a professional dance group committed to cooperative politics and politically engaged artistic work. Daniel Payero Zaragoza, a dancer and choreographer from the northeastern province of Santa Fe, was one of the first new members to join Nuevos Rumbos and stay on once it became the CNDC.[50] He trained at the San Martín Theater's Taller de Danza Contemporánea (Contemporary Dance Workshop) and danced with the Ballet Contemporáneo before joining the CNDC in solidarity with the group's mission. In our conversation, Payero Zaragoza explained that his work *Retazos pequeños* (and his broader interest in joining the CNDC) arose from his desire to explore how choreographed movement might intervene in the frenzy of everyday life and create possibilities for reflecting on the politics of the past as well as the present.[51] Though the work's primary referent is the last military dictatorship, Payero Zaragoza revealed that the titular qualifier "of our most recent history" reflects the last military dictatorship's place in a longer continuum of state violence in Argentina as well as his desire to transmit Argentine cultural memory through contemporary dance.[52] *Retazos pequeños* exemplifies how the CNDC fostered artistic work that extended Bailarines Organizados' danced memory entrepreneurship as post-2001 labor activism onto the concert stage.

Retazos pequeños is an evening-length piece for ten dancers (five men and five women). The work premiered in November 2010 at the Cervantes National Theater, a frequent venue for CNDC performances. I had the opportunity to view the work live during this initial run. The technically demanding movement vocabulary maintains clear markings of Payero Zaragoza's—and his fellow company members'—training. The musical score includes a medley of songs that draw on *chamamé*, a folkloric music genre from northeastern Argentina. To locate the historical context of the last military dictatorship, the piece draws heavily on the archive of authoritarianism. Citing Argentine and European histories of terror, the work directly references Argentine dictatorship-era speeches and announcements, the Madres de Plaza de Mayo, and the German Third Reich. The choreography does not attempt a literal or narrative interpretation of these citations, but rather dialogues with and comments on them as archival references.[53] The work is layered and nuanced, and deserving of extended analysis; however, in this discussion I would like to highlight selections that emphasize how it mobilizes memory on the post-2001 concert stage.[54]

Retazos pequeños begins as a solo female dancer carefully steps over a series of overturned chairs scattered about the stage. As the Cervantes's ornate curtain lowers, she moves onto the thin strip of stage space that remains. Her movements are soft, fluid, and deliberate. Moving within the constraints of a narrow space, she rolls across the stage, pausing occasionally on her back or seat, glancing into the space around her. Eventually her body finds stillness, and she begins to call out names. A glance at the program reveals that these are the names of her co-performers. This opening invokes the practice of naming as an act of presenting those no longer physically here—activist groups frequently recite the names of *desaparecidos* during gatherings. This inaugural spoken gesture signals an act of solidarity with the victims of state violence. It also marks an effort to inscribe the dancers' names, and by extension personal histories of exclusion, into a broader legacy of memory and activism. The gesture recalls the "Ballet of Terror" poster as it again draws together the experiences of economic and political disappearance. *Retazos pequeños*, however, also keeps the distances between these experiences in close view. While the named dancers are alive, well, and about to take the stage, the remainder of the piece explores the violence inflicted on political prisoners and the presence of their absence.

One episode in particular theorizes how dancing bodies might call attention to the absences that the state's violent actions and discourses created (video clip 5.1 ▶). The audio score plays fragments of Videla's statements on human rights and disappeared persons in response to a journalist's question during a 1979 press conference:

> In a Christian vision of human rights, life is fundamental, freedom is important, as is work, family, home, etc., etc. Argentina attends to human rights in this comprehensive manner. I speak concretely because I know your question refers not to this comprehensive vision of human rights, but specifically to the man who is detained without process, that is one case, or the disappeared person, which is another. In the case of a disappeared person, it is an unknown. If the person appears, OK, he or she will have X treatment, and if the disappearance becomes proof of the person's death, then the person will have Z treatment. But while the person is disappeared—no, no, no—he or she cannot have any special treatment, the person is an unknown, disappeared, without entity, not here, not alive nor dead, disappeared.[55]

As the recording plays, the five female dancers and one male dancer take the stage. Forming pairs, they gently embrace. One dancer in each pair initiates a movement series as his or her partner repeats the movement with a brief delay. The movements are rounded and soft, characterized by sweeping limbs, circular arms, and spinal curves. The initial shadowing gives way to tender weight sharing and partnered lifts as the audio recording repeats and overlaps the phrase "the person is an unknown, disappeared, without entity, not here, not dead nor alive, disappeared" (figure 5.3). The repetition of the movements counters the repetition of Videla's phrase, offering bodies where he insists there are none, and presence where his words negate the reality of state violence and government culpability. *Retazos pequeños*'s choreographies of gentle bodily care, juxtaposed with Videla's violent rhetorical and physical disappearance of bodies, move otherwise as they resist violence's divisive effects. As an act of memory and continued protest, movement as care and connection contravenes Videla's words.

Following the choreography set to Videla's statement, the sound score once again drives *Retazos pequeños*'s action, this time as it summons the Madres de Plaza de Mayo. The female dancers recite fragments from television coverage of one of the group's demonstrations in 1978. This footage has particular significance. Shot by international newscasters who were in Argentina to cover the World Cup, it helped draw international attention to the Madres' cause:

> They won't tell us if they are alive, if they are dead. Why don't they tell us? If we are looking for this, nothing more. That they answer us, nothing more./ [The government] lies. It lies!/My daughter was five months pregnant when they took her. My grandson must have been born in August of last year. I still don't know anything about him./We only want to know where our children are, whether dead or alive. We are anguished, because we don't know if they are sick,

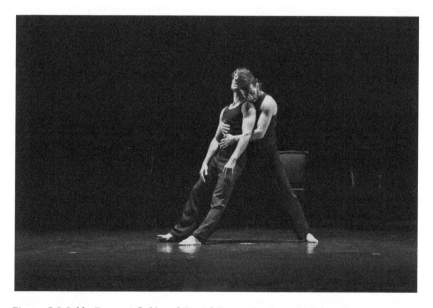

Figure 5.3 Pablo Fermani (left) and Daniel Payero Zaragoza (right) in *Retazos pequeños de nuestra historia más reciente*, 2010. Photograph: Alejandra Viviana Aranda. Courtesy of photographer.

cold, hungry, we don't know anything. And we are desperate, sir, because we don't know who to appeal to.[56]

The women sit down on chairs arranged in a line upstage as the male dancer steps into a pool of light. As the women's shouts fade, a violin sounds as he slowly raises his arms until outstretched at his sides, horizontal with the floor. The dancer executes a lower body-based choreography composed of runs in deep plié and small leaps. He maintains extended arms as the audio score shifts to the sound of lapping waves and a humming engine (video clip 5.2 ⓹). Referencing the military practice of tossing drugged but living bodies from planes into the Río de la Plata bordering Buenos Aires, the dancer's outstretched arms poignantly suggest the plane's wings. When I first saw the piece live, this moment stole my breath. The juxtaposition between the tenderness of the dancer's movement quality and subtle choreographic invocations of one of the dictatorship's most infamously brutal practices exemplified how dance can remember violence gently, in a way that sparks the hope of redress.

As the male soloist exits, the female dancers arrange the chairs in a semicircle. Moving now to the original recording of the Madres' words, which like Videla's speech is arranged so particular phrases repeat and overlap, the dancers stomp feet, raise fists, and fall to the ground—evoking the Madres' decades-long struggle for and dedication to the slow process of juridical reclamation. In citing the Madres, who according to Jelin are the inaugural generation of memory entrepreneurs, *Retazos pequeños* dialogues with politicized memory practice and inscribes the piece into a tradition of living with and critically engaging the past as a call for change in the present. The fragile, childlike quality of the dancer's outstretched arms as a citation of the death flights interpolates spectators into the Madres' refrain that their disappeared children are indeed all of "our" children. The physical evocation of the Madres' struggle, captured by the women's labored movements, choreographically memorializes and transmits their activist legacy through a new generation of bodies—a generation who put their bodies in the street to fight for their rights as cultural workers. As it honors the Madres, *Retazos pequeños* links the traumatic past with its continued traces in the present.

Because Payero Zaragoza joined the CNDC and choreographed *Retazos pequeños* on the heels of Bailarines Organizados' labor movement, his work is in part a testament to the translation of the movement's spirit into socially engaged choreographic work. However, as the dust of the labor movement settled and the CNDC began to grow in size and audience, the group was faced with the complex task of developing a sustainable, cooperative artistic and administrative structure that functioned within the Ministry of Culture's vertical bureaucracy. This ongoing work is the subject of Julia Martinez Heimann and Konstantina Bousmpoura's elegant documentary, *Trabajadores de la danza* (*Working Dancers*, 2017).[57] In the documentary, founding members Chacón

Oribe, Victoria Hidalgo, Pablo Fermani, and Quintá describe the process of learning how to occupy leadership roles that departed significantly from their experiences as Ballet Contemporáneo dancers, including running the company and determining formats for group decision-making. While Chacón Oribe, Quintá, and Hidalgo co-directed the company for several years following its establishment, in 2013 company members voted to employ an external artistic director to help relieve administrative demands. At the same time that the CNDC made the choice to name a director, they also re-committed to maintaining what Chacón Oribe characterizes as a "group consciousness."[58] Company meetings, which include dancers as well as technical crew and union representatives, became the primary sites for collectively discussing and voting on pressing issues. The documentary features multiple meetings in which the dancers confront the limits, possibilities, and contradictions of cooperative labor within a state-funded dance company: What is the role of the individual in the collective? Are efficiency and collective deliberation irreconcilable? Can a company that values a high level of technical rigor also respect the unique physical needs and artistic interests of its members? Is horizontality fundamentally incompatible with the verticality of state bureaucracy?[59]

While the challenges—and privileges—the CNDC experiences are in some ways unique to the organization's state-funded structure, the questions they confront are also broadly resonant with the tensions inherent to cooperative initiatives. However, as the company continues to grow and shift—as of this writing under Macri's conservative, neoliberal federal government that does not include memory politics or a robust cultural politics within its purview—their commitment to "group consciousness" and choreographic investments in charting historical patterns of injustice (like *Retazos pequeños*) remains more important than ever, even if their management structure now resembles that of a traditional company. Their commitment to a cooperative model—and willingness to adapt and change its form as new generations of dancers join the company—testifies to the long-term efficacy and influence of post-2001 mobilization. Additionally, the company has lent their support to other Argentine dance labor movements, including the Ley Nacional de Danza (National Dance Law) considered in the introduction, as well as to protests against the government's elimination of the Ballet Nacional Danza (Dance National Ballet 2013–17), which aimed to make classical ballet accessible to a broad public.

Ultimately, Bailarines Organizados' labor movement and the CNDC's creative work manifest both the historical connections and precarious corporeal conditions that tie neoliberalism and the last military dictatorship. Through an embrace of cooperative politics, both moved otherwise to social, political, and artistic logics and practices predicated on worker dispensability and individualist ethics. At the same time, Bailarines Organizados' ultimate appeal to a liberal conception of worker rights and the CNDC's ongoing attempts to nest a horizontal structure within a vertical one (the state) evidence how ideas like horizontality and self-management interact with—and sometimes revert to—dominant social and political structures. I now turn to Bailarines Toda la Vida, a community dance collective equally invested in recuperating the link between economic and political disappearance through cooperative labor on and off the concert stage. Like the CNDC, Bailarines Toda la Vida is connected to a labor movement, albeit one not directly related to dance. While the federally supported CNDC created the artistic infrastructure for extending Bailarines Organizados' movement onto the concert stage, as an independent community dance project, Bailarines Toda la Vida sustained itself through a symbiotic relationship with the worker-run Grissinopoli factory. Unlike the CNDC, however, Bailarines Toda la Vida de-emphasizes physical virtuosity and envisions inclusivity as central to its cooperative ethics. In the next section, I demonstrate how the group's movement methodology developed in tandem with that of the factory's cooperative labor initiative, negotiating horizontal artistic and pedagogical relationships by extending creative agency, quite literally, to all bodies.[60]

NEW HOPE AT THE FACTORY: BAILARINES TODA LA VIDA AND THE RECUPERATION OF MOVEMENT'S GRACE

I first saw Bailarines Toda la Vida perform in November 2010 in the Our Children Cultural Space (Espacio Cultural Nuestros Hijos, ECuNHi) located in the former Navy Petty-Officers School of Mechanics (Escuela de Suboficiales de Mecánica de la Armada, ESMA) detention center. In this haunting space, surrounded by buildings in which *desaparecidos* sustained brutal physical and psychological torture during the last military dictatorship, I watched the group's director Aurelia Chillemi take the stage. In her quiet and steady voice, she explained the community nature of the dance project and its genesis alongside the Grissinopoli factory's La Nueva Esperanza labor cooperative. Bailarines Toda la Vida, she emphasized, is open to all participants regardless of dance background and physical ability, and collective creation generates embodied dialogue around labor rights, human rights, and possibilities for intimacy and connection in contemporary urban life.[61] The project was founded in 2002 when Chillemi, a dance professor at the National Arts University and psychotherapist, responded to the institution's call for community extension projects.[62] With funding in place, a colleague recommended that she consider joining the cultural programming at Grissinopoli, where the group rehearsed until early 2018. While community theater has a rich history in Argentina, Bailarines Toda la Vida was one of the first dance groups of its kind in the country and inspired a number of projects nationally.[63]

Despite the setting, neither work presented that November evening spe-cifically treated dictatorship themes. However, Chillemi's description of *La ruptura* (*The Rupture*, 2005) during her introduction piqued my interest. The work explores social conflicts, particularly the mechanization of bodies within everyday urban life. The dance, she stated, proposes a basis for breaking away from this "alienating system."[64] The choreography moved between renderings of struggling, labored bodies and abstract sections based on physical contact between dancers.[65] During this first encounter, I admittedly paid less atten-tion to whether the choreography achieved what Chillemi described in her introduction. I found myself more interested in the diversity of bodies moving on stage (age, ability, physical appearance) and the palpable sense of invest-ment that united them. Both made for startlingly compelling viewing. As a community group, Bailarines Toda la Vida emphasizes process over product. However, the apparent integrity of their process, palpable in the moment of performance, seemed to unsettle the unspoken (and at times spoken) as-sumption that community work is not as interesting to watch as professional work, or that the performance of community work is incidental to the process. My own spectatorial experience, and the testimonies of the many spectators I would come to meet, suggested otherwise.

Upon my return to Buenos Aires in February 2011, I eagerly took up the invitation Chillemi extended to audience members on that November eve-ning to attend the company's weekly rehearsals at Grissinopoli—those first three hours turned into nearly a year as a member of the collective. Every Friday evening when I arrived for rehearsal at the small factory, I squeezed through the gate that opens into the first-floor production area (figure 5.4). Just inside, a "National Movement of Worker Recuperated Factories" poster immediately announced the success of Grissinopoli's cooperative labor model. The late Norma Pintos, a member of La Nueva Esperanza who acted for many years as the dance collective's liaison, would greet me from the small front office. Norma remained at the factory for the duration of the three-hour rehearsals—long after the other workers had gone home—to lock up once practice was complete.

The life of the factory permeated the weekly rehearsal experience. Upon ar-rival, dancers met the presence or absence of the heat of the ovens with joy or dismay depending on the season, chatted with the bakers, worked with them to locate the brooms necessary for cleaning the dance space, and sampled from the open sacks full of broken, discarded breadsticks. Bailarines Toda la Vida shared the third-floor space with the factory's storage area; the costume collection and a small seating area brushed up against pieces of machinery and dusty stockpiles of shipping boxes. During my time with the group, between fifteen and twenty-five participants were present on a weekly basis for re-hearsal, though collective members (past and present) total in the hundreds.[66] Labor at Grissinopoli, from the machinations of industrial food production to

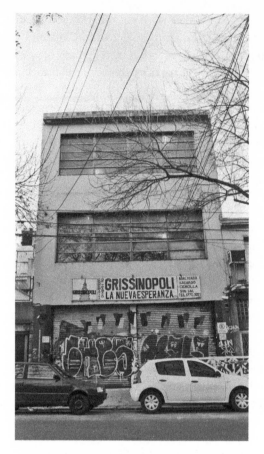

Figure 5.4 The Grissinopoli factory viewed from the front, 2016. Photograph by author.

the preparation of space for creative practice, blurred traditional boundaries between industry and art.

Bailarines Toda la Vida's unification of dance and factory labor recalls the efforts of US modern dancers in the 1930s to engage workers in "mass dance" that dealt with labor rights issues and sought to make of dance a "weapon in the class struggle" during the Depression years, a project itself inspired by worker's theater in Germany and Russia.[67] While distant temporally and geographically, Bailarines Toda la Vida shares their interest in embodying political consciousness through dances whose movement vocabularies and themes are broadly accessible and legible. The unification of creative and manual labor also resonates with more recent local projects. As considered in chapter 2, the late 1960s and early 1970s saw the development of an artistic vanguard that held at its core a commitment to working-class revolution. Recall also that Ana Kamien's 1970 *Ana Kamien*, discussed in chapter 1, asserted dance as a form of valuable cultural labor in the midst of an increasingly volatile political climate, decades before Bailarines Organizados launched their movement.

At the same time that Bailarines Toda la Vida echoes these historical precedents, their installation in a worker-run factory/cultural center was a decidedly post-2001 Argentine phenomenon. Following the 2001 crisis, artists' presence in worker-run factories such as Grissinopoli served a critical space-keeping function. As police and previous owners attempted to intervene in transitions to worker management, artists mobilized networks of support and attracted media attention. Prominent cultural theorist Beatriz Sarlo describes the worker-run factory/cultural center phenomenon:

> The factory-cultural center is fundamentally a concept: where there is production, the workers take charge according to cooperative ideals based on a model as horizontal as the work process permits. Added to this labor reorganization initiative . . . is the idea of an alliance between the cultural and the productive that forms part of the socialist or libertarian imagination. The factory does not become a cultural center because the industrial building offers an attractive setting for artistic activities, but rather because intellectual and manual labor, separated by the capitalist mode of production, encounter new combined modalities in this urban island. As if it were possible to revitalize the figure of the worker who grasps the artist's hand, which seemed to break down various times in the twentieth century, beginning with the misfortunes of the Russian Revolution.[68]

Following her apt description of the worker-run factory/cultural center concept, Sarlo's closing commentary links the phenomenon to an outdated socialism—at the same time that it questions whether such a union between worker and artist is, in fact, tenable. (Ghosting behind her discussion is perhaps agitprop art that has presumably forsaken aesthetic rigor for a political agenda.) She goes on to suggest that the majority of workers who aligned themselves with bourgeois political/cultural movements post-crisis were those too old to be viable in the labor market. For Sarlo, the "cultural factory" represents a "reconciled moment of the relationship between the working and middle classes in a time when culturalization is the trend and the style." [69] She argues that the "cultural factory" needs to be read as part of a broader post-crisis marketing of Buenos Aires to tourists as a "cultural city," an important point that demonstrates how cooperative initiatives, particularly creative ones, can in fact articulate with market forces.[70] Her concerns echo broader skepticism, in colloquial as well as academic contexts, around the long-term efficiency or sustainability of post-crisis political strategies.[71]

Bailarines Toda la Vida, however, was not initially designed with Grissinopoli (or even labor rights issues) in mind. Instead, once located there, the community dance project developed in tandem with the factory's principles of cooperative labor. This process—one of the longest lasting worker-run factory/artistic partnerships—not only challenged Sarlo's skepticism but also exceeded "culturalization" as a market trend. Furthermore, as a member of the collective, I witnessed class (not to mention, age, gender, sexuality, national, and ethnic) diversity in the dance collective as well as among the factory workers that Sarlo's assessment forecloses.[72] Bailarines Toda la Vida is more productively understood through Marcela Fuentes's invitation to reconsider the idea of political "returns" in the wake of collective forms of protest and art making in post-crisis Argentina. In response to both sociological research that measures the success of social movements in structural change and speculative finance's emphasis on "investments toward returns," Fuentes argues that, "symbolic practices enable us to explore the new political subjectivities and modes of action at work within market conditions."[73]

At Grissinopoli, the alliance between the cultural and productive was not limited to space sharing and themes in the group's works.[74] Bailarines Toda la Vida reciprocated monetarily to the factory, paying La Nueva Esperanza members for time spent keeping the factory open during rehearsals and sharing funds earned from paid performances and the weekly contributions of participants to an oversized *mamadera* (a baby bottle used to collect contributions). Though anyone is free to participate at no charge, those who can afford to do so are asked to contribute weekly. During my time with the group, dancers were asked to contribute extra money to help fund factory repairs required by a recent inspection, and we scheduled a series of performances to support this cause. In addition to monetary support, Bailarines Toda la Vida hosted regular *peñas*, or gatherings with music and dance, where dancers and workers had opportunities to mingle in a relaxed social environment.[75] By fostering a symbiotic relationship between cultural and manual labor under the same roof of this small factory, cooperative management and artistic models—both difficult to sustain long term—became tenable.

Ultimately, it was the group's commitment to supporting Grissinopoli's ongoing survival that prompted Chillemi to move rehearsals to the Mutual Sentimiento's Sexto Kultural (itself a cooperative initiative also located in the factory's Chacarita neighborhood) in March 2018.[76] Under successive conservative city governments, the Grissinopoli factory had become the target of increased inspections. When inspectors took issue with Bailarines' use of the factory for rehearsals, Chillemi determined that relocating was the best way to ensure the factory would not be closed down. Though weekly rehearsals moved, Chillemi kept her university courses related to the project at the factory, emphasizing the centrality of the space to the group's history, political alignments, and creative practice.[77]

Cooperative labor shapes Bailarines Toda la Vida on artistic as well as logistical levels. Each rehearsal begins with a warm-up followed by structured improvisation based on *expresión corporal* (corporal expression) principles.

Developed by Argentine dancer Patricia Stokoe in the 1950s, *expresión corporal* aims to access the body's "inner" movement creativity through improvisation, freeing it from the confines of codified techniques.[78] Chapter 3 demonstrated how during the last military dictatorship, the practice of *expresión corporal* functioned, in part, as a response to the physical censure of bodies occurring in everyday life. Following the 2001 crisis, Bailarines Toda la Vida adapted *expresión corporal* as a way of moving otherwise to economic disappearance. Maintaining Stokoe's core objective—to put "dance within everyone's reach"—Chillemi's pedagogical emphasis is twofold.[79] First, classes focus on improvisations that not only invite an individualized exploration of the body's movement, but also foster group dynamics. Secondly, Chillemi designs improvisation exercises with the aim of addressing social and political themes vis-à-vis movement. Movements generated through group improvisations then form the basis for dance works, and the final portion of weekly rehearsals is dedicated to either choreography development or readying existing repertory for upcoming performances.

This improvisatory movement process is the cornerstone of Bailarines Toda la Vida's work in response to, as Silvia Buschiazzo puts it in her writing on the group, "the necessity to recompose a social network fragmented by a political-social system that did not attend to the needs of the community."[80] In a conference paper, Chillemi theorizes how movement circulates during group improvisations, recomposing the networks fractured by neoliberal disjunction. Referring specifically to her frequent prompt for dancers to experiment with "mirroring," or taking on movement generated by other dancers in a given improvisation, she writes:

> As movement circulates, when someone is capable of recuperating the movement's grace, they are able to share it, transmitting and retransmitting it as in the structure of a rhizome . . . . Taking on borrowed movement in group improvisation allows for the construction of another movement language that enriches one's own, offering new subtleties. This movement that circulates is a common good that sustains the individual and supports the group identity. Every group improvisation is a common good . . . it is not necessary to sign contracts or agreements, but simply to be present, with the tactic accord of solidarity in shared doing.[81]

Enacting cooperative labor through the creative process, Chillemi's notion that the movement generated through group improvisations is a "common good" challenges the single-authorship choreography model fundamental to concert dance's survival in a capitalist market. Dance, here, is not a commodity but rather a practice and artistic product that are both common goods.

I argue that shared movement not only constitutes a certain identity, as Chillemi signals, but also opens the body to new modes of sociality beyond neoliberalism's—and professional dance's—emphasis on individual achievement and ownership. Movement as a common good establishes the kinesthetic conditions of possibility for connections to other bodies and experiences vis-à-vis the social and political issues addressed in improvisation prompts. Chillemi's notion of "recuperating movement's grace" that attends dance as a "common good" articulates with movement theorist Erin Manning's concept of relational movement. Echoing Chillemi's conception of how movement-as-grace connects bodies, Manning asserts that the "essence of relational movement is the creation of a virtual node, an in-between that propels the dance, that in-forms the grace that is not strictly of the body but of the movement itself."[82] Reading Chillemi through Manning, movement's grace—and the act of recuperating it—is the ability to cooperatively generate an impulse that spills into a movement or movements that, circulating through bodies yet autonomous from them, become the basis for connection to other bodies present—and past. Recuperating movement's grace in the recuperated factory generated powerful ways of relating through shared doing.

Chillemi and Manning's concept of relational movement's grace becomes evident not only through group improvisations when the "virtual node" emerges among bodies, but also when, solidified into choreography, movement's grace enters the repertoire. During my time dancing with Bailarines Toda la Vida, the group researched and developed a new work titled . . . *Y el mar* (. . . *And the Sea*). The piece is dedicated to family members of *desaparecidos*, and drew inspiration from the life and death of Azucena Villaflor, a founder of the Madres de Plaza de Mayo in search of her son, who was disappeared herself in December 1977. A victim of the dictatorship's death-flight method of disposing bodies—which is so poignantly rendered in Payero Zaragoza's *Retazos pequeños*—Villaflor's remains washed up on the beaches of Santa Teresita in the Buenos Aires province the same month as her disappearance. Her remains were identified via forensic analysis in 2005. As we worked on the piece in May 2011, several former military officials were arrested in conjunction with her disappearance and death as part of the ongoing trials the Kirchner administration had reopened.[83] Inspired by Villaflor's memory, improvisations for the work centered on the traces (both physical and affective) left by *desaparecidos*, the violent yet tender movements of the sea, the act of witness, and persistence over time.

Asked to work in pairs on the idea of the trace, my partner and I found our virtual node, or our "in-between that propels the dance."[84] During my early rehearsals with Bailarines Toda la Vida, I often struggled with the openness characteristic of and required by Chillemi's *expresión corporal*-based method. Muddling through the baggage of my structured technical training in modern dance, I initially feared the cue to wordlessly locate a partner. Intent to corporeally listen and respond to his or her body, I would become frustrated by my own subsequent attempts to escape the grasp of "technique," and the defined repertoire of movements it implied, over my body. The trace improvisation, however, marked my first encounter with the graceful common good that is in-formed (to recall Manning's construction) movement.

That day, we began our practice following a group discussion of a moving interview with Villaflor's daughter published around the March 2011 anniversary of the coup that began the last military dictatorship. My partner and I first began working with the lower body, experimenting with how far we could stretch our legs forward before losing balance. Coordinating our bodies required a shared physical investment in playing with the paradox of wanting to remain and advance at the same time. Our agreement was not determined verbally, but rather felt out through attention to the pace and suspension of the other's movements. The pull of the leg extending before us eventually morphed, releasing into a deep lunge—our extended supporting legs still firmly rooted in place. Kinesthetically agreeing it was time, we slowly shifted forward, dragging our extended legs to bring our feet together, slowly rolling up the spine. With repetition, the initiation of our slow, sustained sequence took on a faint militarized quality. Oppositional legs and arms formed right angles before stretching and pulling forward into the lunge and beginning the sequence once more.

As Chillemi arranged the choreography from the movement generated by participants during improvisations, my partner and I were asked to teach our sequence to a group of dancers. Though my partner stopped coming to rehearsals soon after the staging process began, I performed the movement sequence with the group for the remainder of my time with the collective.[85] During one of my final rehearsals with the group before leaving for the United States, I taught the sequence and narrated the history of its relational genesis to a dancer who would take my place in upcoming performances. Watching the piece for the first time as a spectator, I experienced not only a mournful release of the movement but also joy as I watched the steps literally "put" another body into a painful, yet hope-filled, reflection on what it means to remember that which can never be whole. In that moment, I experienced movement as a common good not only in the sense of cooperative creation, but also in the sense of its graceful circulation between bodies over time. A movement born of an in-formed improvisation, the repeated phrase was now a corporeal chronotope in Judith Hamera's sense, or a codified movement that holds bodies in a "both-and relationship to here and now, there and then," activating both the historical memory that the movement strove to connect with as well as the steps of dancers (recently) past.[86] Just several months after I returned to the United States, Bailarines Toda la Vida shot a video dance of . . . Y el mar on the beaches of Santa Teresita, where Villaflor's body surfaced over forty years ago, with the official support of the Abuelas de Plaza de Mayo (video clip 5.3 ⓑ).[87]

While Bailarines Toda la Vida's collaborative creation method evidences how their creative practice complemented the work of the La Nueva Esperanza labor cooperative and articulated with the broader post-2001 context, their repertory also offers a site for reading how they, like the CNDC, connect histories of economic disappearance to political disappearance. In the following, I offer analysis of the stage (2006) and video dance (2009) versions of *La oscuridad* (*The Darkness*). Dedicated to those disappeared during the last military dictatorship, this long-standing piece in the group's repertory exemplifies how Bailarines Toda la Vida moves otherwise in performance.[88]

BREADSTICKS AND MEMORIES: *LA OSCURIDAD* (2006)

In addition to weekly rehearsals, Bailarines Toda la Vida maintains a lively performing schedule throughout the capital and Buenos Aires province, appearing in independent theaters, cultural centers, schools, and open-air spaces at cultural and political events. During my time with the group, we performed . . . *Y el mar* and other works at the Carlos Gardel Cultural Center in Grissinopoli's neighborhood, the Jorge Donn Dance School No. 2 (a public secondary school and site of Alicia Muñoz's tactical negotiations of the dictatorship climate recounted in chapter 3), and the Argentine Metalwork and Plastics Industries (Industrias Metalúrgicas y Plásticas Argentina, IMPA), another worker-run factory/cultural center. We also performed in La Plata's Plaza Italia to commemorate the 2006 redisappearance of Jorge Julio López (initially detained during the last military dictatorship) when he was serving as a key witness in the trial against former police officer Miguel Etchecolatz. López's disappearance has yet to be accounted for despite extensive activist actions—a chilling reminder of the persistence of the authoritarian past.

La oscuridad is the group's most regularly performed piece borne of their cooperative creation method.[89] As was the case for Bailarines Organizados and the CNDC, Bailarines Toda la Vida's emphasis on memory of the last military dictatorship signals membership within a broader activist and artistic field that links memory politics with progressive politics. Where Bailarines Organizados/CNDC acted as memory entrepreneurs, strategically deploying dictatorship symbols and activist tactics (like *escraches*) to help secure a specific set of labor rights, Bailarines Toda la Vida's creative focus on histories of political violence invites its long-term and transitory members alike to choreographically integrate their bodies into the ongoing history of moving otherwise that their repertoire, and the group's time in the Grissinopoli factory, represent. A twelve-minute work, *La oscuridad* weaves fragmentary

movement explorations of authoritarian violence with possibilities for physical connection and care. Group improvisations began with ideas around
power, persecution, order, fear, loss, and clashing ideologies. As improvised
movement crystallized into set choreography, it generated narratives with
more specific reference to the dictatorship. They include scenarios around the
dynamics of 1970s leftist militant organizations and different experiences of
the regime, such as persecution, support of the military, and blindness or in-
difference to violence. Circulating during rehearsals as cue shorthand, these
narratives are used to introduce the movement to new participants. Thus,
newer collective members learn the dance with these established narratives;
however, the stories passed down by group pedagogy often draw attention to
the kinesthetic marks left by former dancers on both the narratives and the
movement itself. These traces—like the ones I transmitted through . . . Y el
mar—emphasize the piece as living and continually evolving, reflecting the
composition of the group itself.

In 2009, Bailarines Toda la Vida collaborated with videographer Adolfo
Cabanchik (who also directed . . . Y el mar) on a video dance of La oscuridad
set in the factory with La Nueva Esperanza workers, featuring the piece's
original choreography alongside the choreography of breadstick making
(video clip 5.4 ⏵).[90] My analysis of La oscuridad here is based primarily on
the video dance; however, I mark the points where it departs from the stage
version, which I performed on numerous occasions during my time with the
group. Perhaps more so than any other Bailarines Toda la Vida work, the La
oscuridad video dance visually and choreographically connects histories of political and economic disappearance. The film has been shown in a variety of
venues throughout Buenos Aires and its success in fact inspired the . . . Y el
mar video dance.

The La oscuridad video dance opens with a scene of labor (figure 5.5). It
features the workers on the second floor of the factory (both the first and
second floors of the factory are production areas), removing freshly baked
breadsticks from the conveyor belts and packing them in cardboard boxes. The
dancers, costumed in the royal blue skirts or pants and tops also used for live
performances of the piece, stand gathered close together beside the bakers. In
stillness, they closely watch the workers' motions with keen absorption and
focus. The scene changes, and the dancers are lined up among the workers
along the conveyor belts. The collective members perform the workers' choreography of scooping, straightening, and removing the breadsticks from
the belt, embodying their movements without physically touching the
breadsticks.[91]

As resident musician Osvaldo Aguilar's drum-based score begins to play,
the scene cuts to the dancers performing the original La oscuridad choreography in the otherwise empty second-floor production space. Transporting
the viewer temporally to the trauma of dictatorship violence, three groups

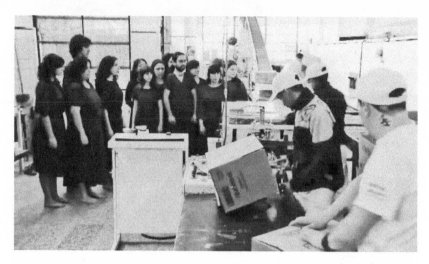

Figure 5.5 Bailarines Toda la Vida in the video dance *La oscuridad*, 2009. Courtesy of Adolfo Cabanchik.

perform movements that correspond to different experiences of dictator-ship violence. "Repressors" point and strike the air while the "persecuted"—yet resistant—dancers protect themselves and stand their ground. A third group—attempting to block out the struggle happening around them—embody the impulse to disconnect, covering their faces with their hands and skipping through the space.[92]

Following a musical interlude, the Grissinopoli workers re-enter the second-floor space, followed by the dancers. Once more lining up along the conveyor belts, the dancers slowly bend their torsos toward and away from the belts in slow and mournful movement, with several performers re-citing the labor movements of scooping, straightening, and removing the breadsticks from the belt. The video dance then cuts to Bailarines Toda la Vida's third-floor re-hearsal space, where the dancers enact *La oscuridad*'s only unison sequence. In this segment, the dancers stand tightly clumped together in wide stances with legs bent in plié. Raising one fist and leg at a time, the dancers stomp their feet to the floor, bending their elbows and clasping their fists as if pulling down on a heavy lever. As they stomp and pull, the dancers call out "ha!" to punctuate their effort. Inspired by the 1970s political movements that fought for a dif-ferent socioeconomic order than the one that contextualized the group's foun-dation, dancers call the sequence *la montonera*, a reference to female members of one of the most visible leftist militant groups during the late 1960s and early 1970s, the Montoneros. *La montonera* transitions into an episode that invokes the terror of persecution. In the stage version of the piece, dancers run from one set of wings to the other, crossing only when they make eye contact with a dancer on the other side willing to receive them. In the video dance, however, the performers run chaotically through the machinery in the darkened second floor. The final scene returns the viewer to the third-floor rehearsal space. *La oscuridad* ends with a choreography of embrace. First moving blindly with closed eyes throughout the space, upon encountering another body, the dancers embrace, swaying softly to the closing instrumental score.

Throughout, but particularly in the opening, the video dance stages labor as choreography and choreography as labor.[93] Or, in other words, the movement opens the possibility of the artist grasping the worker's hand, given that the roles in the scene are interchangeable. Situating the costumed bodies as engrossed spectators and even students, the opening scene asks the video viewer to consume manual labor as artistic endeavor. While the dancers' citation of the choreography of scooping, straightening, and removing the breadsticks from the belt further renders these actions "art" within the representational frame of the video dance, these embodiments do not constitute nonproductive mimetic meditations on the kinesthetic dynamics of factory work. Rather, enacted with the choreography reflecting on the last military dictatorship, these danced labor movements establish the conditions of possibility for connections to bodies now (post-2001 cooperative workers) and then (those subjected to exclusionary dictatorship violence). By layering the embodied invocation of dictatorship violence, captured in the episodes invoking persecution, terror, and political struggle, with post-2001 labor movements, the video dance manifests the elements of continuity—while marking the differences—between histories of political and economic disappearance. Furthermore, performing the piece in the factory activates another level of historical memory. Considering labor unions and factories hotbeds of "subversion," the military government specifically targeted the former and raided the latter.

The linkages that the video dance enacts also evidence the broader modes of embodied sociality that Bailarines Toda la Vida makes possible. In one sense, the group's repertory and methodology intervene in a particular post-crisis climate by connecting it to its past—that is, by recuperating the relationship between economic violence and political violence. More broadly, the collaborative practice and product of this community dance project define political possibility through the unification of creative and manual labor, engendering new steps in the choreography of labor movements. While Bailarines Toda la Vida emerged as part of a series of ad hoc practices responding to a particular historical juncture of neoliberal crisis, the practice extended beyond this moment and continues to use collaborative movement as the basis for alternative ways of relating to others in a globalized urban context. The name of the group—Dancers for Life—echoes the temporal mandate to carry on the labor of making cooperative labor possible in the face of persistent neoliberal policies and government changeovers. Doing so in fact required them to stop rehearsing at Grissinopoli in order to protect the very labor cooperative that sustained and inspired their creative practice. Carrying on, however, also takes the form of the group's ongoing transmission of the memory of Argentina's histories of political and economic violence through the mobilization of bodies in motion, in open rehearsals and on Buenos Aires's stages, to recuperate, again and again, the need for cooperative alternatives to free-market demands.

(CO)-LABORING ON

This chapter has demonstrated how Bailarines Organizados/CNDC and Bailarines Toda la Vida, post-crisis initiatives that center the memory of the last military within their cooperative practices, refigure the hold of the neoliberal market over the body in artistic as well as quotidian spaces. The Bailarines Organizados movement mobilized dictatorship memory to make claims for dancers' rights to labor rights. In the wake of the dancers' political mobilization, the initially cooperatively-run CNDC created a platform for artistic work, like Payero Zaragoza's *Retazos pequeños*, that extended the spirit of the movement onto the stage through a focus on social-justice themes. Bailarines Toda la Vida's movement methodology worked in tandem with the Grissinopoli's factory's cooperative labor initiative, as the company's repertoire interpolates its ever-fluctuating ensemble into a living history of memory and resistance through works like . . . *Y el mar* and *La oscuridad*. Both initiatives imagine new and resistive ways of making dance within neoliberal configurations while maintaining present the violence of the recent past.

In prominent geographer David Harvey's 2007 *A Brief History of Neoliberalism*, he mused, "it is unthinkable but not impossible that the US will become like Argentina in 2001 overnight."[94] In the years following the publication of his study, the cracks in neoliberal economic models in the global north continually widened, giving rise to grass-roots political mobilization across the globe. The US Occupy Wall Street and Spain-based Indignados (Indignants) movements in 2011, as well as riots in Greece in 2012, decried the austerity measures and economic inequality that accompany neoliberalism. The Argentine economic crisis is no longer a cautionary tale; rather, this chapter demonstrates how its telling might be productive and instructive as the global north and south alike grapple toward ways of moving otherwise. And in the Argentine national context, the work of the initiatives considered here have taken on new urgency amid the re-entrenchment of neoliberal approaches under the presidency of Mauricio Macri (2015–). Bailarines Organizados/CNDC and Bailarines Toda la Vida also prefigured Argentina's recent, large-scale struggle for federal dance legislation: see this book's introduction for more about the activism occurring around the proposed National Dance Law, which would provide infrastructure for supporting dance production across the country. As the struggle for dance labor rights continues, Bailarines Organizados/CNDC and Bailarines Toda la Vida offer models for understanding dance not only as a form of labor in and of itself, but also as a rich site for exploring the politics of the laboring body within broader social and political configurations.[95] Offering cooperation against social disjunction, and care and community against precarity, post-crisis contemporary dance moved and continues to move otherwise.

Epilogue

The History of Memory

As described in the preface, early inspiration for *Moving Otherwise* grew out of my experience viewing the March 24, 2006, human rights march on the thirtieth anniversary of the coup that began Argentina's last military dictatorship. On the National Day of Memory for Truth and Justice (Día Nacional de la Memoria por la Verdad y la Justicia), the demonstrators' moving mass powerfully called attention to the absence of those forcibly disappeared three decades earlier. That event prompted me to question how movement in dance studios and on stages both reflected Argentine activist histories and responded to quotidian choreographies of physical harm that accompanied periods of military dictatorship and economic crisis from the mid-1960s to the mid-2010s. The chapters of this book analyze a myriad of ways in which Buenos Aires-based contemporary dance practices "moved otherwise"—that is, how they offered alternatives to, and sometimes directly critiqued, the patterns of movement and bodily comportment that shaped everyday life in periods marked by violence. *Moving Otherwise* frequently emphasizes how their interventions fell outside of established modes of activism (like the human rights march) and political performance. As chapters 2 and 3 in particular demonstrate, it was sometimes dance's presumed apoliticism and relative marginality that actually facilitated moving otherwise in contexts of leftist political militancy and the last military dictatorship.

To conclude, however, I want to return to the impressive scale and hypervisibility of the annual human rights march and consider how dance found a role in it. In March 2006, I first glimpsed the potentialities of dance and movement to reflect on and shape politics in Argentina, but that day I happened to not be on the street where the members of Oduduwá Danza Afroamericana (Oduduwá Afro-American Dance) were preparing to lead a group of dancing volunteers as their contribution to the demonstration. Between 2005 and 2012, Oduduwá brought together hundreds of people to perform choreography that blended elements of Orishá dance vocabularies with gestural movements. Orishá dance originated in Yoruban religious practices and is practiced throughout the African diaspora (most notably in Cuba, Haiti, and Brazil). Oduduwá followed a secularized approach that invoked the symbolism of Yoruban Orishá gods while removing the steps from a religious context. In 2011, I moved from witness to participant, and danced in the march as one of Oduduwá's volunteers. Though Oduduwá ceased to organize volunteers following the dissolution of their dance company, in 2015 members once again began to organize participation in the march through a group called Colectivo Danza Afro (Afro Dance Collective).[1]

Orishá dance's Yoruban origins and linkage to the African diaspora make it an unexpected addition to a demonstration commemorating Argentina's last military dictatorship. Despite significant activist and scholarly work that aims to move toward a more complex understanding of race in Argentina, the construction of Argentina as exceptionally white and European among Latin American nations remains deeply entrenched. The year I participated, volunteers (like the company members and myself) were indeed predominately young, middle-class white women. Oduduwá, however, strove to make an embodied connection between Orishá dance's link to the violence of the trans-Atlantic slave trade and Argentina's history of political disappearance, as well as to the country's own historical erasure of black bodies and cultural influences.[2] Though contemporary dance's negotiation of racial difference has not been the central point of inquiry in this book, Oduduwá's practice nuances questions about how memories are lived and transmitted through dances, and to what ends. Locating their work alongside the practices considered in the book also contributes, if only briefly, to cross- and interdisciplinary efforts to locate Argentina "more firmly within the vibrant scholarly conversations on race and nation in the Americas and beyond."[3] As a point of conclusion for this book and a point of departure for future scholarly inquiry, the conjunction of movement, recent histories of political violence, and longer histories of global atrocity reiterates the importance of taking dance—in studios, on stages, and in streets—seriously as a political praxis and site for tracing histories of violence from national and transnational perspectives.

Oduduwá was founded in the late 1990s by women whose commitments to Orishá dance and Argentine memory movements ultimately led them to "a different way of putting the body [*poner el cuerpo*] to evoke other bodies that are no longer present and to express what the voice is often tired of yelling."[4] Oduduwá members recruited participants for the march from their student populations as well as through a general call circulated among the city's arts venues and human rights organizations.[5] Oduduwá and their volunteers were able to participate in the human rights component of the march—which generally is limited to formally recognized groups like the Madres de Plaza de Mayo and H.I.J.O.S.—because of company members' relationships and work with these groups.[6] In 2011, Oduduwá company members advocated to march directly before the Madres, arguing that this coveted position would allow the dancers to properly "open" the space for the Madres to make their way to the Plaza de Mayo.

Through physical and symbolic work like holding space for this revered human rights group, founding member Alejandra Vassallo proposed Oduduwá's participation as a critical complement to the work of established human rights groups. Vassallo drew on her scholarly training in history as well as dance when she co-directed the 2015 documentary *Piedra Libre: Women Dance Memories*, a documentary film on Oduduwá's participation in the march. In our interview, she argued:

> We are constructing history, the history of memory. Much has been said, discussed, and written about what constitutes the memory and history of Argentina's recent past . . . . Personally, I would like to expand this discussion beyond academia to say there are certain practices that do not occur because of a political party or particular group. They do not happen because of a stable community, but rather for reasons far more specific and ephemeral. They are ephemeral communities, like what happens March 24 when a group, through ancestral dance, intervenes in memory discourses.[7]

If memory is the past summoned through embodied practice in the present, Vassallo's understanding of Oduduwá's construction of a history of memory can be read in three connected ways.

First, Oduduwá aimed to extend the practice of Orishá dance as always already about performing identity in the face of the generational ruptures caused by large-scale violence. Orishá practices historically have transmitted conceptions of ancestral identity in the face of colonial and neocolonial configurations that have sought to systematically denigrate African diasporic culture in the Americas.[8] Moreover, by literally positioning their dancing—and often the thematic content of the march choreography—in relationship to human rights groups like the Madres, Oduduwá saw its work as chronicling a national history of memory practice around political disappearance. And finally, as anthropologist and Oduduwá member María Balmaceda argues in her written scholarship, the company's use of Orishá dance as part of a history of remembering the disappeared also registered the erasure of the Afro-Argentine population from the national body.[9] There are various and debated hypotheses on the late-nineteenth and early-twentieth-century decline of the Afro-Argentine population. Prominent explanations include the outbreak of yellow fever; heavy causalities during the War of the Triple Alliance (1864–70), in which

Afro-Argentines formed a disproportionate part of the frontlines; and emigration to Uruguay and Brazil.[10] What is clear, however, is the vigor with which post-independence nation-building projects promoted and crafted a white Argentina. As part of these projects, the government forged statistics that artificially accelerated a decline in Afro-Argentine demographics to support narrations of Argentina as a nation of European immigrants.[11] Audiences at the march—and volunteer dancers—may not have registered this reflection on the historical erasure of blackness and contemporary racism in Argentina and may indeed have engaged with it as a further exotification and/or othering of African diasporic culture. Nonetheless, Balmaceda's argument evidences Oduduwá's own understanding of how their work recognized and critically engaged with Afro-Argentine history.

Vassallo's statement, however, also stakes a broader claim for the intervention that the volunteer dancers' "ephemeral community" made into the history of memory practice. Outside of any official group or long-term agenda, Oduduwá offered a way for any willing participant to dance the past into the present alongside some of the most significant groups in recent Argentine history. In addition to "putting" their bodies to work in the name of continual calls for juridical action, participants also inscribed their own bodies, regardless of background, party affiliation, or personal connection to political violence, into the history of memory. While Vassallo refers specifically to the march, her words also apply more broadly to many of the practices considered across *Moving Otherwise*'s chapters. In most cases, dancers' politics did not constitute part of a formally articulated political program—Bailarines Organizados' labor movement, discussed in chapter 5, perhaps comes closest. Rather, the possibilities of moving otherwise arose through the "specific and ephemeral" impacts of stage works and quotidian danced negotiations that addressed histories of political and economic violence. Oduduwá's practice, in turn, evidences how dance's particular ability to enact politics lived within the traditionally political format of the march.

In early March 2011, I joined scores of dancers on the grass in front of the Buenos Aires Planetarium to learn Oduduwá's choreography under the early autumn sun. Each year that they marched, the group developed an accessible phrase, which could be repeated and reasonably sustained across the multiple hours of the march. The choreography addressed recent human rights developments, and the choreographers were careful to explain the movement's symbolism and relationship to the Orishás. They also assigned a color theme—red and black in 2011—for participants to wear. In 2011, the choreography expressed concern that the aging Madres and Abuelas might not be able to put their bodies in the streets much longer. Trials of military officials, although underway, were long, arduous, and ongoing. In an email to march participants, Oduduwá wrote:

Even though justice is arriving, it should be sped up. We have waited too long and our Madres and Abuelas' long history of resistance is coming to an end. Furthermore, judgement and punishment is owed without delay to the victimizers on behalf of the whole society. We must accelerate the times of truth. This advance is possible only in movement, in the comings and goings and changes of direction that seem contradictory, but in reality produce the beginning of the action, the push forward, the opening of new paths that until now were closed to us.[12]

Oduduwá choreographed steps and sequences aimed at speeding up the pursuit of justice. During the march, dancers waited for hand signals from group leaders that indicated which sequence to perform next—in that way the dance created for the march was simultaneously choreographed and improvised. One segment included a diagonally travelling cross step, accompanied by an arm slicing across the body from above the head to below the hip, that captured the sense of advance and the need to open the new paths articulated in their statement. This step, along with a series of turns and direction changes expressing the nonlinear nature of justice's arrival, formed part of a sequence inspired by the Orishá Exú, the trickster deity of crossroads. A sequence the choreographers associated with Xangó, the powerful Orishá of thunder, called for long-delayed government redress.[13] Returning to the cross step, dancers continued to move forward in space as they struck imagined staffs, as if held in each fist, against the ground. This gesture in particular issued a powerful demand for the arrival of justice, now.

The gestural components of the choreography were based on photographer Oscar Santiago Palmas's 2011 testimony in which he described photographing corpses, later identified as Azucena Villaflor (a founding Madre de Plaza de Mayo) and others, at the request of local police after the bodies washed up on the beaches of Santa Teresita in the Province of Buenos Aires in December 1977.[14] Villaflor's activism following her son's disappearance and her own subsequent disappearance inspired Bailarines Toda la Vida's 2011 . . . Y el mar, discussed in chapter 5. Like Bailarines, Oduduwá found choreographic motivation in the sea both as the final resting place of lost loved ones and in the continual movement of its rolling waves. For both groups, the sea's continual movement symbolized the ongoing nature of trauma as well as the slow pace of government recognition. In a sequence referred to as the "detention," Oduduwá's dancers slowly spiraled to the ground and rolled toward surrounding bodies to form a mound of intertwined limbs and torsos. These formations of still, tangled bodies scattered over the pavement functioned to memorialize and make visible an event—the resurfacing of violated and violently disposed bodies—that few had initially witnessed. In performance, this portion of the choreography cast a still and quiet over the otherwise animated and noisy crowd around us.

On the day of the march, my partner accompanied me downtown. We came out of the subway and into a vast sea of circulating bodies, pounding drums, and waving flags. As we pushed our way through the crowd to find Oduduwá's meeting point on one of the streets leading to the Plaza de Mayo, crowds of spectators mingled with marchers readying for their cue. Once we located Oduduwá and La Chilinga—the drummers who accompanied us in the march—I took my place in line (figure E.1).[15]

While witnessing the mass movement of the 2006 march gave me insight into why movement matters to claims for justice, dancing in the 2011 march exemplified *poner el cuerpo* as an act of physical endurance. As we danced, progressing down the street in lines kept organized as best we could, ensuing chaos meant that the struggle of simply making it to the Plaza de Mayo became as important as successfully executing Oduduwá's thoughtfully crafted choreography. At a post-march gathering, company members and volunteer dancers alike agreed that the 2011 march was particularly tumultuous. At one point, a student group tried to break into the demonstration with a force that nearly toppled dozens of dancers. In the chaos of the march, we stopped dancing at another point to allow the Madres to pass through, ostensibly due to the late running time. The march for political parties that took place before the human rights march took nearly an hour and half longer than anticipated. As the Madres moved down the center of the street, the dancers linked arms

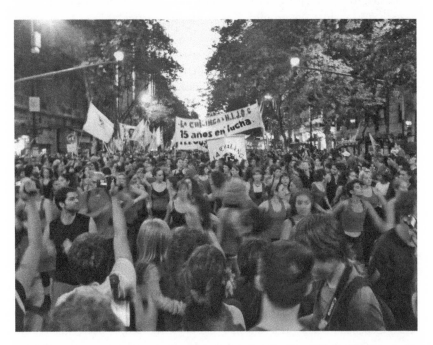

Figure E.1 Oduduwá Danza Afroamericana dancers and volunteers participating in the March 24, 2011, human rights march. Photograph by author.

on the periphery to form a protective chain, later lowering to the ground and fanning outstretched arms in a gesture of honor. Though we kept progressing toward the Plaza de Mayo even after the Madres passed by, Oduduwá's dancing bodies had succeeded in opening and holding space for the group.

When the Plaza de Mayo finally came into sight in the shadowy glow of sunset, the march again surprised us. As we approached, a large bulbous object I could not quite make out came into view. As we moved closer, it become clear: a giant inflatable head of former President Néstor Kirchner, ostensibly to commemorate his death in October 2010. The enormous balloon not only called on spectators to remember Kirchner's presidency (2003–7), but also staked a bold claim for his role, and that of his successor and wife, President Cristina Fernández de Kirchner (2007–15), in reopening the federal conversation around memory of the last military dictatorship. It, quite literally, positioned the late President Kirchner as part of the history of memory. Due to factors related but not exclusive to the space occupied by the inflated head, the Oduduwá dancers were not able to enter the plaza that day. Yet as we lowered to the ground, pounding our flattened palms against the concrete to honor the lives we were there to commemorate and to bring our dancing to a close, the work nevertheless felt complete (figure E.2).

While I was startled in the moment of seeing Kirchner's head, upon later reflection, it actually brought into sharp relief the multiple meanings

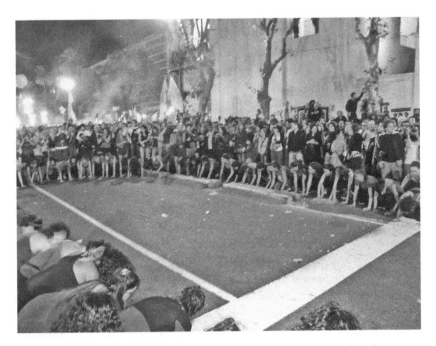

Figure E.2 Oduduwá Danza Afroamericana dancers and volunteers concluding their participation in the March 24, 2011, human rights march. Photograph by author.

articulated through our danced march. Memory—like movement—is unruly. Both often summon more than properly pertains to any given body, time, or place, and frequently improvise to negotiate claims to community, identity, and possible futures. The presence of Néstor's head joined the other ostensibly imperfect "fits" that mark this story, like Oduduwá's repurposing of a racially marked practice as well as the presence of a foreign researcher committed to what performance ethnographer Dwight Conquergood has called "co-performative witnessing," or as D. Soyini Madison summarizes, "a politics of the body deeply in action with Others."[16] The collective presence of these apparent excesses to the aim of the march made clear, as Diana Taylor has argued, that "performed, embodied practices make the past available as a political resource in the present by simultaneously enabling several complicated multilayered processes."[17] On March 24, 2011, masses of dancers performing Orishá-based choreography, the giant inflatable head of a late political leader, and multitudes of other bodies scripted themselves into a multivalent history of memory that spanned the generational ruptures caused by the last military dictatorship and the trans-Atlantic slave trade, racial erasure in Argentina, a recent presidential administration, and likely many others.

The multilayered nature of memory and movement politics at work in the march also has characterized the histories of moving otherwise documented in this book. As they moved otherwise, these dance practices activated "complicated multilayered processes" like the ones circulating in the march. Under Juan Carlos Onganía's dictatorship in the late 1960s, Susana Zimmermann's *Polymorphias* called on the memory of the Holocaust to critique the current political climate, while Ana Kamien's self-titled piece connected the ongoing retraction of resources and spaces for artistic expression with increases in state and revolutionary violence alike. At the same time that Silvia Hodgers and Alicia Sanguinetti crossed repertoires of dance and political militancy in the early 1970s, Estela Maris's *Juana Azurduy* echoed militant groups' frequent practice of invoking independence-era heroes to give meaning to current political struggles. In the waning years of the last military dictatorship, Renate Schottelius's *Paisaje de gritos* summoned the Holocaust once again. In the post-dictatorship period, Hodgers, Silvia Vladimivsky, and Susana Tambutti choreographed works that approached the individual and collective trauma of the last military dictatorship through the tango's history of articulating the displacement that marked the context of its early-twentieth-century development. As the fifth chapter demonstrated, Bailarines Toda la Vida and the Compañía Nacional de Danza Contemporánea linked histories of 1970s and 1980s political disappearances with the experiences of economic disenfranchisement that marked the 1990s and 2000s. Told through the story of moving otherwise, the history of danced memory is fundamentally "multidirectional," to re-cite Michael Rothberg's name for "the convoluted, sometimes historically unjustified, back-and-forth movement of seemingly distant collective memories . . . [that] traverse sacrosanct borders of ethnicity and era."[18] Oduduwá's march, then, is part of the extended history of dancing memory analyzed in *Moving Otherwise*.

In addition to capturing the history of danced memory's multidirectional moves, the march also echoed the ways in which many of the practices considered in *Moving Otherwise* took place in spaces not traditionally associated with contemporary dance. For Ana Kamien, navigating the transgressive "crazy block" (*manzana loca*) where the Di Tella Institute stood was as important for her experience of artistic, social, and political mobility as creating the works she presented on its state-of-the-art stage. Political prisoners danced through the halls of the Rawson Penitentiary in 1972 as part of their carefully planned, but ultimately ill-fated, prison escape. Audience members flooded the sidewalks outside of the Bambalinas Theater to enter Danza Abierta in 1981. Bailarines Organizados occupied Corrientes Avenue during their demonstrations in front of the San Martín Theater. Bailarines Toda la Vida rehearsed weekly in the Grissinopoli breadstick factory between 2002 and early 2018. Considered as part of this multivalent story of movement, Oduduwá's participation in the human rights march is not so much an "entrance" of the dance community into the streets, but rather part of a rich history of moving otherwise beyond the studio and the stage.

And finally, Oduduwá's transnational imagination of the history of memory through Orishá dance also highlights Buenos Aires-based contemporary dance's own global past and present. Though rooted in Buenos Aires, the practices detailed throughout this book also map broader genealogies—of migration, exile, and belonging—that live in concert dances, techniques, and pedagogies passed down between bodies and across borders. As it intervenes in the quotidian choreographies that map bodies' movements in urban space, contemporary dance also charts alternate routes for understanding the relationship of Buenos Aires-based dance to networks across the global north and south. As Buenos Aires contemporary dance continues its travels across local and international stages and streets it will surely imagine new modes of sociality attuned to the stakes of political histories and transnational connections. This book is an attempt to honor, document, and argue for contemporary dance practices' extensive—and richly complex—history of moving otherwise.

NOTES

PREFACE

1. Throughout the text, the names of dance companies, concert works, techniques, festivals, and some organizations (that are objects of extended analysis) are named in the original Spanish, while institutions, theaters, and other organizations are listed in English with the original Spanish accompanying the first mention. Acronyms, when used, reflect the original Spanish. All translations by author, unless otherwise noted.

2. Jennifer Muller, "Bailar es una experiencia, y no debería ser un juicio," interview by Analía Melgar, *Página/12*, December 24, 2004, https://www.pagina12.com.ar/diario/espectaculos/6-45186-2004-12-24.html. The General San Martín Municipal Theater is subsequently referred to as the San Martín Theater.

3. As of July 15, 2008, the official website of the Abuelas de Plaza de Mayo, https://www.abuelas.org.ar, featured a page titled "Concurso Danza x la Identidad" ("x" here stands for "por," or "for") that described the outcome of the 2004 call in the cited language: "no logró la temática propuesta." It also named four finalists, though the festival did not advance the pieces to production: Vilma Emilia Rúpolo's *Madres* (Mothers), Paulina Ossona's *Mater dolorosa*, Claudia Barretta's . . . *de nudos y desnudos . . .* (. . . *of knots and nudes . . .*), and Julieta Eskenazi's *Restos de oscuras* (*Pieces of Darkness*). This web page has been discontinued.

4. Unpublished poem, n.d., Private Collection of Nora Codina. "En todo hecho cotidiano, por insignificante que sea, vive el inagotable germen de la emoción. La danza debe encenderlo hasta provocar una explosión." Cited with Codina's permission.

INTRODUCTION

1. The law is based, in part, on the Argentine National Theater and Music Laws, which established the National Theater and Music Institutes, respectively.

2. "Quienes somos," Movimiento por la Ley Nacional de Danza, accessed December 29, 2016, http://www.leynacionaldedanza.com/p/quienes-somos.html. In the mid-1980s, contemporary choreographer Susana Zimmermann spearheaded legislation for federal dance support that included the creation of national companies dedicated to genres including folklore, classical ballet, and contemporary dance. "Propugnan la creación del Ballet Nacional," *Tiempo Argentino*, September 28, 1984, 6, Private Collection of Susana Zimmermann.

3. The Argentine National Congress, the nation's bicameral legislative branch, is made up of a 72-seat Senate and a 257-seat Chamber of Deputies.

4. Prodanza, or the law that provides municipal support in the form of competitive grants to independent choreographers, passed into law in 2000.

5. For the version of the proposed law as of 2016, see "Proyecto de Ley–Versión 2016," Movimiento por la Ley Nacional de Danza Argentina, accessed January 2, 2017, http://www.leynacionaldedanza.com/p/descargar-el-proyecto-completo.html.

6. For footage of and additional information on the events of April 29, 2014, see Julia Martinez Heimann and Konstantina Bousmpoura's documentary, *Trabajadores de la danza* (Buenos Aires and Athens: Kinsi, 2016), streaming video courtesy of directors. See also "29A eventos de apoyo a la presentación de la Ley Nacional de Danza 2014," last modified March 31, 2015, https://www.youtube.com/playlist?list=PLzzme7XW1I0sn1oYBWzeSwb-pEOvZKEly.

7. "Postales de apoyo a la Ley Nacional de Danza," last modified March 4, 2016, https://www.youtube.com/playlist?list=PLzzme7XW1I0t-hkR7NiMkeKmuaKpV57C8.

8. "OCTUBREARGENTINADANZA: Unidos por nuestra ley," Movimiento por la Ley Nacional de Danza Argentina, accessed January 3, 2017, http://www.leynacionaldedanza.com/p/octubreargentinadanza-unidos-por.html.

9. Despite mobilization and the law's annual reintroduction, Congress has not taken up the bill for discussion or vote as of 2018. As of this writing, the movement is assessing next steps and has put substantial energy into supporting provincial dance legislation. For a critical analysis of the National Dance Law project, see Paula Rodríguez, "Danza y 'más allá.' Una crónica reflexiva-analítica sobre el Proyecto de la Ley Nacional de Danza," in *VI Jornadas de investigación en danza 2012*, ed. María Eugenia Cadús (Buenos Aires: Universidad Nacional de las Artes, 2016), 198–216.

10. Though English-language scholarship often refers to this period as the "Dirty War," I have chosen to follow Argentine scholars in forgoing use of this term, given its origins in the language of the military junta itself and the false implication that there were two equal "sides" during the dictatorship. Furthermore, the phrase "last military dictatorship" appropriately situates this period within a longer history of alternating military coups and civilian governments in the twentieth century.

11. Déborah Kalmar, interview by author, Buenos Aires, Argentina, August 17, 2011. "[Es] como que el que se mueve es otro. Por algo todos los caminos de represión más explícitos o implícitos o más encubiertos tienen que ver con frenar el cuerpo."

12. Hannah Arendt, *The Origins of Totalitarianism* (San Diego: Harcourt, 1973), 465.

13. While Kalmar inspired the use of "moving otherwise" in this book, similar terminology has appeared in recent dance scholarship. Judith Hamera, drawing on Leonard C. Hawes, employs a related construction in the essay "Becoming-Other-Wise: Conversational Performance and the Politics of Experience," *Text and Performance Quarterly* 18, no. 34 (1998): 273–99, as does Emily E. Wilcox in her essay "Women Dancing Otherwise: The Queer Feminism of Gu Jiani's *Right & Left*," in *Queer Dance: Meanings & Makings*, ed. Clare Croft (New York: Oxford University Press, 2017), 67–82. Both essays analyze how dance practices imagine alternate ways of being.

14. Rob Nixon, *Slow Violence and the Environmentalism of the Poor* (Cambridge: Harvard University Press, 2011), 2.

15. Historians Valeria Manzano and Karina Felitti analyze the rise of the term among youth in activist circles in the 1960s and 1970s. Both trace the relationship between the term's roots in activist practices and broader shifts in gender and sexual norms. See Valeria Manzano, *The Age of Youth in Argentina: Culture,*

Politics, and Sexuality from Perón to Videla (Chapel Hill: The University of North Carolina Press, 2014), 193–94, and Karina Felitti, "Poner el cuerpo: género y sexualidad en la política revolucionaria de Argentina en las décadas de los sesenta y setenta," in *Political and Social Movements During the Sixties and Seventies in the Americas and Europe*, ed. Avital H. Bloch (Colima: Universidad de Colima, 2010), 70.

16. Barbara Sutton, *Bodies in Crisis: Culture, Violence, and Women's Resistance in Neoliberal Argentina* (New Brunswick, NJ: Rutgers University Press, 2010), 161–62.

17. For Foucault's discussion of how states exercise control over citizens' bodies, see *"Society Must Be Defended" Lectures at the Collège de France 1975–1976*, trans. David Macey (New York: Picador, 2003), 239–63. In his work on the Holocaust, Agamben argues that biopolitics taken to its logical extreme produces a continual state of exception where "bare life"—citizens denied political and legal representation and subjected to devastating violence—produces the authority of the state. See Giorgio Agamben, *Homo Sacer: Sovereign Power and Bare Life*, trans. Daniel Heller-Roazen (Stanford, CA: Stanford University Press, 1998), 6. Also reformulating Foucauldian biopolitics, Mbembe argues that modern political power is more accurately characterized by the term "necropolitics," or a politics of death predicated on the "maximum destruction of persons." See "Necropolitics," trans. Libby Meintjes, *Public Culture* 15, no. 1 (2003): 40. For a comprehensive consideration of violence and modernity in Latin America, see Jean Franco, *Cruel Modernity* (Durham, NC: Duke University Press, 2013).

18. Andrew Hewitt, *Social Choreography: Ideology as Performance in Dance and Everyday Movement* (Durham, NC: Duke University Press, 2005), 3.

19. Jacques Rancière, *Dissensus: On Politics and Aesthetics*, trans. Steven Corcoran (London: Bloomsbury, 2010), 36.

20. Ibid., 37.

21. André Lepecki, "Choreopolice and Choreopolitics: or, the task of the dancer," *TDR* 57, no. 4 (2013): 19.

22. Ibid., 20.

23. Randy Martin offers a related concept in his notion of the "kinestheme." Adapting the Foucauldian notion of the episteme, kinesthemes are "the regularization of bodily practices, the moment of power by and through which bodies are called—and devise responses—to move in particular ways." Randy Martin, *Knowledge LTD: Toward a Social Logic of the Derivative* (Philadelphia: Temple University Press, 2015), 158.

24. Lepecki, "Choreopolice and Choreopolitics: or, the task of the dancer," 20.

25. Erin Manning, *Politics of Touch: Sense, Movement, Sovereignty* (Minneapolis: University of Minnesota Press, 2007), 65.

26. Book-length studies include Diana Taylor, *Disappearing Acts: Spectacles of Gender and Nationalism in Argentina's "Dirty War"* (Durham, NC: Duke University Press, 1997); Jean Graham-Jones, *Exorcising History: Argentine Theater under Dictatorship* (Cranbury, NJ: Bucknell University Press, 2000); Ana Puga, *Memory, Allegory, and Testimony in South American Theatre: Upstaging Dictatorship* (New York: Routledge, 2008); Brenda Werth, *Theatre, Performance, and Memory Politics in Argentina* (New York: Palgrave Macmillan, 2010); Philippa Page, *Politics and Performance in Post-Dictatorship Argentine Film and Theatre* (Woodbridge, UK: Tamesis, 2011); and Noe Montez, *Memory, Transitional Justice, and Theater in Postdictatorship Argentina* (Carbondale: Southern Illinois University Press, 2017).

27. Taylor, *Disappearing Acts*, 123.

28. See Diana Taylor, *The Archive and the Repertoire: Performing Cultural Memory in the Americas* (Durham, NC: Duke University Press, 2003), 161–89.

29. This distinction is drawn out in the introductions of three recent anthologies dedicated to examining the relationship between dance and politics. See Alexandra Kolb, "Cross-Currents of Dance and Politics: An Introduction," in *Dance and Politics*, ed. Alexandra Kolb (Bern: Peter Lang, 2011), 1–36; Gerald Siegmund and Stefan Hölscher, introduction to *Dance, Politics & Co-Immunity*, ed. Gerald Siegmund and Stefan Hölscher (Zürich: Diaphanes, 2013), 11; and Rebekah J. Kowal, Gerald Siegmund, and Randy Martin, introduction to *The Oxford Handbook of Dance and Politics*, ed. Rebekah J. Kowal, Gerald Siegmund, and Randy Martin (New York: Oxford University Press, 2017), 3–4.

30. For book-length discussions of leftist dance in New York City in the 1930s, see Ellen Graff, *Stepping Left: Dance and Politics in New York City, 1928–1942* (Durham, NC: Duke University Press, 1997) and Mark Franko, *The Work of Dance: Labor, Movement, Identity in the 1930s* (Middletown, CT: Wesleyan University Press, 2002). For extended consideration of how this movement intersected with Jewish identity in particular, see Naomi M. Jackson, *Converging Movements: Modern Dance and Jewish Culture at the 92nd Street Y* (Middletown, CT: Wesleyan University Press, 2000), 55–74. See also Stacey Prickett's analysis of Edith Segal's dances with workers in *Embodied Politics: Dance, Protest and Identities* (Alton, UK: Dance Books, 2013), 11–53.

31. Recent studies that emphasize dance's relationship to state politics include Rebekah J. Kowal's, *How To Do Things with Dance: Performing Change in Postwar America* (Middletown, CT: Wesleyan University Press, 2010); Jens Richard Giersdorf's *The Body of the People: East German Dance Since 1945* (Madison: University of Wisconsin Press, 2013); and Clare Croft's *Dancers as Diplomats: American Choreography in Cultural Exchange* (New York: Oxford University Press, 2015). Also see Susan Manning's foundational *Ecstasy and the Demon: Feminism and Nationalism in the Dances of Mary Wigman* (Berkeley: University of California Press, 1993). The analysis of how racialized and gendered identities intersect with national and transnational political economies is a rich and fast-growing area of research. Among others, see Ann Cooper Albright, *Choreographing Difference: The Body and Identity in Contemporary Dance* (Middletown, CT: Wesleyan University Press, 1997); Susan Manning, *Modern Dance/Negro Dance: Race in Motion* (Minneapolis: University of Minnesota Press, 2004); Jacqueline Shea Murphy, *The People Have Never Stopped Dancing: Native American Modern Dance Histories* (Minneapolis: University of Minnesota Press, 2007); Yutian Wong, *Choreographing Asian America* (Middletown, CT: Wesleyan University Press, 2010); Ramón H. Rivera-Servera, *Performing Queer Latinidad: Dance, Sexuality, Politics* (Ann Arbor: University of Michigan Press, 2012); Melissa Blanco Borelli, *She is Cuba: A Genealogy of the Mulata Body* (New York: Oxford University Press, 2015); and Anthea Kraut, *Choreographing Copyright: Race, Gender, and Intellectual Property Rights in American Dance* (New York: Oxford University Press, 2016). For studies that center on philosophical approaches to dance, politics, and protest, see Randy Martin, *Critical Moves: Dance Studies in Theory and Politics* (Durham, NC: Duke University Press, 1998); André Lepecki, *Exhausting Dance: Performance and the Politics of Movement* (New York: Routledge, 2005); Manning, *Politics of Touch*; Dana Mills, *Dance & Politics: Moving Beyond Boundaries* (Manchester: Manchester University Press, 2017); and Lucía Naser Rocha, "La Politización de la danza a la dancificación de la política" (PhD diss., University of Michigan, 2017).

32. Mark Franko, "Dance and the Political: States of Exception," *Dance Research Journal* 38, no. 1–2 (2006): 6.
33. For an anthology focused on danced engagements with war, including discussions of work from and about the global south, see Gay Morris and Jens Richard Giersdorf, eds., *Choreographies of 21st Century Wars* (New York: Oxford University Press, 2016). For consideration of the relationship between dance practices and political violence within a human-rights framework, see the essays in *Dance, Human Rights, and Social Justice: Dignity in Motion*, ed. Naomi Jackson and Toni Shapiro-Phim (Lanham, MD: Scarecrow Press, 2008).
34. Rachmi Diyah Larasati, *The Dance That Makes You Vanish: Cultural Reconstruction in Post-Genocide Indonesia* (Minneapolis: University of Minnesota Press, 2013), 16.
35. For a succinct overview of the consolidation of modern dance during Juan Perón's first two presidential terms, see María Eugenia Cadús, "La consolidación de la práctica de la danza escénica durante el primer peronismo," *Revista Afuera: Estudio de crítica cultural* no. 17–18 (2016–17), http://revistaafuera17-18.blogspot.com.ar/p/blog-page.html.
36. This strategy roughly mirrors Argentine dance scholar Susana Tambutti's approach in her foundational article, "100 años de danza en Buenos Aires," *Funámbulos: Revista bimestral de teatro y danza alterativos* 12, no. 3 (2000): 23–32. Marcelo Isse Moyano, however, privileges "modern" in his English-language entry "Argentina—Modern Dance," in *The International Encyclopedia of Dance*, ed. Selma Jeanne Cohen (Oxford Reference, 2005), accessed January 15, 2017, http://www.oxfordreference.com/view/10.1093/acref/9780195173697.001.0001/acref-9780195173697.
37. Marcelo Isse Moyano, *Cuadernos de Danza III* (Buenos Aires: Facultad de Filosofía y Letras–UBA, 2002), 5. For two central articulations of the debate in US dance studies about modern versus postmodern dance, see Susan Manning, "Modernist Dogma and Post-modern Rhetoric: A Response to Sally Banes' *Terpsichore in Sneakers*," *TDR* 44, no. 4 (1988): 32–9 and Sally Banes, "Terpsichore in Combat Boots," *TDR* 33, no. 1 (1989): 13–15.
38. For recent studies that critically engage these categories in the European context, see Bojana Cvejić, *Choreographing Problems: Expressive Concepts in European Contemporary Dance and Performance* (Hampshire, UK: Palgrave Macmillan, 2015) and Ramsay Burt, *Ungoverning Dance: Contemporary European Theatre Dance and the Commons* (New York: Oxford University Press, 2017). For a comparative look at the United States and Europe, see André Lepecki, *Singularities: Dance in the Age of Performance* (New York: Routledge, 2016).
39. Laura Falcoff's "La danza moderna y contemporánea," in *Historia general de la danza en la Argentina*, ed. Beatriz Durante (Buenos Aires: Fondo Nacional de las Artes, 2008), 231–321, constructs a historical narrative around what she identifies as influential tours of US and European artists. For published oral histories, see Marcelo Isse Moyano, *La danza moderna argentina cuenta su historia* (Buenos Aires: Ediciones Artes del Sur, 2006) and Analía Melgar, ed., *Puentes y atajos: Recorridos por la danza en Argentina* (Buenos Aires: Editorial De Los Cuatro Vientos, 2005).
40. The anthology, Gabily Anadón, ed., *El milagro al borde del estado: Discursividades políticas en cuerpos de danza* (Buenos Aires: Centro Cultural de la Cooperación, 2011), is dedicated to examining the relationship between contemporary dance and politics in theory and practice. For comprehensive critical analysis of Argentine concert dance during the first two administrations of Juan Perón

(1946–55), see María Eugenia Cadús, "La danza escénica durante el primer Peronismo: Formación y práctica de la danza y políticas del estado" (PhD diss., University of Buenos Aires, 2017). In addition to her other publications, Susana Tambutti's *fichas de cátedra*, or unpublished texts used for the University of Buenos Aires course "Reflexiones sobre la danza escénica en Argentina Siglo XX" ("Reflections on Concert Dance in Argentina in the Twentieth Century") also approach dance history through a critical lens. Beyond the field of concert dance studies, anthropologist Silvia Citro, whose research focuses on indigenous dance practices in northern Argentina, has published multiple volumes that examine theories and methods of critical dance ethnography. See Silvia Citro, *Cuerpos Significantes: Travesía de una etnografía dialéctica* (Buenos Aires: Biblos, 2009) and *Cuerpos en Movimiento: Antropología de y desde las danzas*, ed. Silvia Citro and Patricia Aschieri (Buenos Aires: Biblos, 2012).

41. Among others, see Suki John, *Contemporary Dance in Cuba: Técnica Cubana as Revolutionary Movement* (Jefferson: McFarland & Company, Inc., Publishers, 2012); Victoria Fortuna, *"Poner el cuerpo*: Buenos Aires Contemporary Dance and the Politics of Movement" (PhD diss., Northwestern University, 2013); Lester Tomé, "'Music in the Blood': Performance and Discourse of Musicality in Cuban Ballet Aesthetics," *Dance Chronicle* 36, no. 2 (2013): 218–42; Cristina F. Rosa, *Brazilian Bodies and Their Choreographies of Identification: Swing Nation* (New York: Palgrave Macmillan, 2015); Jose Luis Reynoso, "Racialized Dance Modernisms in Lusophone and Spanish-Speaking Latin America," in *The Modernist World*, ed. Stephen Ross and Allana Lindgren (New York: Routledge, 2015), 392–400; Sofie Narbed, "The Cultural Geographies of Contemporary Dance in Quito, Ecuador" (PhD diss., Royal Holloway, University of London, 2016); Elizabeth Schwall, "Dancing With the Revolution: Cuban Dance, State, and Nation, 1930–1960" (PhD diss., Columbia University, 2016); and Stephanie Sherman "(Dis)Plazas and (Dis)Placed Danzas: Space, Trauma, and Moving Bodies in Mexico City" (PhD diss., University of California, Berkeley, 2016).

42. For analyses of the historical development of tango, see Marta Savigliano, *Tango and the Political Economy of Passion* (Boulder, CO: Westview Press, 1995) and Robert Farris Thompson, *Tango: The Art History of Love* (New York: Vintage Books, 2006). For ethnographies that focus on contemporary practices of tango, see Julie Taylor, *Paper Tangos* (Durham, NC: Duke University Press, 1998) and Carolyn Merritt, *Tango Nuevo* (Gainesville: University of Florida Press, 2012).

43. Book-length studies include Barbara Browning's *Samba: Resistance in Motion* (Bloomington: Indiana University Press, 1995); John Charles Chasteen, *National Rhythms, African Roots: The Deep History of Latin American Popular Dance* (Albuquerque: University of New Mexico Press, 2004); Ruth Hellier-Tinoco, *Embodying Mexico: Tourism, Nationalism & Performance* (New York: Oxford University Press, 2011); and Paul A. Scolieri, *Dancing the New World: Aztecs, Spaniards, and the Choreography of Conquest* (Austin: University of Texas Press, 2013). For an influential collection of essays, see Celeste Fraser Delgado and José Esteban Muñoz, eds., *Everynight Life: Culture and Dance in Latin/o America* (Durham, NC: Duke University Press, 1997). The recent collection of essays, Pablo Vila, ed., *Music, Dance, Affect and Emotions in Latin America* (Lanham, MD: Lexington Books, 2017), considers both popular and concert forms of music and dance.

44. For a critical discussion of world dance as a category, see Susan Leigh Foster, "Worlding Dance—An Introduction" in *Worlding Dance*, ed. Susan Leigh Foster (New York: Palgrave Macmillan, 2009), 1–13.

45. Emily E. Wilcox, "When place matters: Provincializing the 'global,'" in *Rethinking Dance History: Issues and Methodologies*, ed. Geraldine Morris and Larraine Nicholas (New York: Routledge, 2018), 166.

46. Susan Manning, "Dance History," in *The Bloomsbury Companion to Dance Studies*, ed. Sherril Dodds (London: Bloomsbury, Forthcoming 2019).

47. Anna Tsing, *Friction: An Ethnography of Global Connection* (Princeton: Princeton University Press, 2005), 3–4.

48. Jody Weber, *The Evolution of Aesthetic and Expressive Dance in Boston* (Amherst, NY: Cambria Press, 2009), Kindle edition, ch.7.

49. Ibid., ch. 8.

50. John Martin, "The Dance: Ambassadors Miriam Winslow and Foster Fitz-Simons As Good Neighbors in South America," *New York Times*, July 13, 1941.

51. For a discussion of early Argentine ballet culture and influential tours, see Enrique Honorio Destaville, "Mirada sobre el siglo XIX y el siglo XX en sus primeros años," in *Historia General de la danza en la Argentina*, ed. Beatriz Durante (Buenos Aires: Fondo Nacional de las Artes, 2008), 13–49. For an examination of the early years of the Colón Theater Ballet, see Carlos Manso, "Cuatro décadas del cuerpo de baile del Teatro Colón," in *Historia General de la danza en la Argentina*, ed. Beatriz Durante (Buenos Aires: Fondo Nacional de las Artes, 2008), 51–141. See also Inés Malinow, *Desarrollo del ballet en la Argentina* (Buenos Aires: Ediciones Culturales Argentinas, 1963).

52. *Facundo* and Juan Bautisa Alberdi's *Bases y puntos de partida para la organización de la República Argentina* (*Bases and Starting Points for the Organization of the Argentine Republic*, 1852) were foundational nation-building texts influential in drafting the Argentine Constitution of 1853. Both texts reacted to post-independence challenges to unifying the nation and the conflicts resulting from Argentina's organization as a confederation without a head of state (1831–52). For a comprehensive discussion of the nation-building era, see Tulio Halperín Donghi, *Proyecto y construcción de una nación (1846–1880)* (Buenos Aires: Emecé, 2007).

53. Adrián Gorelik, *Miradas sobre Buenos Aires* (Buenos Aires: Siglo XXI Editores, 2004), 74.

54. For a historical overview of the construction of Argentine racial exceptionalism and the role scholarship has played in upholding narratives of whiteness, see Paulina L. Alberto and Eduardo Elena, "Introduction: The Shades of the Nation," in *Rethinking Race in Modern Argentina*, ed. Paulina L. Alberto and Eduardo Elena (New York: Cambridge University Press, 2016), 1–23.

55. For an analysis of the role that indigenous-themed ballets produced between the early and mid-twentieth century played in this process, see Victoria Fortuna, "Dancing Argentine Modernity: Imagined Indigenous Bodies on the Buenos Aires Concert Stage (1915–1966)," *Dance Research Journal* 48, no. 2 (2016): 44–60. For broader consideration of this period, see also Susana Tambutti, "El 'nosotros' europeo," (course text, Reflexiones sobre la danza escénica en Argentina Siglo XX, Facultad de Filosofía y Letras, Universidad de Buenos Aires, 2011).

56. See Giersdorf's chapter on Chilean choreographer Patricio Bunster in *The Body of the People*, 157–78. Bunster trained in Chile with members of Kurt Jooss's company who, exiled in Chile during World War II, founded a dance department at the

University of Chile. Bunster was then exiled to East Germany between 1973 and 1985 during Augusto Pinochet's dictatorship.

57. Michelle Clayton's "Modernism's Moving Bodies," *Modernist Cultures* 9, no. 1 (2014): 27–45—which traces the movements of figures including Charlie Chaplin, Vaslav Nijinsky, and Tórtola Valencia—offers a model for charting the transnational circulation of dance modernisms in Latin America. Prarthana Purkayastha's study of the development of modern dance in India likewise emphasizes how the practices she examines developed in parallel with European and North American modernisms across the twentieth century: *Indian Modern Dance, Feminism, and Transnationalism* (New York: Palgrave Macmillan, 2014).

58. Winslow's date of return to Argentina is often cited as 1944; however, newspaper clippings held in the Miriam Winslow Papers suggest that she in fact returned in 1943 and presented work. Jerome Robbins Dance Division, New York Public Library for the Performing Arts, Folder 52.

59. Weber, *The Evolution of Aesthetic and Expressive Dance in Boston*, ch. 8.

60. Susana Tambutti, "Miriam Winslow como nexo entre la danza moderna norteamericana y el surgimiento de la danza moderna en Argentina" (course text, Reflexiones sobre la danza escénica en Argentina Siglo XX, Facultad de Filosofía y Letras, Universidad de Buenos Aires, 2011).

61. Weber, *The Evolution of Aesthetic and Expressive Dance in Boston*, ch. 8.

62. In a letter dated November 15, 1948, Winslow writes to concert manager Rhea Powers, "I have almost done what I set out to do—form a company and take it back to the States. I have the company—now to the States!!" Miriam Winslow Papers, Jerome Robbins Dance Division, New York Public Library for the Performing Arts, Folder 20.

63. Weber, *The Evolution of Aesthetic and Expressive Dance in Boston*, ch. 8.

64. Susan Manning terms this "metaphorical minstrelsy" in relationship to female dancers performing Negro spirituals in the 1920s, *Modern Dance/Negro Dance*, 10. A breadth of additional dance scholars have also analyzed how white, early modern dancers—including Isadora Duncan, Ruth St. Denis, and Martha Graham—represented non-white others. See Jane Desmond, "Dancing Out the Difference: Cultural Imperialism and Ruth St. Denis's 'Radha' of 1906," *Signs: Journal of Women in Culture and Society* 17, no. 1 (1991): 28–49; Ann Daly, *Done into Dance: Isadora Duncan in America* (Bloomington: Indiana University Press, 1995); and Priya Srinivasan, *Sweating Saris: Indian Dance as Transnational Labor* (Philadelphia: Temple University Press, 2011).

65. For thorough documentation of Ana Itelman's prolific career see Rubén Szuchmacher, *Archivo Itelman* (Buenos Aires: Eudeba, 2002).

66. See Cadús, "La danza escénica durante el primer Peronismo."

67. Margarita Bali, interview by author, Buenos Aires, May 5, 2011, and Susana Tambutti, interview by author, Buenos Aires, July 22, 2011.

68. The designation is notably invoked in one of the few English-language texts on Argentine modern dance, Stephanie Reinhart's "Renate Schottelius: Dance at the Bottom of the World in Argentina," in *Dancing Female: Lives and Issues of Women in Contemporary Dance*, ed. Sharon E. Friedler and Susan Glazer (London: Taylor & Francis, 1997), 45–58.

69. Susana Tambutti, *Patagonia trío* (Coral Gables, FL: VI International Hispanic Theater Festival, June 1991), DVD, Private Collection of Susana Tambutti.

70. Tambutti, interview by author. The Podestá brothers' circus is credited with the genesis of the *criollo* theatrical tradition that blended *rioplatense* (Argentine and

Uruguayan) traditions with Italian and Spanish influences. Famous skits initiated in the circus include Pepino el 88, a *cocoliche* character who spoke a mix of Italian and Spanish, and *Juan Moreira* by Eduardo Gutiérrez, a pantomime based on the life of the mythic gaucho outlaw. For analyses of this performance tradition, see Chasteen, *National Rhythms*, 51–70, and Manuel Maccarini, *Teatro de identidad popular: Los géneros sainete rural, circo criollo y radioteatro argentino* (Buenos Aires: Inteatro, 2006).

71. Tambutti, *Patagonia trío* and interview by author.

72. Tambutti, interview by author. "La idea de *Patagonia trío* en realidad surgió . . . porque me acuerdo cuando estaba en Europa me causaba no sé si gracia es la palabra como mucha gente de Sudamérica (inclusive los veo ahora también), tocando la quena en la esquina del Saint-Michel, o sea la idea del artista sudamericano que intenta hacer lo mejor que puede un show digno pero que en realidad es el antihéroe, o sea que trata de vender lo folklórico pero desde una mirada turística. Inclusive la idea era poner un nombre inglés que después no se lo pusimos pero el primer nombre fue *The Patagonia Song and Dance Team* a propósito, después terminó siendo *Patagonia trío* porque teníamos miedo justo a la auto-censura que cuando lo hiciéramos acá la gente creyera que le poníamos ese título en inglés porque nosotros andábamos mucho de gira, entonces que nos hicieran una crítica en contra diciendo: 'ay mira ponen nombres en inglés.'"

73. Ananya Chatterjea, "On the Value of Mistranslations and Contaminations: The Category of 'Contemporary Choreography' in Asian Dance," *Dance Research Journal* 45, no. 1 (2013): 11.

74. See Tambutti, "100 años de danza en Buenos Aires," 31–2.

75. "Por el dinero," Alternativa Teatral, accessed November 10, 2016, http://www. alternativateatral.com/obra28427-por-el-dinero. "*Por el dinero* es un estudio, o análisis, acaso un retrato festivo del bolsillo de los artistas en nuestra país, del absurdo rol del artista en el mercado, pero también un retrato de la perversa relación entre los fondos europeos y los artistas en la periferia."

76. Luciana Acuña and Alejo Moguillansky, *Por el dinero*, General San Martín Cultural Center, Buenos Aires, Argentina, July 12, 2014 and Luciana Acuña, interview by author, Buenos Aires, Argentina, July 23, 2014. My movement description here is supplemented by video documentation of the work from Acuña's private collection.

77. Acuña and Moguillansky, *Por el dinero*.

78. Ibid.

79. Marta Savigliano, "Worlding Dance and Dancing Out There in the World," in *Worlding Dance*, ed. Susan Leigh Foster (New York: Palgrave MacMillan, 2009), 170.

80. During the early 2000s, the South American Dance Network (Red Sudamericana de Danza)—which aims to connect practitioners and researchers across the Southern Cone and, more recently, dance communities across the global south— emerged as a principal forum for exchange and dialogue.

81. Savigliano, *Tango and the Political Economy of Passion*; Shea Murphy, *The People Have Never Stopped Dancing*; and Rebecca Rossen, *Dancing Jewish: Jewish Identity in American Modern and Postmodern Dance* (New York: Oxford, 2014).

82. Susan Leigh Foster argues for attending critically to the embodied nature of archival research in the introduction to *Choreographing History*, ed. Susan Leigh Foster (Bloomington: Indiana University Press, 1995), 3–21.

83. D. Soyini Madison, *Acts of Activism: Human Rights as Radical Performance* (Cambridge: Cambridge University Press, 2010), 23.

84. For a case study relevant to chapter 5, see Victoria Fortuna, "Between the Cultural Center and the *Villa*: Dance, Neoliberalism, and Silent Borders in Buenos Aires," in *The Oxford Handbook of Dance and Politics*, ed. Rebekah J. Kowal, Gerald Siegmund, and Randy Martin (New York: Oxford University Press, 2017), 371–94. As of this writing, I am developing a case study relevant to chapter 4 for separate publication tentatively titled, "Dancing Exclusion: Performance and the Politics of Exile in Fernando Solanas's *Tangos: El exilio de Gardel* (1985)," commissioned for inclusion in the volume *Theatre After Empire*, edited by Harvey Young and Megan Geigner.

CHAPTER 1

1. The Torcuato Di Tella Institute is subsequently referred to as the Di Tella.

2. For a historical discussion of this period, see María Estela Spinelli, *Los vencedores vencidos: El antiperonismo y la "revolución libertadora"* (Buenos Aires: Biblos, 2005).

3. Laura Podalsky, *Specular City: Transforming Culture, Consumption, and Space in Buenos Aires, 1955–1973* (Philadelphia: Temple University Press, 2004), 50.

4. Ibid., 150.

5. Jorge D'Urbano, "Sin crisis en el alma," *Panorama*, December 1966, 57. "Mientras los economistas hablaban de iliquidez y retracción del mercado, los argentinos hacíamos de la cultura un importante bien de consumo."

6. Manzano, *The Age of Youth in Argentina*, 100.

7. Ibid., 98. See also Isabella Cosse, *Pareja, sexualidad y familia en los años sesenta: Una revolución discreta en Buenos Aires* (Buenos Aires: Siglo XXI Editores, 2010).

8. Catalina H. Wainerman and Rebeca Barck de Raijman, *Sexismo en los libros de lectura de la escuela primaria* (Buenos Aires: IDES, 1987), 85–86.

9. Susana Zimmermann, *Cantos y exploraciones: Caminos de teatro-danza* (Buenos Aires: Editorial Balletin Dance, 2007), 96. "Estado de alerta."

10. While the movement vocabularies and choreographic strategies of *Polymorphias* and *Ana Kamien* drew on modern dance, they do not fall neatly into this category. As noted in this volume's introduction, the category of "contemporary" does not gain broader usage until the 1970s; however, the hybrid influences and experimental components of *Polymorphias* and *Ana Kamien* merit consideration under the term's broad umbrella. While her terminology shifts throughout the decade, Zimmermann notably used the category "danza contemporánea" in her 1964 article, "El mundo de la danza contemporánea." Featured in the March-April edition of *Mundo de la Danza* magazine, the piece describes Argentine contemporary dance as the "large group of dancers, choreographers, and teachers that desire to find new forms to express the emotions and sentiments of contemporary man" ("[el] grupo numeroso de bailarines, coreógrafos y maestros, deseosos de encontrar nuevas formas para expresar las emociones y sentimientos del hombre contemporáneo"), n.p., Private Collection of Estela Maris.

11. For a detailed discussion of *Tucumán Arde*'s featured works and testimonials of participants, see Ana Longoni and Mariano Mestman, *Del Di Tella a "Tucumán Arde": Vanguardia artística y política en el 68 argentino* (Buenos Aires: Eudeba, 2010), 178–236.

12. Ana Kamien, interview by author, Buenos Aires, July 5, 2011 and Susana Zimmermann, interview by author, Buenos Aires, March 20, 2011.

13. For an overview of Schottelius's career, see Victoria Fortuna, "Schottelius, Renate (1921–1998)," in *The Routledge Encyclopedia of Modernism* (New York: Taylor and Francis, 2016), https://www.rem.routledge.com/articles/schottelius-renate-1921-1998.

14. Kamien, interview by author. A prominent figure in the Argentine dance community, María Fux trained in classical ballet and midcentury modernist techniques. She studied in the United States with figures including Martha Graham, Louis Horst, and Merce Cunningham. In addition to her work in the concert dance field, Fux was central to the development of dance therapy in Argentina and has published extensively on the topic. See María Fux, *Primer encuentro con la danzaterapia* (Buenos Aires: Paidós, 1982).

15. According to Zimmermann's autobiography, Hoyer's classes incorporated intensive explorations of the body as a conduit of emotional drives. *Cantos y exploraciones*, 44. They emphasized what Susan Manning terms the expressionist principle of *Gestalt im Raum*, or "configuration of energy in space," Manning, *Ecstasy and the Demon*, 41.

16. Kamien, interview by author. Other participants included Oscar Araiz, Iris Scaccheri, Ana Labat, Estela Maris, and Doris Petroni, among others. For further discussion of Hoyer's classes and her impact on Argentine dancers, see Patricia Dorin, "Legados y continuidades: Derivaciones de una danza de expresión en Argentina," in *Pensar con la danza*, ed. Carlos Eduardo Sanabria Bohóriquez and Ana Carolina Ávila Pérez (Bogotá: Ministerio de Cultura de Colombia, Universidad de Bogotá Jorge Tadeo Lozano, Facultad de Ciencias Sociales, Departamento de Humanidades, 2014), 123–28.

17. Zimmermann, *Cantos y exploraciones*, 53.

18. Ana Kamien performed in the theater's inaugural performance in María Fux's contribution to the program. Kamien, interview by author.

19. A relatively prolific area of press coverage in the late 1950s and early 1960s, articles outlining the debate between definitions of modern dance versus ballet include Torres Pereyra, "La danza moderna: ¿Puede ser popular?," *Teatro Popular*, September 1958, 12, Private Collection of Estela Maris; "Danza moderna y danza clásica," *El Mundo*, June 23, 1960, n.p., Renate Schottelius Papers, Documentation Center of the General San Martín Municipal Theater; "La danza clásica y la danza moderna," *La Nación*, June 15, 1961, 24, Renate Schottelius Papers, Documentation Center of the General San Martín Municipal Theater; and "Polémica entre la danza clásica y moderna," *La Nación*, June 22, 1961, 24, Private Collection of Estela Maris.

20. Zimmermann, interview by author. "Clásico, neoclásico, [y] moderno, no un moderno ultra renovador, pero moderno."

21. For a historical narrative of the development of AADA, descriptions of important works, and reproductions of programs, see Silvia Kaehler, *Asociación Amigos de la Danza, 1962–1966* (Buenos Aires: Eudeba, 2013). Choreographers Oscar Araiz, Estela Maris, Rodolfo Dantón, Ana Itelman, Cecilia Bullaude, Ana Labat, Juan Falzone, Beatriz Amábile, Doris Petroni, and others presented work through AADA. In addition to producing original works, the organization also supported restaging works by Miriam Winslow and Dore Hoyer.

22. Croft, *Dancers as Diplomats*, 66. Though AADA works tended toward universalism, programs indicate that several ballet and modern dance pieces featured Argentine tango and rural themes, including Amalia Lozano's *Tango para una ciudad* (*Tango for a City*, 1962) and *La nueva tierra* (*The New World*, 1963, based on the conquest

narrative), Program for AADA, Buenos Aires: General San Martín Municipal Theater, June 11, 1962, Private Collection of Estela Maris; and Program for AADA, Buenos Aires: General San Martín Municipal Theater, November 25, 1963, Private Collection of Estela Maris. See also Beatriz Amábile and Doris Petroni's *El Tango* (1966) and Néstor Roygt's *La cautiva* (*The Captive*, 1966, based on Esteban Echeverría's 1837 epic poem, which depicted a white woman's capture by indigenous peoples on the rural plains), Program for AADA, Buenos Aires: General San Martín Municipal Theater, October 17, 1966, Private Collection of Estela Maris; and Program for AADA, Buenos Aires: General San Martín Municipal Theater, 1966, Documentation Center of the General San Martín Municipal Theater.

23. Though José Limón's company did not perform in Argentina during their 1954 South American State Department tour, the company later returned in 1960. See Melinda Copel, "The 1954 Limón Company Tour to South America: Goodwill Tour or Cold War Cultural Propaganda?," in *José Limón: The Artist Re-viewed*, ed. June Dunbar (New York: Routledge, 2003), 97. The Paul Taylor Dance Company performed in Buenos Aires under the auspices of the State Department in 1965.

24. Croft, *Dancers as Diplomats*, 66–67. See also Kowal, *How to Do Things with Dance*, 19–51.

25. Isse Moyano, *La danza moderna argentina cuenta su historia*, 97. "Se bailaban los grandes temas de la humanidad: la angustia, el dolor, el sufrimiento, era una cosa de post-guerra. Se bailaba Bach, Vivaldi, eran grandes temas, grandes gestos, grandes coreografías . . . . Empezamos a querer derribar todo eso, a hacer otras cosas. En parte porque yo no tenía acceso a ese mundo."

26. Quoted in Falcoff, "La danza moderna y contemporánea," 266.

27. Alberto Calvo, "Danza: Ana Kamien, la silla, el escobillón y los talentos," *Panorama*, November 10–16, 1970, 56, and Kamien, interview by author.

28. Isse Moyano, *La danza moderna argentina cuenta su historia*, 86.

29. Manzano, *The Age of Youth in Argentina*, 101.

30. Zimmermann, interview by author. "Concretar a través de acciones algo de lo que había estudiado."

31. For a comprehensive history of the Di Tella, see John King, *El Di Tella y el desarrollo cultural argentino en la década del sesenta* (Buenos Aires: Asunto Impreso Ediciones, 2007). For in-depth consideration of theater production at the Di Tella, see María Fernanda Pinta, *Teatro expandido en el Di Tella* (Buenos Aires: Biblos, 2013). For examinations of the Di Tella's visual arts production within the broader political context of the 1960s, see Inés Katzenstein and Andrea Giunta, eds. *Listen, Here, Now! Argentine Art of the 1960s: Writings of the Avant-Garde* (New York: The Museum of Modern Art, 2004); Andrea Giunta, *Avant-Garde, Internationalism, and Politics: Argentine Art in the Sixties*, trans. Peter Kahn (Durham, NC: Duke University Press, 2007); and Longoni and Mestman, *Del Di Tella a "Tucumán Arde."*

32. Longoni and Mestman, *Del Di Tella a "Tucumán Arde,"* 43.

33. Podalsky, *Specular City*, 138.

34. Kamien, interview by author. Roberto Villanueva, the director of the Di Tella's Audiovisual Experimentation Center, also noted the phenomenon of women waiting to put on miniskirts until they arrived at the Di Tella. See Podalsky, *Specular* City, 142.

35. According to Podalsky, in the early 1960s only women associated with the Di Tella wore miniskirts. See Podalsky, *Specular City*, 188.

36. Other notable dance works performed at the Di Tella include Oscar Araiz's *Crash* (1967) and Iris Scaccheri's *Oye, humanidad* (*Listen, Humanity*, 1969). Though

the Di Tella's visual arts, musical, and theatrical works have generated significant scholarly interest, few scholars have addressed its dance productions. For a brief discussion of *Danse Bouquet* in relationship to the broader development of pop art in the 1960s, see María Fernanda Pinta, "Pop! La puesta en escena de nuestro 'folklore urbano,'" *Caiana: Revista de Historia del Arte y Cultural Visual del Centro Argentino de Investigadores de Arte* 4 (2014): 3. In the same essay, Pinta also considers Graciela Martínez's *Jugamos en la bañera*? (1966), a solo piece performed entirely in a porcelain bathtub, within the Di Tella's vanguard tradition (45). Notably, Kamien and Marini were included in the catalog of artists featured in the exhibition *Radical Women: Latin American Art, 1960–1985*, curated by art historians Cecilia Fajardo-Hill and Andrea Giunta and presented at UCLA's Hammer Museum (September 15–December 31, 2017) and the Brooklyn Museum (March 16–July 8, 2018). In 2017, Ana Caterina Cora, Sofía Kauer, and Nicolás Licera Vidal presented *Danza actual, danza en el Di Tella (1962-1966)* at the Cooperation Cultural Center in Buenos Aires, a documentary and stage work that explores the work of dance artists at the center.

37. Ana Kamien and Marilú Marini, Program Notes for *Danse Bouquet*, Buenos Aires: Torcuato Di Tella Institute, September 23, 27, and 30 and October 4, 7, 14, and 18, 1965, Torcuato Di Tella Institute Archives, Torcuato Di Tella University, Audiovisual Experimentation Center. "Evitar todos los amaneramientos: los de la danza clásica y los de la moderna."

38. Ibid. The program uses the term "music hall," the British variety-show genre popular from the mid-1800s through the 1960s, to describe the piece's structure. In our interview, Kamien also cited the premiere of the Broadway musical comedy *Hello, Dolly!* in Buenos Aires as inspiration for *Danse Bouquet*. Kamien, interview by author.

39. Calvo, "Danza: Ana Kamien, la silla, el escobillón y los talentos," 57.

40. "Un ballet para 007," *Primera Plana*, September 21, 1965, 63.

41. Ibid. "Cursi."

42. "Vestida de novia," *Danse Bouquet*, Photograph by Leone Sonnino, Private Collection of Ana Kamien.

43. *Oh! Casta Diva* included a sketch called *Cascaflores (Flowercracker)* that playfully parodied Kamien's background in classical ballet. Set to a musical collage that included snippets of Tchaikovsky's "Waltz of the Flowers" from *The Nutcracker* (hence the clever title), Kamien performed a series of grand jetés (leaps with both legs extended in a split) clad in pointe shoes and a white tutu. After a few successfully executed jumps, she began to stumble and fall in comedic fashion, playfully calling attention to classical ballet's emphasis on technical perfection. Kamien, interview by author.

44. For a foundational study of the New York City-based work most closely associated with the postmodern turn, see Sally Banes, *Democracy's Body: Judson Dance Theatre, 1962–1964* (Durham, NC: Duke University Press, 1993).

45. In addition to her work as a dancer and choreographer with AADA, during the mid-1960s Zimmermann also performed with and presented works as part of the group Ballet de Hoy (Ballet of Today) that she cofounded with Oscar Araiz and Ana Labat.

46. Zimmermann, *Cantos y exploraciones*, 75.

47. Ibid., 74–75. "No se me hubiera ocurrido presentarlo en Amigos de la Danza, porque ese era un santuario en el que el lenguaje era más formal."

48. King, *El Di Tella*, 108.

49. Podalsky, *Specular City*, 142.

50. Ezequiel Lozano, *Sexualidades disidentes en el teatro: Buenos Aires, años 60* (Buenos Aires: Editorial Biblos, 2015), 170.

51. Other notable instances of censorship during Onganía's government included the banning, by municipal decree, of the opera *Bomarzo* in July 1967 on the basis of scenes containing sexual content. Alberto Ginastera, a well-respected composer who directed the Di Tella's music department, wrote the opera. It premiered in Washington, DC, in May 1967, though the Argentine government banned the work prior to its scheduled national premiere at the Colón Theater in August. For an extended discussion of these events, see Esteban Buch, *The Bomarzo affair: Ópera, perversión y dictadura* (Buenos Aires: Adriana Hidalgo Editora, 2003). In 1967 Onganía's government also recommended the removal of Oscar Araiz's acclaimed *La consagración de la primavera* (*The Rite of Spring*, 1966) from the Colón's repertoire, once again on the basis of sexual content, though the government did not issue an official decree. Onganía saw the work at the Colón Theater on May 17, 1967, at a performance in honor of Japanese Prince Akihito and Princess Michiko's visit to Buenos Aires. For discussions of the censorship of Araiz's *Consagración*, see Victoria Fortuna, "Dancing Argentine Modernity," 49–54. For a consideration of the *Consagración* case alongside Ana Itelman's *Phaedra*, see Juan Ignacio Vallejos, "Dance, Sexuality, and Utopian Subversion Under the Argentine Dictatorship of the 1960s: The Case of Oscar Araiz's *The Rite of Spring* and Ana Itelman's *Phaedra*," *Dance Research Journal* 48.2 (2016): 61–79. For a broader overview of the explicit and implicit valences of censorship between 1966 and 1973 in Buenos Aires, see Podalsky, *Specular City*, 198–207.

52. For additional discussion of the censure of Plate's *Baño* and the Di Tella's response, see Podalsky, *Specular City*, 143; Pinta, *Teatro expandido*, 152–62; and Lozano, *Sexualidades disidentes*, 171–73.

53. Zimmermann, *Cantos y exploraciones*, 93.

54. Susana Zimmermann, *El laboratorio de danza y movimiento creativo* (Buenos Aires: Editorial Hvmanitas, 1983), 37. "Es un lugar donde se prueba, se experimenta, se analiza, se transforma y finalmente se crean nuevas esencias, nuevas materias."

55. Ibid., 37–38. "Una exploración profunda del cuerpo." In the text, Zimmermann foregrounds her discussion of her improvisation methods with a survey of philosophical texts, physical practices (including hatha yoga and massage), and dance forms that have been influential in her conception of the body.

56. Zimmermann, *Cantos y exploraciones*, 76–77.

57. Ibid., 76–77.

58. Ibid., 76.

59. Ibid., 77. "compromiso ético-político."

60. Susana Zimmermann and Laboratorio de Danza, Program Notes for *Polymorphias*, Buenos Aires: Torcuato Di Tella Institute, 1969, Torcuato Di Tella Institute Archives, Torcuato Di Tella University, Audiovisual Experimentation Center. "Es recuperar la capacidad de creación humana, rompiendo el esquema tradicional: coreógrafo-intérprete-público como tres entes separados e integrar estos tres elementos en una nueva interpretación dinámica . . . se propone crear-entre-todos-un-idioma-nuevo-para-un-hombre-nuevo."

61. See Che Guevara, *El socialismo y el hombre en Cuba* (Atlanta: Pathfinder Press, 1992). Argentine cultural historian Hugo Vezzetti aptly points out that the notion of the "new man" extends beyond Latin American revolutionary discourse.

He locates the phrase's roots in Christian rhetoric, particularly the replacement of the "old man" (the fall of Adam and Eve) with the "new man" baptized in the church. See *Sobre la violencia revolucionaria: Memorias y olvidos* (Buenos Aires: Siglo XXI Editores, 2009), 174.

62. It is worth noting that as Zimmermann's Laboratorio de Danza echoed Cuban revolutionary language to shape its work, in Cuba *técnica cubana*, or Cuban contemporary dance, developed following the Revolution as part of the mandate to create national culture that supported the Revolution's principles. For a comprehensive discussion of the rise and development of the form, see John, *Contemporary Dance in Cuba*.

63. Andrea Andújar, prologue to *De minifaldas, militancias y revoluciones: Exploraciones sobre los 70 en la Argentina*, ed. by Andrea Andújar, et al. (Buenos Aires: Ediciones Luxemburg, 2009), 11. "Conceptos y palabras tales como revolución, socialismo en sus diferentes variantes, la unidad en la acción, liberación, victoria, entre otras, se incorporaron de manera definitiva al lenguaje de la época."

64. For a discussion of partnerships between artists and political groups in the late 1960s, see Giunta, *Avante-Garde*, 234–78, and Longoni and Mestman, *Del Di Tella a "Tucumán Arde*,*"* 302–16. For a discussion of the politicization of theater during this time period, see Lorena Verzero, *Teatro militante: Radicalización artística y política en los años 70* (Buenos Aires: Editorial Biblos, 2013), 47–68.

65. Giunta, *Avant-Garde*, 272.

66. Longoni and Mestman, *Del Di Tella a "Tucumán Arde*,*"* 304. "La transformación de la sociedad (inscribiéndose en la oleada revolucionaria) y al mismo tiempo a la del campo artístico (destruyendo el mito burgués del arte, el concepto de la obra única para el goce personal, etc.)."

67. The Di Tella, notably, was not immune from critique following the politicized shift in the art field. Some members of the left accused the Di Tella of acting as an instrument of imperial and capitalist control, given its close relationship with elite art circles in the United States and Europe and its national relationship to private industry—which is how leftist filmmakers Fernando Solanas and Octavio Getino depicted the Di Tella in the 1968 documentary *La hora de los hornos* (*The Hour of the Furnaces*). See Podalsky, *Specular City*, 142–44.

68. Zimmermann, *El laboratorio de danza*, 37. "una mejor relación consigo mismo y con el otro."

69. Zimmermann, *Cantos y exploraciones*, 87, and Zimmermann, interview by author. Upon her return to Buenos Aires, Zimmermann was invited to join the first, though short-lived, city-supported contemporary dance company. Housed in the San Martín Theater and directed by Oscar Araiz, the Ballet del San Martín (San Martín Ballet, 1968–71) represented contemporary dance's first permanent residency in a public theater and employed many of AADA's most talented dancers. For an overview of Araiz's prolific career, see Victoria Fortuna, "Araiz, Oscar (1940–)" in *The Routledge Encyclopedia of Modernism* (New York: Taylor and Francis, 2016), https://www.rem.routledge.com/articles/araiz-oscar-1940.

70. "Polyzimmermann: todos para todos," *Panorama*, April 29–May 5, 1969, 57; Emilio Stevanovitch, "Polymorphias," *Talía*, 1969, 3, Private Collection of Susana Zimmermann; "Un llamado patético," *La Razón*, April 28, 1969, n.p., Private Collection of Susana Zimmermann.

71. Zimmermann, *Cantos y exploraciones*, 96. "La historia de la comunicación—incomunicación." The score is reprinted in its entirety in this book.

72. Ibid. "Masa anónima."

73. Susana Zimmermann, *Teatro-danza creaciones*, Buenos Aires: Los Teatros de San Telmo, July 1981, DVD, Private Collection of Susana Zimmermann.
74. Zimmermann, *Cantos y exploraciones*, 96–97.
75. Zimmermann, *Teatro-danza creaciones*.
76. Zimmermann, *Cantos y exploraciones*, 97. "hambre, sed o miedo."
77. Zimmermann, interview by author.
78. Anonymous letter, Private Collection of Susana Zimmermann. "Al final, en Dies Irae, cuando bajan y se juntan con nosotros y piden ayuda, me pasó una cosa muy extraña. Uno de los muchachos entro en mi fila y la fue recorriendo muy despacio. Era desesperante verlo con las manos abiertas pidiendo, exigiendo otra mano . . . . Al lado mío había un tipo de traje gris, corbata, zapatos lustrados con su señora gorda. Se paró delante de él . . . . El hombre del traje gris los miraba y bajaba los ojos, las manos le temblaban . . . . Estaba lívido, hubiera dado cualquier cosa por estar a un millón de kilómetros. No pude más. Le alargué yo mi mano y el pibe se agarró con fuerza . . . . En ese momento no pensé en nada solamente sentí. Yo tenía que ayudarlo porque si no él, yo y todos nos íbamos al pozo."
79. Zimmermann, *Cantos y exploraciones*, 96. "Estado de alerta."
80. Michael Rothberg, *Multidirectional Memory: Remembering the Holocaust in the Age of Decolonization* (Stanford, CA: Stanford University Press, 2009), 17.
81. The Di Tella also presented *Polymorphias* in 1970 when Penderecki visited Buenos Aires. Alberto Ginastera, the Argentine composer who directed the Di Tella's music department, arranged the performance. Zimmermann, *Cantos y exploraciones*, 95.
82. Zimmermann, interview by author.
83. Manuel Román and Adolfo Tessari, "Instituto Di Tella: ¿Muerte o transfiguración?" *Panorama*, June 30-July 6, 1970, 48. "Las cosas han sido planteadas a nivel económico, y, analizándolas así, tienen razón. Analizando las cosas a nivel cultural, no sé si conscientemente o no, la supresión de Florida [el Instituto] implica la destrucción de un estilo de vida."
84. N. C., "Por amor al arte," *Clarín Revista*, March 25, 1973, 10–11.
85. Ibid.
86. Kamien, interview by author; Estela Maris, interview by author, Mar del Plata, September 25, 2011; and Silvia Kaehler, interview by author, Buenos Aires, September 22, 2011. A 1973 write-up of the CCGSM programming also emphasized the cramped quarters, N. C. "Por amor al arte," 11.
87. Kamien, interview by author. "Una modernidad mía, ese lenguaje, no hecho de Graham."
88. Ibid., "El otro mundo de la danza."
89. Ibid., and *Expodanza 70*, Arranged by Leone Sonnino, 1970, mp3, Private Collection of Ana Kamien. "Destajo."
90. A strong advocate for dance, Freixá also facilitated the establishment of the contemporary dance companies of the San Martín Theater in 1968 and 1977.
91. *Expodanza 70*. "Yo, lamentablemente, lo que sé desde que ocupo de la Secretaría de la Cultura es que no tengo tiempo realmente para la cultura."
92. For a discussion of an earlier representation of dancers as workers, in this case Colón Theater Ballet dancers in the 1949 film *Mujeres que bailan*, see María Eugenia Cadús, "'¿Dejarás el baile por mí?': La representación de la bailarina como trabajadora en *Mujeres que bailan* de Manuel Romero," *Cultura: Debates y perspectivas de un mundo en cambio* 9 (2015): 49–65.

93. "Sigue 'Expodanza' su positivo desarrollo," no publication visible in clipping, May 28, 1970, n.p., Private Collection of Ana Kamien. "Símbolo de los medios puestos a su disposición."
94. Calvo, "Danza: Ana Kamien, la silla, el escobillón y los talentos," 57. "¡Hasta cuándo van a seguir quejándose!"
95. Kamien, interview by author.
96. Stewart O'Nan, "Songs," in *The Vietnam Reader: The Definitive Collection of American Fiction and Nonfiction on the War*, ed. Stewart O'Nan (New York: Anchor Books, 1998), 282.
97. Kamien, interview by author. "Tomo el escobillón y me lo pongo acá y me paseo como si fuera un centinela que se está paseando por el cuartel haciendo guardia. Y después los pelos del escobillón los apunto para atrás y me dirijo al público y el palo se convierte en un arma. Todo esto con la "Marcha fúnebre" . . . . En un determinado momento lo dejo en mitad del escenario [y] yo me sentaba [y] yo empiezo a marchar así también, pero sentada en el piso con las piernas extendidas como el paso de ganso alemán y voy rodeando el escobillón que esta paradito ahí. Me empiezo a apurar y cuando llego al centro que está el palo me quedo amarrada así. Fue escobillón, fue arma, fue muleta y fue mi cruz. Porque me agarré del palo, enlacé las manos con el escobillón, yo me voy de espaldas al público y me voy para el fondo. Y entonces avanzo y voy marchando y se siente el apunten, ¡fuego! Y apagón y me fusilan, no me puedo escapar."
98. Calvo, "Danza: Ana Kamien, la silla, el escobillón y los talentos," 57. "el objeto más célebre que acompañó a la Kamien en sus zapatetas fue el escobillón que enarboló—cruz, fusil, muleta, acaso también símbolo de los gobernantes autoritarios—en su espectáculo para Expodanza."
99. This stipulation was listed in the Montoneros official communication regarding the execution. See "Comunicado 3," *La Causa Peronista* 9, September 3, 1974, 30, *El Topo Blindado*, accessed February 10, 2018, http://eltopoblindado.com/opm-peronistas/montoneros/montoneros-prensa/la-causa-peronista-n-9/.
100. For a discussion of the cultural and memory politics around Aramburu's assassination, see Beatriz Sarlo, *La pasión y la excepción: Eva, Borges y el asesinato de Aramburu* (Buenos Aires: Siglo XXI Editores, 2009). See also, Donna J. Guy, "Life and the Commodification of Death in Argentina: Juan and Eva Perón," in *Death, Dismemberment and Memory: Body Politics in Latin America*, ed. Lyman L. Johnson (Albuquerque: University of New Mexico Press, 2004), 245–72.

CHAPTER 2

1. *Panorama*, March 28–April 3, 1972. "¿Qué cara tiene la izquierda Argentina?"
2. Ibid., "La nueva ofensiva de la guerrilla."
3. See Sebastián Carassai's analysis of the middle class's growing disapproval of militant movements across the early 1970s, *The Argentine Silent Majority: Middle Classes, Politics, Violence, and Memory in the Seventies* (Durham, NC: Duke University Press, 2014), 102–50.
4. Here we might recall the Montoneros' kidnapping and later execution of former President Pedro Eugenio Aramburu that occurred within days of the premiere of Ana Kamien's *Ana Kamien* on May 29, 1970.
5. See Hugo Vezzetti, *Pasado y presente: Guerra, dictadura, y sociedad en Argentina* (Buenos Aires: Siglo XXI Editores, 2002), 121–28, and *Sobre la violencia revolucionaria*, 44–53.

6. In this chapter "militate" refers primarily to acting on behalf of defined political organizations, but it is worth noting that the term was and is employed more broadly to signal commitment to and activist action on behalf of a range of causes and interests.

7. Verzero, *Teatro militante*, 127. "Experiencias culturales afines en su ideario revolucionario o social."

8. Vezzetti, *Sobre la violencia revolucionaria*, 105. "¿Qué actos, conductas, decisiones, pasiones, deben ser legítimamente incluidos en el rubro de una obra o una acción militante revolucionaria?"

9. Giunta, *Avant-Garde*, 272, and Longoni and Mestman, *Del Di Tella a "Tucumán Arde,"* 303–4.

10. Larasati, *The Dance That Makes You Vanish*, xxii.

11. Heinrich photographed many famous national and international subjects, including Eva Perón, singer Mercedes Sosa, film actress Tita Merello, and dancer Katherine Dunham, among others.

12. Gabriel Rot, "Entrevista a Alicia Sanguinetti," in *El Devotazo: Alicia Sanguinetti Fotografías*, comp. Gabriel Rot (Buenos Aires: El Topo Blindado, 2013), 13.

13. Ana Longoni, "El FATRAC, frente cultural del PRT/ERP," *Lucha Armada en la Argentina* no. 4 (2006): 21.

14. The FATRAC's documented activities were linked most closely with the visual art community. For a discussion of their interventions, see Longoni "El FATRAC" and Longoni and Mestman, *Del Di Tella a "Tucumán Arde,"* 135–39.

15. For an extensive documentary on the history of the PRT-ERP, see Aldo Getino, Laura Lagar, Omar Neri, Mónica Simoncini, and Susana Vázquez, *Gaviotas blindadas: historias del PRT-ERP* (Córdoba: Mascaró Cine Americano, 2007).

16. Alicia Sanguinetti, interview by author, Buenos Aires, October 7, 2011.

17. "A Miembros de una célula extremista dictan prisión," *Clarín*, September 7, 1971, 42. Unfortunately, I was unable to interview Maucieri. Hodgers and Sanguinetti indicate that they lost touch with her. Her dance background is equally unclear, though programs indicate that she was a member of María Fux's dance group in 1965, María Fux, Program for Recital, November 22, 1965, Buenos Aires: General San Martín Municipal Theater, Documentation Center of the General San Martín Municipal Theater.

18. There are conflicting reports as to whether they intended to destroy the stage the night before as a symbolic act, or during the parade itself. *Clarín*'s report on the group's arrest states that they were planning to attack during the parade, "A Miembros de una célula extremista dictan prisión," 42. In interviews, Sanguinetti maintains that they planned to destroy the stage the evening before the parade. See Rot, "Entrevista a Alicia Sanguinetti," 14, and Daniel Enzetti, "Instantáneas de una época en la que lo única irreal eran las rejas," *Tiempo Argentino*, August 19, 2013, http://www.infonews.com/nota/92807/instantaneas-de-una-epoca-en-la-que-lo. The plan is also recounted in Santiago Garaño and Werner Pertot, *Detenidos-aparecidos: presas y presos políticos desde Trelew a la dictadura* (Buenos Aires: Biblos, 2007) 32–33, though in that source President Juan María Bordaberry (1972–76) is incorrectly listed as then president of Uruguay.

19. Enzetti, "Instantáneas."

20. In our interview, Hodgers stated that she was incarcerated with Maucieri, as well as Sanguinetti, at Villa Devoto in 1971. Silvia Hodgers, Skype interview by author, Geneva and Oberlin, August 9, 2014. Sanguinetti did not specifically mention Maucieri in our interviews, but in Rot's published interview she states that the

whole group involved in the plan ended up at Villa Devoto. See Rot, "Entrevista a Alicia Sanguinetti," 14.

21. Laura Lifschitz, "Silvia Hodgers: La danza y la militancia política," *Tiempo Argentino*, October 24, 2010, accessed September 9, 2011, http://tiempo. elargentino.com/notas/danza-y-militancia-politica (site discontinued).

22. Hodgers, interview by author.

23. Ibid.

24. Ibid., "Si la tienen que torturar, tortúrenla pero no la violen."

25. It remains unclear whether Maucieri was released from Villa Devoto prior to the others' transfer.

26. Mariana Arruti, *Trelew: La fuga que fue masacre* (Buenos Aires: Fundación Alumbrar, 2004), DVD.

27. Ibid. The documentary features the testimonies of imprisoned militants of various associations (many high-ranking leaders)—including Hodgers and Sanguinetti (the only female militants represented)—and local collaborators to narrate the formulation, execution, and ultimate failure of the escape plan. Throughout the documentary, the former militants are identified by organizational affiliation alone; no professions or personal histories beyond militancy (and militant couples) are mentioned, a narrative choice that reflects militant organizations' emphasis on anonymity and total dedication to the revolutionary cause.

28. Hodgers, interview by author.

29. Arruti, *Trelew: La fuga que fue masacre*.

30. Ibid., and Hodgers, interview by author.

31. *Zamba* is a form of folkloric music and dance. For a historical overview of its development and adaptation as a national form in Argentina, see Saúl Domínguez Zaldívar, *La música de nuestra tierra la zamba: Historia, autores, y letras* (Buenos Aires: Imaginador, 1998). For a discussion of militant *zamba* songs, see Carlos Molinero and Pablo Vila, "A Brief History of the Militant Song Movement in Argentina," in *The Militant Song Movement in Latin America: Chile, Uruguay, and Argentina*, edited by Pablo Vila (Lanham, MD: Lexington Books, 2014), 193–228.

32. Arruti, *Trelew: La fuga que fue masacre*. "'¿Con qué armas pelearemos? Con las que les quitaremos,' dicen que gritó."

33. Ibid. "Había que generar en el penal determinados tipos de movimientos que no llamaran la atención fundamentalmente de la guardia interna. Se empezó a hacer cosas que no se hacían habitualmente, peñas, guitarreadas, y cánticos. Así que cuando se produjera la fuga, para ellos fuera normal que en el penal hubiera bullicio, canto, movimiento."

34. Katrina Hazzard-Gordon, *Jookin': The Rise of Social Dance Formations in African American Culture* (Philadelphia: Temple University Press, 2010), 34.

35. Hodgers, interview by author.

36. Alicia Sanguinetti, interview by author, Buenos Aires, July 21, 2014. "Gimnasia común."

37. Arruti, *Trelew: La fuga que fue masacre*.

38. Ibid., "La marcha agachada."

39. Susana Barco, a woman imprisoned at Villa Devoto during these years, describes these performances in some detail in her testimony featured in Viviana Beguán, ed., *Nosotras, presas políticas* (Buenos Aires: Nuestra America, 2006), 332–33.

40. Garaño and Pertot, *Detenidos-aparecidos*, 31.

41. Ibid., 31–32.

42. Arruti, *Trelew: La fuga que fue masacre*.

43. Francisco Urondo, *La patria fusilada* (Buenos Aires: Ediciones de Crisis, 1973), 46. See also Tomás Eloy Martínez, *La pasión según Trelew* (Buenos Aires: Granica Editor, 1973), 66–67.

44. Garaño and Pertot, *Detenidos-aparecidos*, 53–55.

45. Martínez, *La pasión según Trelew*, 70–75.

46. Urondo, *La patria fusilada*, 54–56.

47. Ibid., 91. See also the diagram of the cells in Martínez, *La pasión según Trelew*, 98.

48. Urondo, *La patria fusilada*, 103. Berger, Camps, and Haidar were all disappeared during the last military dictatorship. A career military official, Sosa was sentenced to life in prison for the Trelew murders on October 15, 2012, and he died under house arrest in 2016.

49. Rot, "Entrevista a Alicia Sanguinetti," 15.

50. For an account of the Ezeiza Massacre, see Horacio Verbitsky, *Ezeiza* (Buenos Aires: Editorial Planeta Argentina, 1995).

51. Sanguinetti, interview by author, 2011.

52. Hodgers, interview by author. Fernández Baños worked in the intelligence sector of the PRT-ERP.

53. Verzero, *Teatro militante*, 127. "Experiencias culturales afines en su ideario revolucionario o social."

54. Vivian Luz, Olkar Ramirez, and Milka Truol continued careers in contemporary dance and Filiberto Mugnani became a successful photographer.

55. For a discussion of theater projects, see Verzero, *Teatro militante*, 219–64. For a discussion of the visual arts, see Ana Longoni, *Vanguardia y revolución: Arte e izquierdas en la Argentina de los sesenta-setenta* (Buenos Aires: Ariel, 2014). For discussions of popular music's intersections with militancy in Argentina, Uruguay, and Chile, see Pablo Vila, ed., *The Militant Song Movement in Latin America: Chile, Uruguay, and Argentina* (Lanham, MD: Lexington Books, 2014).

56. Vivian Luz, interview by author, Buenos Aires, November 3, 2010. "Nos juntó a cinco personas entre veinte y treinta años, a expresar esa inquietud que teníamos, que era en ese momento del imperialismo yanqui, la guerra de Vietnam, todas las preocupaciones de nuestra época y que estábamos muy imbuidos."

57. Cuca Taburelli, Skype interview by author, Bogotá and Oberlin, September 12, 2014.

58. Ibid.

59. Milka Truol, interview by author, Buenos Aires, April 9, 2011.

60. Pulso Cinco Danza Teatro, Photographs from *Preludio para un final*, Buenos Aires: Teatron, November 1973, Private Collection of Cuca Taburelli.

61. Pulso Cinco Danza Teatro, Program for *Preludio para un final*, Buenos Aires: Teatron, November 1973, Private Collection of Vivian Luz.

62. Cuca Taburelli, email message to author, September 25, 2014. "Removiendo el pasado."

63. Taburelli's autobiographical text, *Una valija de vida: cuarenta años de danzateatro* (Bogotá: Goethe-Institut Kolumbien, 2010), 17, features several photographs of the restaged work. In a revision of the original version, dancers clad in colorful unitards read and sift through shreds of newspapers scattered throughout the stage.

64. Their daughters, Federica Pais and Ernestina Pais, are noted television anchors. In our interview, Truol mentioned that she choreographed a dance based on the loss of her husband as a method of mourning; however, she did not recall the details of the piece itself. Truol, interview by author.

65. Maris, interview by author.
66. *Perfiles* also included pieces choreographed by Rodolfo Dantón and performed by Maris. Based on the programs, *Juana Azurduy* was presented as an individual work in December 1973 on a shared program with Rodolfo Dantón at the Buenos Aires Municipal Theater located in the Palermo Rose Garden. Estela Maris, Program for Recitales en el Lago, December 20, 1973, Buenos Aires: Buenos Aires Municipal Theater, Private Collection of Estela Maris.
67. Maris, interview by author. "La mujer de nuestra historia que me parece más ejemplar."
68. Asunción Larvin, "Juana Azurduy de Padilla (c. 1780–1862)," in *The Oxford Encyclopedia of Women in World History* (Oxford University Press, 2008), accessed October 29, 2016, http://www. oxfordreference.com/view/10.1093/acref/9780195148909.001.0001/ acref-9780195148909-e-71?rskey=PFy5U4&result=61.
69. Ibid.
70. For a discussion of the history and politics of replacing the Columbus statue with one of Azurduy, see Luis Padín, ed., *El vuelco latinoamericano: De Cristóbal Colón a Juana Azurduy* (Buenos Aires: Ediciones de la UNLa, 2015). Under President Maurico Macri's administration (December 2015–), the statue was moved to the Plaza del Correo.
71. Maris, interview by author, and Isse Moyano, *La danza moderna argentina cuenta su historia*, 69.
72. Estela Maris, Program for Recitales en el Lago. In our interview, Maris was not able to recall more specific details of the movement of the piece.
73. Estela Maris, Photograph from *Juana Azurduy*, Buenos Aires: General San Martín Cultural Center, June 1973, Private Collection of Estela Maris.
74. Fernando de Toro, "Ideología y teatro épico en *Santa Juana de América*," *Latin American Theatre Review* 14, no. 1 (1980): 57.
75. Andrés Lizárraga, *Santa Juana de América* (Havana: Casa de las Américas, 1968), 124. "Esta guerra no terminó!"
76. De Toro, "Ideología y teatro épico en *Santa Juana de América*," 62. "Incita directamente a la acción armada como única vía revolucionaria."
77. "Heroica muerte de Padilla," *Estrella Roja*, no. 25, September 21, 1973, 21–22, *Ruinas Digitales*, accessed September 4, 2016, http://www.ruinasdigitales.com/ revistas/EstrellaRoja%2025.pdf.
78. For discussion of how militant groups invoked independence-era heroes, see Jennifer L. Schaefer, "Rebels, Martyrs, Heroes: Authoritarianism and Youth Culture in Argentina, 1966–1983" (PhD diss., Emory University, 2015), 220.
79. Berta Wexler, *Juana Azurduy y las mujeres en la revolución altoperuana* (Sucre: Centro "Juana Azurduy," 2002), 79. "Justificar su carácter varonil."
80. Ibid., 84.
81. Ibid. "Esta incorporación oficial y la incorporación de la madre tierra como la Pachamama, es hacer el imaginario de 'un nosotros' con la figura de la madre."
82. Andújar, prologue to *De minifaldas, militancias y revoluciones*, 12–13.
83. Marta Vassallo, "Militancia y transgresión," in *De minifaldas, militancias y revoluciones*, ed. Andrea Andújar et al. (Buenos Aires: Ediciones Luxemburg, 2009), 26. "'Célula básica' de afecto y acción." Militant groups privileged constructions of virile masculinity (with Guevara as the main referent) and explicitly rejected homosexuality. The experience of gay and lesbian militants in the Latin American left remains an under-researched area. For an analysis of the Brazilian context, see

James N. Green, "'Who is the Macho Who Wants to Kill Me?' Male Homosexuality, Revolutionary Masculinity, and the Brazilian Armed Struggle of the 1960s and 1970s," *Hispanic American Historical Review* 92, no. 3 (2012): 437–69.

84. Isabella Cosse, "Infidelities: Morality, Revolution, and Sexuality in Left-Wing Guerilla Organizations in 1960s and 1970s Argentina," *Journal of the History of Sexuality* 23, no. 3 (2014): 419.

85. Cosse, *Pareja, sexualidad y familia en los años sesenta*, 146.

86. Felitti, "Poner el cuerpo," 77.

87. For a collection of testimonies of female militants, see Marta Diana, *Mujeres guerrilleras: La militancia de los setenta en el testimonio de sus protagonistas* (Buenos Aires: Planeta, 1996). For specific consideration of gender and sexuality in the PRT-ERP, see Paola Martínez, *Género, política y revolución en los años setenta: Las mujeres del PRT-ERP* (Buenos Aires: Imago Mundi, 2009).

88. Maris, interview by author and Vassallo, "Militancia y transgresión," 26.

89. Maris, interview by author.

90. Vezzetti, *Pasado y presente*, 121–28, and *Sobre la violencia revolucionaria*, 44–53.

91. Zimmermann, interview by author.

92. Alicia Muñoz, "Por la desaparición de casi todos sus elencos, los bailarines piden auxilio," *Clarín*, April 3, 1975, n.p., Private Collection of Estela Maris.

CHAPTER 3

1. "La fantástica guerra del cuerpo humano contra sus enemigos," *Gente*, June 30, 1977, 26.

2. Ibid.

3. As considered in the previous chapter, practices of forced disappearance and torture had already begun during the early 1970s through the Triple A; however, the scale and intensity of state violence increased dramatically following the 1976 coup.

4. Quoted in Amnesty International, *Report on an Amnesty International Mission to Argentina 6–15 November 1976* (Middlesex: Hill and Garwood Ltd, 1977), 34–35, accessed June 14, 2016, https://www.amnesty.org/en/documents/amr13/083/ 1977/en/.

5. For thorough historical analysis of this period, see David Rock, *Authoritarian Argentina: The Nationalist Movement, Its History and Its Impact* (Berkeley: University of California Press, 1993).

6. Ana María Stekelman, interview by author, Buenos Aires, May 30, 2011. "Es ese temor que te mete por los poros."

7. Taylor, *Disappearing Acts*, 123.

8. Francine Masiello, "La Argentina durante el Proceso: Las múltiples resistencias de la cultura," in *Ficción y política: la narrativa argentina durante el proceso militar*, ed. Daniel Balderston (Buenos Aires: Alianza Editorial, 1987), 13. "La ventaja del espacio marginal."

9. Ibid.. "Un refugio seguro tanto para las oposiciones espontáneas como para las planificadas."

10. Recall the instances of censorship under Juan Carlos Onganía's "Argentine Revolution" (1966–70), particularly the recommended removal of Araiz's acclaimed *La consagración de la primavera* (*The Rite of Spring*, 1966) from the Colón Theater's repertoire in 1967. See Fortuna, "Dancing Argentine Modernity," and Vallejos, "Dance, Sexuality, and Utopian Subversion Under the Argentine Dictatorship of the 1960s."

11. Tambutti, interview by author. "¿Quién va a perseguir a tres coreógrafos que quieren bailar en un cuarto?"
12. Isse Moyano, *La danza moderna argentina cuenta su historia*, 154. "La intensidad política que había acompañado a nuestra generación se iba a transformar en una asfixiante dictadura militar que nos pondría en suspenso, y ante aquella mezcla de perplejidad, incredulidad y terror se tornaba necesario encontrar un significado y un sentido para quienes no habíamos asumido un lugar en la lucha política. Lo que ocurrió en esos años tuvo aquel oscuro telón de fondo. Comenzamos a buscar un sentido en ésta, nuestra minúscula historia como grupo de danza independiente . . . . En pequeños teatros como el Teatro Payró, el Teatro Planeta, y otros similares, nos fuimos creando un refugio del horror."
13. Ana Kamien, interview by author.
14. Isse Moyano, *La danza moderna argentina cuenta su historia*, 103. "Los estudios de la danza eran lugares relativamente seguros. Creo que más seguros que los lugares de teatro donde se usa la palabra y se dicen cosas. Eran lugares de reunión, los estudios estaban llenos de chicos. Aunque parezca raro estaban llenos de muchachos; los muchachos se sentían seguros, era un lugar donde estaban aceptados en forma y condición. Los chicos sentían que podían expresarse, que podían estar, que se podían mostrar de todas formas posibles. Eran, yo creo, asilos culturales y de expresión, era un gran boom." While "muchachos" can be inclusive of men and women, the context and language of this quote strongly suggest that Kamien is referring to men.
15. Graham-Jones, *Exorcising History*, 17.
16. Masiello, "La Argentina durante el Proceso," 13.
17. Dance scholars trace the anxiety around the male body on the Western concert stage to the rise of the European middle classes around the turn of the nineteenth century. Where men dominated classical ballet in the pre-Romantic era, by the late 1840s, the bourgeois decadence that ballet signaled conflicted with dominant conceptions of "virile" middle- and working-class masculinity. See Ramsay Burt, *The Male Dancer: Bodies, Spectacle, Sexualities* (New York: Routledge, 1995) and Lynn Garafola, ed. *Rethinking the Sylph: New Perspectives on the Romantic Ballet* (Middletown, CT: Wesleyan University Press, 1997).
18. Judith Hamera, *Dancing Communities: Performance, Difference and Connection in the Global City* (New York: Palgrave, 2007), 117.
19. Taylor, *Disappearing Acts*, 96.
20. Frank Graziano, *Divine Violence: Spectacle, Psychosexuality, and Radical Christianity in the Argentine "Dirty War"* (Boulder, CO: Westview Press, 1992), 68.
21. Taylor, *Disappearing Acts*, 156.
22. Alicia Muñoz, interview by author, Buenos Aires, December 13, 2010. "Respirar un poco."
23. Ibid. "Todavía no hemos logrado la revolución. Todavía no hemos logrado la libertad."
24. Ibid. "Los docentes decían que mi escuela era un oasis."
25. Ibid. "Un día me llamaron por teléfono para pedirme los nombres de los docentes que habían hecho un paro, entonces yo les dije, señor, yo no tengo ningún inconveniente en darle los nombres, yo creo que usted me entienda, que por teléfono yo no sé si usted es quien dice que es, a mí me encantaría, yo no tengo ningún problema, yo le voy a dar los nombres de las personas pero ¿por qué usted no se presenta en la escuela?"

26. Ibid. "En ese sentido vas manejando las cosas, pero te digo realmente cada vez que yo salía de la escuela yo me fijaba si no había un [Ford] Falcon parado."

27. Rivera-Servera, *Performing Queer Latinidad*, 141.

28. One of the theater's longest-serving directors, Staiff held this position from 1971–73, 1976–89, and 1998–2010. The company became known as the Ballet Contemporáneo in the late 1980s. In this chapter I employ the name, Grupo de Danza Contemporánea, in use during the period under consideration.

29. Stekelman, interview by author. "ser coreógrafa y hacer mi grupo porque somos personas criadas en el miedo."

30. Mónica Fracchia, interview by author, Buenos Aires, October 21, 2010. "El lugar era una especie de reducto intocable donde no teníamos censura, o nos subestimaban."

31. Stekelman, interview by author. "Isla."

32. Ibid. "No era la realidad que había afuera. Lo que ellos querían decir es que estemos atentos."

33. Fracchia, interview by author, and Ana Deutsch, interview by author, Buenos Aires, May 12, 2011.

34. Deutsch, interview by author. "Ahora lo pienso que fue también un refugio la actividad."

35. Lepecki, "Chorepolitics and Choreopolice," 16.

36. Larasati, *The Dance That Makes You Vanish*, 16.

37. "Expresión corporal, la nueva fiebre de los porteños," *Clarín Revista*, May 30, 1982, 10–11.

38. Patricia Stokoe, "Historia y antecedentes de esta corriente, según la experiencia de su creadora," appendix in *Qué es la expresión corporal*, by Déborah Kalmar (Buenos Aires: Lumen, 2005), 132. "La danza al alcance de todos."

39. In London, Stokoe studied ballet at the Royal Academy of Dance and modern dance with Agnes de Mille, Catherine de Vos, and Sigurd Leeder.

40. For a comparative analysis of training in classical ballet, contemporary dance, and *expresión corporal* in Argentina, see Ana Sabrina Mora, "El cuerpo en la danza desde la antropología. Prácticas, representaciones y experiencias durante la formación en danzas clásicas, danza contemporánea y expresión corporal" (PhD diss., National University of La Plata, 2010).

41. Patricia Dorin, interview by author, Buenos Aires, September 13, 2011. While *expresión corporal* classes depend largely on the individual instructor, movement is generally based on prompts focused around energy, explorations of planes in space, affective intensities, and other dynamics. The literature on *expresión corporal* is extensive. For encompassing descriptions of the mechanics of the practice and its pedagogical approaches, see Patricia Stokoe, *Expresión corporal: Arte-salud-educación* (Buenos Aires: ICSA-Hvmanitas, 1987) and Déborah Kalmar, *Qué es la expresión corporal: A partir de la corriente de trabajo creada por Patricia Stokoe* (Buenos Aires: Lumen, 2005).

42. "Historia," *UNA Artes del Movimiento*, accessed June 1, 2017, http://movimiento.una.edu.ar/contenidos/historia_12492.

43. Kalmar, interview by author.

44. Ibid.

45. Kalmar, *Qué es la expresión corporal*, 18. "Una propuesta frente a la necesidad de nuevas pautas de relación entre las personas, una búsqueda que ayude a reencontrar la alegría de vivir a través del baile, después de tanta muerte y destrucción."

46. Kalmar, interview by author. "Ha salido como respuesta vital para preservar la vida con lo que tiene de esencial de posibilidad de desplegarse como vida en la relación con los otros ante épocas con diferentes formas de violencia que las que hay hoy, que las hubo en el Proceso, que las hubo durante la segunda guerra mundial; lo nombro por la historia de Patricia que ella a sus dieciocho años atravesó los bombardeos en Londres, yo a los dieciocho años, el Proceso o sea, toda la época de salir al mundo, de mayor vitalidad y con toda esa energía creadora pero también con todo lo que significa la represión. . . . Para mí siempre la danza unida a la vida, aunque esté hablando del dolor más grande."

47. Maralia Reca, a former member of the Argentine La Plata Theater Ballet (Ballet Estable del Teatro Argentina de La Plata) and trained dance therapist, explored dance as the preservation of life from an explicitly therapeutic perspective. For a detailed account of how Reca located and worked with torture survivors during and after the last military dictatorship, see Maralia Reca, *Tortura y trauma: Danza/ movimiento terapia en la reconstrucción del mundo de sobrevivientes de tortura por causas políticas* (Buenos Aires: Biblos, 2011).

48. Kalmar, interview by author. "[Es] como que el que se mueve es otro. Por algo todos los caminos de represión más explícitos o implícitos o más encubiertos tienen que ver con frenar el cuerpo."

49. Osvaldo Aguilar, interview by author, Buenos Aires, October 11, 2011.

50. Ibid.

51. Patricia Stokoe, "Grupo Aluminé, antecedentes e historia," appendix in *Qué es la expresión corporal*, by Déborah Kalmar (Buenos Aires: Lumen, 2005), 139.

52. Beatriz Doumerc and Ayax Barnes, *La línea* (Buenos Aires: Ediciones del Eclipse, 2003), digitized by Roberto Boote, last modified August 20, 2007, accessed July 20, 2012, https://www.youtube.com/watch?v=vbR_l1VnKm4. "Donde viva el hombre nuevo." The line in this video is blue, a modification made in the 2003 reprint of the book on which the video is based. See Graciela Bialet and Ángel Luis Luján, "Censura y LIJ durante la dictadura argentina de 1976–1983," in *Censuras y literatura infantil y juvenil en el siglo XX (En España y 7 países latinoamericanos)*, eds. Pedro C. Cerrillo and M. Victoria Sotomayor (Cuenca: Ediciones de la Universidad de Castilla-Mancha, 2016), 298.

53. Guevara, *El socialismo y el hombre en Cuba*.

54. Stokoe, "Grupo Aluminé, antecedentes e historia," 139. Despite their inability to premiere this particular work, Grupo Aluminé did present a number of other works during the last military dictatorship including *Collage* (1976–78), *Este es nuestro canto* (*This Is Our Song*, 1980, an exploration of Argentine identity featuring music by Mercedes Sosa), and *Recoged, esta voz* (*Pick Up, This Voice*, 1982). Stokoe, "Grupo Aluminé, antecedentes e historia," 137–40.

55. Larasati, *The Dance That Makes You Vanish*, 61.

56. Stokoe, "Grupo Aluminé, antecedentes e historia," 139. "Una coreografía madura tras tantos años de aprendizaje."

57. *Patricia Stokoe "Con los ojos del corazón . . . " (imágenes y recuerdos)*, Estudio Kalmar Stokoe, n.d., DVD.

58. Ibid.

59. Doumerc and Barnes, *La línea*. "Línea: Sucesión de puntos. Historia: Sucesión de hechos. Los puntos hacen la línea. Los hombres hacen la historia."

60. *Patricia Stokoe "Con los ojos del corazón . . . " (imágenes y recuerdos)*.

61. Doumerc and Barnes, *La línea*. "Contra la historia."

62. *Patricia Stokoe "Con los ojos del corazón . . . " (imágenes y recuerdos)*.

63. For a discussion of the gender politics of the Madres de Plaza de Mayo's protest performance, see Taylor, *Disappearing Acts*, 183–222.

64. Notably, in Chile women danced the traditionally partnered cueca alone in protest of disappearances under the dictatorship of Augusto Pinochet (1972–90). For discussions of the practice, see Marjorie Agosín, "The Dance of Life: Women and Human Rights in Chile," in *Dance, Human Rights, and Social Justice: Dignity in Motion*, ed. Naomi Jackson and Toni Shapiro-Phim, trans. Janice Molloy (Lanham, MD: Scarecrow Press, 2008), 296–303, and Karolina Babic, "Todavía Bailamos la cueca sola: From Local Protest Practice against Chile's Dictatorship to (Trans)national Memory Icon" (PhD diss., University at Albany, State University of New York, 2014).

65. Organized by playwright Osvaldo Dragún, the festival included other well-known dramatists, including Diana Raznovich, Griselda Gambaro, Roberto Cossa, and Ricardo Monti, among others. In addition to Danza Abierta, Teatro Abierto also inspired Música Siempre (Music Always), Cine Abierto (Open Film), Poesía Abierta (Open Poetry), and a youth version of Teatro Abierto. For extended discussions of Teatro Abierto in English, see Graham-Jones, *Exorcising History*, 89–122, and Taylor, *Disappearing Acts*, 223–54. See also Juana A. Arancibia and Zulema Mirkin, *Volumen II: Teatro argentino durante el Proceso (1976–1983): ensayos críticos-entrevistas* (Buenos Aires: Instituto Literario y Cultural Hispánico, 1992).

66. Graham-Jones, *Exorcising History*, 89.

67. Ibid., 91–92.

68. Napoleón Cabrera, "Un comienzo a toda danza," *Clarín*, November 22, 1981, 7, and Lucía Fernández Mouján, "Danza Abierta: Open Dance against Oppression in Buenos Aires" (MA thesis, University of Amsterdam, 2003), 18, Documentation Center of the San Martín Municipal Theater.

69. Tambutti, "100 años de la danza en Buenos Aires," 30.

70. "Ciclo de Danza abierta," *La Prensa*, October 30, 1981, n.p., Private Collection of Alicia Muñoz; "Mañana comienza 'Danza Abierta,'" *Clarín*, November 19, 1981, 6; and "Danza Abierta: Los nuevos caminos de la libertad," *Clarín Revista*, November 22, 1981, 8.

71. Mouján, "Danza Abierta: Open Dance against Oppression in Buenos Aires," 20.

72. Danza Abierta Flyer, 1981, Private Collection of Vivian Luz. "¿Qué es? Danza Abierta. Un movimiento espontáneo; sin fines de lucro, organizado por artistas representativos de la danza argentina, preocupados en demonstrar la vigencia y vitalidad de la danza en nuestro país. ¿Por qué? Porque necesitamos hacer saber que la danza no es un arte de élite, sino una de las más bellas y populares expresiones del espíritu y queremos hacerla llegar—con precios muy accesible en las localidades, alta calidad y gran cantidad de creadores—a nuestra comunidad."

73. This spirit of radical inclusivity prompted debates around the quality of the dancing presented. The ensuing discussion among choreographers and in the press resulted in the imposition of selection criteria in the 1983 festival. Silvia Vladimivsky, interview by author, Buenos Aires, Argentina, July 7, 2009, and Muñoz, interview by author.

74. Tambutti, interview by author. "Otro que recién empezaba y hacía su primer coreografía tres minutos estaba bárbaro, estaba todo muy bien y nosotros que teníamos ya un poquito de nombre . . . estábamos todos ahí."

75. Nora Codina, interview by author, Buenos Aires, April 12, 2011. "Fue apoteósico . . . fue un momento que dio auge a la danza contemporánea . . . y bailaba todo el mundo que quería bailar."

76. Muñoz, interview by author. "No hubo la más mínima selección: vos querías bailar, nadie te preguntaba si habías bailado, no habías bailado, entrabas a bailar. Está bien, ante tanta cosa amordazada, ante tanta falta de expresión."

77. "Un comienzo a toda la danza," 7; Néstor Tirri, "'Danza Abierta' siguió con fervor y desniveles," *Clarín*, November 23, 1981, n.p., Private Collection of Susana Zimmermann; and "'Danza abierta' y su favorable eco popular," *La Nación*, November 28, 1981, n.p., Private Collection of Alicia Muñoz.

78. "Danza Abierta: Los nuevos caminos de la libertad," 9.

79. Isse Moyano, *La danza moderna argentina cuenta su historia*, 103.

80. Codina, interview by author.

81. Muñoz, interview by author; Codina, interview by author; Isse Moyano, *La danza moderna argentina cuenta su historia*, 135; and Luz, interview by author.

82. Muñoz, interview by author. "Nunca más sucedió eso, jamás sucedió eso salvo que venga a bailar Baryshnikov o una cosa así."

83. "Danza Abierta: Los nuevos caminos de la libertad," 10. "Kamien acepta también que en los últimos años la mujer y el hombre de la calle se sintieron empujados a preocuparse por el cuerpo, algo que antes no sucedía."

84. Ibid., 9. "La danza en los últimos años ha recibido una gran afluencia de gente—se nota la incorporación de muchísimos hombres que antes tenían prejuicios—y esa gente lo hace porque tiene necesidad de expresarse. Nuestros cuerpos necesitan salir de la solemnidad, del estereotipo. En fin, nosotros mismos buscamos liberarnos y la danza es una manera de buscar esa libertad."

85. Ibid., 10. "Quienes amamos la danza quisiéramos que la gente bailara así como está vestida en la platea. Con traje, pero que hiciera mover su cuerpo."

86. Masiello, "La Argentina durante el Proceso," 13. "Un discurso híbrido."

87. Ibid., 17. "Para aquellos que saben escuchar."

88. This reading converges with Danielle Goldman's understanding of improvised dance as a practice of freedom; see *I Want to Be Ready: Improvised Dance as a Practice of Freedom* (Ann Arbor: University of Michigan Press, 2010), 4–5.

89. Tambutti, interview by author, and Kamien, interview by author, Buenos Aires, August 21, 2008.

90. Vladimivsky, interview by author.

91. Dorin, interview by author.

92. Adriana Barenstein, interview by author, Buenos Aires, October 20, 2011.

93. Dorin, interview by author.

94. Ibid.

95. Vladimivsky, interview by author. "La obra fue hecha casi en la inconsciencia, yo no te puedo decir que yo quise hacer una obra de tinte social."

96. Barenstein, interview by author. "Lo que pasa es que es tan inconsciente . . . . Eso tenía un simbolismo, yo no me daba cuenta en ese momento, pero tenía un simbolismo de, si vos querés, de personas a las que estaban matando."

97. The first season in 1977 included Stekeleman's *Memorias* (*Memories*, 1977); Margarita Bali's *Biósfera* (*Biosphere*, 1977); and two works by Ana Itelman, *Y ella lo visitaba* (*She Was a Visitor*, 1976, originally created for Nucleodanza) and *Casa de puertas* (*House of Doors*, 1962), a work based on Federico García Lorca's *La casa de Bernarda Alba* (*The House of Bernarda Alba*, 1936). The company also presented Doris Humphrey's *New Dance*, set by Ruth Currier. Appendix in *Ballet Contemporáneo: 25 años en el San Martín*, ed. Eduardo Rovner (Buenos Aires: Teatro Municipal General San Martín, 1993), 153.

98. Alejandro Cervera, interview by author, Buenos Aires, August 7, 2009.

99. See Fortuna, "Schottelius, Renate (1921–1998)."

100. "Caminos: Renate Schottelius," *Kiné: La revista de lo corporal*, April/May 1996, 11, Documentation Center of the San Martín Municipal Theater.

101. Ibid. Schottelius's mother did successfully immigrate to Argentina.

102. Renate Schottelius, Program notes for *Paisaje de gritos*, Buenos Aires: General San Martín Municipal Theater, 1981, Documentation Center of the San Martín Municipal Theater. "me compadezco del dolor de millones de personas; y, sin embargo, cuando miro el cielo, pienso que todo eso cambiará y que todo volverá a ser bueno . . . porque sigo creyendo en la bondad innata del hombre."

103. "Hoy, ballet en el San Martín," *Clarín*, March 19, 1981, 5. "No se trata tampoco de una historia sino de . . . vínculos humanos, relaciones."

104. Schottelius, Program notes for *Paisaje de gritos*.

105. Renate Schottelius, *Paisaje de gritos*, n.d., DVD. Private Collection of Oscar Araiz.

106. Throughout the course of her career, critics frequently connected Schottelius's work to German expressionism. Though she had early contact with German modern dance before migrating, her training and choreography are much more closely aligned with US midcentury modernisms. See Pompeyo Camps, "Nuevo espectáculo coreográfico," *La Opinión*, March 25, 1981, 11; Paulina Ossona, "Tres estrenos en el San Martín," *La Prensa*, March 25, 1981, 3; and Silvia Gsell, "Danza para emociones profundas," *La Nación*, May 3, 1993, n.p., Documentation Center of the San Martín Municipal Theater. Notably, choreographer Paula Rosolen's 2012 *Die Farce der Suche* (*The Farce of the Search*), an evening-length work based on archival research on Schottelius's life, included reflection on the largely imagined connection between Schottelius and German expressionism.

107. "Hoy, ballet en el San Martín," 5.

108. Schottelius, *Paisaje de gritos*.

109. The celebrations calculated Oscar Araiz's 1968 company as the founding date.

110. Renate Schottelius, "Renate Schottelius habla sobre 'Paisaje de gritos,'" in *Ballet Contemporáneo: 25 años en el San Martín*, ed. Eduardo Rovner (Buenos Aires: Teatro Municipal General San Martín, 1993), 32. "Antibélica y antifascista," "plena dictadura militar."

111. Like Schottelius, Cervera later chose *Dirección* as his contribution to the now renamed Ballet Contemporáneo on the twenty-fifth anniversary program.

112. Cervera, interview by author. "Decadencia."

113. Taylor, *Disappearing Acts*, 122.

114. Cervera, interview by author. "Cuando me pidieron una obra para el San Martín, yo le dije a Kive Staiff: No puedo hacer otra obra que no sea esta en este momento. Me encantaría hacer otra obra donde la gente baile y todos contentos, pero no podría hacerlo. No sería sincero."

115. Isse Moyano, *La danza moderna argentina cuenta su historia*, 170–71.

116. Ibid., 171. "Apasillado." "Donde uno no puede salir, donde hay una obligatoriedad de seguir siempre para ese mismo lugar."

117. Ibid. "Creo que era lo que le pasaba a uno, no se podía cambiar, digamos."

118. Lepecki, "Choreopolice and Choreopolitcs: or, the task of the dancer," 20.

119. Alejandro Cervera, *Dirección obligatoria*, n.d., DVD. Private Collection of Alejandro Cervera.

120. Juan Ignacio Vallejos, "Danza, política y posdictadura: acerca de *Dirección obligatoria* de Alejandro Cervera," *Revista Afuera: Estudios de crítica cultural* 15 (2015), http://www.revistaafuera.com/articulo.php?id=328&nro=15.

121. Carassai, *The Argentine Silent Majority.*
122. Vallejos, "Danza, política y posdictadura." "La divulgación de los horrores a los que los militares habían sometido a los jóvenes soldados argentinos funcionaron como una alerta para una gran parte de la población que comenzaba a tomar consciencia de la dimensión que había adquirido el terrorismo de estado en esos últimos años." Vallejos highlights the 1984 film *Los chicos de la guerra* (*The Boys of the War*), a film based on Daniel Kon's book of the same title featuring interviews with Malvinas soldiers. For a discussion of how the Malvinas conflict shifted the military government's relationship to other cultural actors, specifically rock musicians, see Pablo Vila and Paul Cammack, "Rock Nacional and Dictatorship in Argentina," *Popular Music* 6.2 (1987): 140–43.
123. Cervera, *Dirección obligatoria.*
124. Masiello, "La Argentina durante el Proceso," 13.
125. Barenstein, interview by author.
126. See Tambutti, "100 años de la danza en Buenos Aires," 31–32.
127. *10 Años: Artes del movimiento* (Buenos Aires: Instituto Universitario Nacional del Arte, 2008), 14.

CHAPTER 4

1. *Nunca más: Informe de la Comisión Nacional sobre la Desaparición de Personas* (Buenos Aires: Eudeba, 2009).
2. Two of the original junta leaders, Jorge Rafael Videla and Emilio Massera, were sentenced to life imprisonment. The third member of the initial junta, Orlando Ramón Agosti, and later leaders received shorter sentences.
3. The 1986 Full Stop Law set a cutoff date for the investigation and prosecution of human rights violations by high-ranking military officials. In 1987, the Due Obedience Law declared that all subordinate military officers were simply following orders and could therefore not be tried legally.
4. Menem also unsuccessfully attempted to demolish the Navy Petty-Officers School of Mechanics (Escuela de Suboficiales de Mecánica de la Armada, ESMA)—the largest former clandestine detention center in Buenos Aires. The Supreme Court overturned this order in 2001. After the military vacated the complex in 2007, the center was converted, by federal order, into a memory site and cultural center run by the Asociación Madres de Plaza de Mayo.
5. As Idelber Avelar argues in his study of postdictatorship Latin American fiction, the legislative imperative to move on, in Argentina as well as other South American nations working to restore democratic processes, was itself inextricably linked to the intensification of neoliberal policies first instituted by dictatorial regimes. See *The Untimely Present: Postdictatorial Latin American Fiction and the Task of Mourning*, (Durham, NC: Duke University Press, 1999), 2.
6. While I focus on works that cite tango in this chapter, a number of other contemporary dance works (not limited to those named here) engage the violence of the last military dictatorship. Mauricio Wainrot's *Anne Frank* (1985) allegorized national violence through a danced telling of the Holocaust memoir. Also in the immediate aftermath of the dictatorship period, Nucleodanza member Nora Codina presented *Vivos* (*Alive*, 1984), a work that engaged her husband's 1977 disappearance, and *Suicida* (*Suicide*, 1984), a piece that reflected the trauma of his disappearance as well as her own experiences of torture and detention, Codina, interview by author. La Plata-based Colectivo Siempre's *Siempre* (*Always*, 2006)

and Gabriela Romero's *Senderos de la memoria* (*Paths of Memory*, 2004) examine memory through a site-specific approach; the former piece was staged in the courtyard of the La Plata Museum of Fine Arts and the latter in the Buenos Aires Memory Park. For a discussion of *Siempre* and the group's broader activist work, see Mariana Estévez and Diana Montequin, "Colectivo Siempre—Danza y activismo," *Universidad Nacional de La Plata* (blog), last updated August 2013, accessed July 17, 2014, http://blogs.unlp.edu.ar/arteaccionlaplataxxi/files/2014/05/2013-colectivo-Siempre.pdf. Julieta Eskenazi's work, *Restos de oscuras* (*Remains of Darkness*, 2002) also engages dictatorship violence. Mónica Fracchia's *Fechas patrias* (*National Holidays*, 2008), Paula Etchebehere's *Nunca estuve en otra parte* (*I Was Never Anywhere Else*, 2004), and Vivian Luz's *Serán otros los ruidos* (*The Noises Will Be Different*, 2010) all choreograph dictatorship trauma within broader narratives of histories of political violence in Argentina and globally, including references to World War II and the Spanish Civil War. For an analysis of Luz's work, see Victoria Fortuna, "An Enormous Yearning for the Past: Movement/Archive in Two Contemporary Dance Works," *e-misférica* 9, nos. 1–2 (2012), http://hemisphericinstitute.org/hemi/en/e-misferica-91/fortuna.

7. Influential choreographer Ana Itelman's 1955 *Esta ciudad de Buenos Aires* (*This City of Buenos Aires*) was the first among many works to blend tango with modern and contemporary dance vocabularies. See Tambutti, "Miriam Winslow como nexo entre la danza moderna norteamericana y el surgimiento de la danza moderna en Argentina." In 1993, prominent contemporary dancer and choreographer Ana María Stekelman founded Tangokinesis, a performing company and movement technique that integrate tango and contemporary dance vocabularies.

8. The prominence of tango themes in postdictatorship dance works paralleled a similar trend in theater works. See Perla Zayas de Lima, *El universo mítico de los argentinos en escena: Tomo 2* (Buenos Aires: Inteatro, 2010), 130.

9. In understanding dance as a mode of transmission, I follow Diana Taylor's definition of cultural memory as "a practice, an act of imagination and interconnection" that is "embodied and sensual." See *The Archive and the Repertoire*, 82.

10. In her discussion of Eiko & Koma's 2007 work *Mourning*, Rosemary Candelario makes a similar argument around how concert dance offers a site for understanding mourning as ongoing, embodied labor rather than a linear process from grief to acceptance. See *Flowers Cracking Concrete: Eiko & Koma's Asian/American Choreographies* (Middletown, CT: Wesleyan University Press, 2016), 129–55. Relatedly, in her elegant chapter on a Cambodian family's practice of Khmer classical dance in Long Beach, California, Judith Hamera demonstrates how dance practice constitutes a kind of "answerability" for the violence of the Khmer Rouge. See Hamera, *Dancing Communities*, 138–71.

11. Cathy Caruth, *Unclaimed Experience: Trauma, Narrative, and History* (Baltimore: Johns Hopkins University Press, 1996), 4.

12. Taylor, *The Archive and the Repertoire*, 165.

13. Ibid.

14. Notable pieces not under consideration in this chapter include Susana Zimmermann's *Dolentango* (1999), which commemorates the Madres de Plaza de Mayo through a movement and sound score imbued with tango citations, and Alejandro Cervera's *Tangos golpeados* (*Coup Tangos*, 2008), which combines a hybrid tango and contemporary dance vocabulary to commemorate not only the 1976 coup, but also the military coups of 1930, 1955, and 1966.

15. In addition to Savigliano's *Tango and the Political Economy of Passion* and Julie Taylor's *Paper Tangos*, notable works in English on the history of tango dance include Simon Collier, Artemis Cooper, María S. Azzi, and Richard Martin, *Tango!: The Dance, the Song, the Story* (London: Thames & Hudson, 1997); Chasteen, *National Rhythms*, 17–33; and Thompson, *Tango: The Art History of Love*. For a consideration of recent trends in the Buenos Aires tango dance scene, see Merritt, *Tango Nuevo*.

16. Savigliano, *Tango and the Political Economy of Passion*, 3; Taylor, *Paper Tangos*, 43; and Thompson, *Tango: The Art History of Love*, 265–71.

17. Ana C. Cara, "Entangled Tangos: Passionate Displays, Intimate Dialogues," *The Journal of American Folklore* 122, no. 486 (2009): 439.

18. Ibid., 440.

19. In the postdictatorship period, the Madres split into two groups: Asociación Madres de Plaza de Mayo (Mothers of the Plaza de Mayo Association) and Madres de Plaza de Mayo Línea Fundadora (Mothers of the Plaza de Mayo Founding Line).

20. For the creators' account of the project as well as critical engagement with it, see Ana Longoni and Gustavo A. Bruzzone, eds., *El Siluetazo* (Buenos Aires: Adriana Hidalgo Editora, 2008).

21. For an analysis of H.I.J.O.S.'s *escraches*, see Taylor, *The Archive and the Repertoire*, 161–89.

22. An estimated five hundred children were taken from their detained biological parents during the last military dictatorship. Teatro por la Identidad supported the Abuelas de Plaza de Mayo's extensive project with the National Genetic Bank to reunite families separated by state violence. For an anthology of plays included on the program, see Herminia Petruzzi, *Teatro por la identidad: antología* (Buenos Aires: Ediciones Colihue SRL, 2009). For a critical discussion of the festival (in particular its genealogical relationship to Teatro Abierto), see Werth, *Theatre, Performance, and Memory Politics in Argentina*, 173–95. Additional notable examples of postdictatorship cultural production include Luis Puenzo's Oscar-winning *La historia oficial* (*The Official Story*, 1985), which told the story of a middle-class mother's dawning realization that her adopted daughter's biological parents were *desaparecidos*. For an analysis of *La historia oficial* as well as broader discussion of postdictatorship cinema, see Tamara L. Falicov, *The Cinematic Tango: Contemporary Argentine Film* (London: Wallflower Press, 2007), 47–74. For additional discussion of postdictatorship cinema, see also Ana Amado, *La imagen justa: Cine argentino y política, 1980–2007* (Buenos Aires: Ediciones Colihue SRL, 2009) and Philippa Page, *Politics and Performance in Post-Dictatorship Argentine Film and Theatre*. On the page, Alicia Partnoy's powerful memoir *La escuelita* (*The Little School*, 1986) recounted her time as a prisoner at a clandestine detention center. For analysis of *La escuelita* and writings by other female survivors, see Edurne M. Portela, *Displaced Memories: The Poetics of Trauma in Argentine Women's Writing* (Lewisburg, PA: Bucknell University Press, 2009). See also Ana Amado and Nora Domínguez, eds., *Lazos de familia: Herencias, cuerpos, ficciones* (Buenos Aires: Paidós, 2004). For a broader view of postdictatorship fiction in the Southern Cone, see Avelar, *The Untimely Present*, and Francine Masiello, *The Art of Transition: Latin American Culture and Neoliberal Crisis* (Durham, NC: Duke University Press, 2001), 177–218.

23. See Cecilia Sosa, *Queering Acts of Mourning in the Aftermath of Argentina's Dictatorship: The Performances of Blood* (Rochester, NY: Tamesis, 2014).

24. See Vallejos's reading of Cervera's *Dirección obligatoria* (analyzed in the previous chapter) as a postdictatorship choreography, "Danza, política y posdictadura: acerca de *Dirección obligatoria* de Alejandro Cervera." In her short piece, Laura Noemí Papa considers the relationship between Argentine contemporary dance and memory. See, "La danza como una instancia de construcción de la memoria," *Colectivo Siempre* (blog), last modified July 23, 2009, accessed August 12, 2010, http://cslecturaspapa.blogspot.com/2009/07/la-danza-como-una-instancia-de.html.

25. My descriptions of *La puñalada* draw on live viewing of the work at the American Dance Festival (ADF) in 2007 as well as video documentation from a 1992 ADF performance. Susana Tambutti, *La puñalada*, American Dance Festival, Duke University Reynolds Theater, Durham, North Carolina, July 9, 2007, and Susana Tambutti, *La puñalada*, in *Nucelodanza and Monica Valenciano presented by ADF 23 June* (Durham, NC: American Dance Festival, 1992), VHS, American Dance Festival Reference Collection, Duke University Archives, David M. Rubenstein Rare Book & Manuscript Library, Duke University.

26. For my analysis of the piece in Spanish, see Victoria Fortuna, "Danza, historia, memoria," in *VI Jornadas de investigación en danza 2012*, ed. María Eugenia Cadús (Buenos Aires: Universidad Nacional de las Artes, 2016), 31–42.

27. Tambutti, "100 años de danza en Buenos Aires," 30.

28. For reflections on the interest in dance theater on Buenos Aires's stages in the mid-1980s, see Julia Elena Sagaseta and Perla Zayas de Lima, comps., *El teatro-danza* (conference proceedings, III Encuentro de Estudios del Teatro, Instituto de Artes del Espectáculo, Facultad de Filosofía y Letras, University of Buenos Aires, September 17–20, 1992).

29. Ana Deutsch also joined and choreographed for the company, but left in the mid-1980s to pursue an independent career, at which point Tambutti and Bali acted as co-directors. In general terms, Bali's choreography is aligned more closely with an interest in visual art, while Tambutti's work emphasizes theatricality. See Tambutti, "100 años de danza en Buenos Aires," 30. For a documentary on their work between 1974 and 1993, see Jorge Coscia, *Danza contemporánea argentina: Nucleodanza, 1974–1993* (Buenos Aires: Films de Colección Blakman, 1994), DVD.

30. Solanas invited Bali and Tambutti to choreograph for the film on the recommendation of a mutual friend, Tambutti, interview by author. The film includes professional tango dancers in addition to Nucleodanza company members; however, many of the scenes feature contemporary dance despite the film's emphasis on the tango. This produced a polemic among critics who felt the choreography was too "Europeanized" and did not reflect the "true" Argentine tango, see Falicov, *The Cinematic Tango*, 56. For an interview with Solanas about the film, see Coco Fusco, "The Tango of Esthetics and Politics: An Interview with Fernando Solanas," *Cineaste* 16, nos. 1–2 (1987–88): 57–59.

31. Tambutti, *La puñalada*, 2007, and Tambutti, *La puñalada*, 1992.

32. Elizabeth Freeman, "Packing History, Count(er)ing Generations," *New Literary History* 31, no. 4 (2002): 728.

33. Simon Collier, "The Birth of the Tango," in *The Argentina Reader: History, Culture, Politics*, eds. Gabriela Nouzeilles and Graciela Montaldo (Durham, NC: Duke University Press, 2002), 196.

34. Jorge Salessi, "Medics, Crooks and Tango Queens: The National Appropriation of a Gay Tango," in *Everynight Life: Culture and Dance in Latin/o America*, ed. Celeste

Fraser Delgado and José Esteban Muñoz, trans. Celeste Fraser Delgado (Durham, NC: Duke University Press, 1997), 151.

35. Savigliano, *Tango and the Political Economy of Passion*, 30–72.
36. Ibid., 31.
37. María Rosa Olivera-Williams, "The Twentieth Century as Ruin: Tango and Historical Memory," in *Telling Ruins in Latin America*, ed. Michael J. Lazzara and Vicky Unruh (New York: Palgrave Macmillan, 2009), 97.
38. Ibid., 96.
39. Sirena Pellarolo, "Queering Tango: Glitches in the Hetero-National Matrix of a Liminal Cultural Production," *Theatre Journal* 60, no. 3 (2008): 410.
40. Salessi, "Medics, Crooks and Tango Queens," 161–62.
41. Ibid., 142.
42. Cecilia Hopkins, "Un encuentro a salas llenas," review of XXII Fiesta Nacional del Teatro, *Página/12*, May 8, 2008, accessed June 10, 2010, https://www.pagina12.com.ar/diario/suplementos/espectaculos/10-9998-2008-05-08.html. "Un pequeño grotesco criollo."
43. Ana Elena Puga, "The abstract allegory of Griselda Gambaro's *Stripped* (*El despojamiento*)," *Theatre Journal* 56, no. 3 (2004): 422.
44. Julie Taylor, "Death Dressed As a Dancer: The Grotesque, Violence, and the Argentine Tango," *TDR: The Drama Review* 57, no. 3 (2013): 118.
45. Ibid.
46. Taylor, *Paper Tangos*, 61, 71–72; Savigliano, *Tango and the Political Economy of Passion*, 12; Taylor, "Death Dressed As a Dancer," 127; and Gustavo Varela, *Tango y política: Sexo, moral burguesa y revolución en Argentina* (Buenos Aires: Ariel, 2016), 187–99.
47. Taylor, *Paper Tangos*, 61.
48. Ibid.
49. Dianne Marie Zandstra, *Embodying Resistance: Griselda Gambaro and the Grotesque* (Lewisberg, PA: Bucknell University Press, 2007), 14. Gambaro's work has received significant critical attention in English. Her work *Antígona furiosa* (1986) is frequently analyzed in relationship to postdictatorship cultural production's attempt to supplement or compensate for lack of juridical action. For a discussion of her work in this frame, see Taylor, *Disappearing Acts*, 207–22; Ana Elena Puga, *Memory, Allegory, and Testimony in South American Theater: Upstaging Dictatorship*, 138–93; Annette Levine, *Cry for Me, Argentina: The Performance of Trauma in the Short Narratives of Aida Bortnik, Griselda Gambaro, and Tununa Mercado* (Madison, NJ: Fairleigh Dickinson University Press, 2008), 75–109; and Werth, *Theater, Performance, and Memory Politics in Argentina*, 34–48.
50. Tambutti, *La puñalada*, 2007, and Tambutti, *La puñalada*, 1992. The wiping of the blade on the leg is more of a cutting motion in the 2007 version of the piece.
51. Taylor, *Disappearing Acts*, 96.
52. Ibid., 156.
53. Tambutti, *La puñalada*, 1992. In the 2007 version of the piece featured on the companion site, the knives were replaced by drumsticks, Tambutti, *La puñalada*, 2007.
54. María Negroni, *Ciudad gótica* (Rosario: Bajo la luna nueva, 1994), 29.
55. Anna Kisselgoff, "Works That Cry for Argentina," review of American Dance Festival, Duke University Reynolds Theater, Durham, North Carolina, *New York Times*, July 1, 1989, http://www.nytimes.com/1989/07/01/arts/review-dance-works-that-cry-for-argentina.html; and Jonathan Probber, "Latin Lovers, Lethal

Props," review of American Dance Festival, Duke University Reynolds Theater, Durham, North Carolina, *The Independent Weekly*, July 6–12, 1989.

56. Hodgers, interview by author.
57. In addition to *María Mar*, Hodgers's work *Con los restos* (*With the Remains*, 2003) also addresses her experiences as a militant and political prisoner.
58. Laura Lifschitz, "Silvia Hodgers: La danza y la militancia política," *Tiempo Argentino*, October 24, 2010, accessed September 9, 2011, http://tiempo. elargentino.com/notas/danza-y-militancia-politica (site discontinued).
59. Unfortunately, neither Hodgers nor Aellig Régnier is in possession of the video of the work used in the making of *Juntos*. Hodgers, interview by author, and Raphaëlle Aellig Régnier, email message to author, March 23, 2016.
60. "Juntos—Un Retour en Argentine," *Swiss Films*, accessed May 1, 2016, http:// www.swissfilms.ch/en/information_publications/festival_search/festivaldetails/ -/id_film/-1499420850.
61. Lifschitz, "La danza y la militancia política."
62. Raphaëlle Aellig Régnier and Norbert Wiedmer, *Juntos: Un Retour en Argentine* (Geneva, Switzerland: RaR and Biograph Film, 2001). https://www.artfilm.ch/ juntos-un-retour-en-argentine.
63. Hodgers, interview by author..
64. Hodgers, *María Mar*, in Aellig Régnier and Wiedmer, *Juntos: Un Retour en Argentine*.
65. Hodgers, interview by author.
66. Ibid.
67. Ibid. "Piel de gallina."
68. Hodgers, *María Mar*, in Aellig Régnier and Wiedmer, *Juntos: Un Retour en Argentine*.
69. Hodgers, interview by author.
70. Taylor, *Disappearing Acts*, 96.
71. Oscar del Priore and Irene Amuchástegui, *Cien tangos fundamentales* (Buenos Aires: Aguilar, 2011), E-Book, chap. "Milongas."
72. Hodgers, interview by author.
73. Manning, *Politics of Touch*, 17.
74. Thank you to Elliot Leffler for this insight.
75. Hodgers, interview by author. "tango à plat ventre."
76. Codina, interview by author. "Mi marido médico desaparece, me llevan como rehén, estoy veinte días. ¿Qué hago para no pensar y poder sobrevivir? ¿Qué es lo que había que hacer allí? Hago coreografía, que nunca la puse en escena pero que fue para mí un recurso a los veinticinco años, así que decidí, para aislarme, para no escuchar, para no nada y eso me ayudó muchísimo."
77. Hodgers, interview by author. "Recuperar mi cuerpo."
78. Ibid. "No sería la que yo soy hoy . . . trabajar la improvisación, sacar los sentimientos para afuera, la expresividad, ver que otros bailarines también trabajaban con lo político."
79. Aellig Régnier and Wiedmer, *Juntos: Un Retour en Argentine*.
80. Ibid. English subtitles of the original French spoken in the documentary.
81. Avelar, *The Untimely Present*, 138.
82. Aellig Régnier and Wiedmer, *Juntos: Un Retour en Argentine*.
83. Ibid. English subtitles of the original French spoken in the documentary.
84. Taylor, *Paper Tangos*, 71.

85. "Sobre Silvia Vladimivsky," accessed April 15, 2016, http://vladimivsky.blogspot. com/p/sobre-silvia-vladimivsky.html.

86. Vladimivsky, interview by author. "Que liga el teatro danza con el tango como expresión cultural argentina." In addition to *El nombre, otros tangos* (and related works detailed in note 91) Vladimivsky's *Azares del Quijote y Gardel* (*The Chance Encounters of Quijote and Gardel*, 2009) also engages tango culture, music, and movement.

87. Ibid.

88. Ibid. "Quedar pegado."

89. Ibid.

90. Ibid.

91. Versions of this work have been presented under a number of names across the years, including *Otros tangos* (*Other Tangos*, 2002), *El nombre* (*The Name*, 2003), and *El nombre, otros tangos II* (*The Name, Other Tangos II*, 2007). I have used *El nombre, otros tangos* as it was the title in use during the 2005–06 period Vladimivsky was filming the documentary.

92. Ivana Bosso and Francesca Gentile, *Alma doble* (Turin: La Sarraz Pictures, 2007).

93. Ibid. English subtitles of the original Italian spoken in the documentary.

94. Vladimivsky, interview by author.

95. The military actively policed and censored theater production, see Graham-Jones, *Exorcising History*, 17.

96. Vladimivsky, interview by author. "El lugar de intentar cerrar yo una situación poéticamente que no cierra ni históricamente ni legalmente."

97. Walter Benjamin, "On the Concept of History," translated by Dennis Redmond, *Marxists Internet Archive*, 2005, accessed April 12, 2016, https://www.marxists. org/reference/archive/benjamin/1940/history.htm.

98. Oren Baruch Stier, *Holocaust Icons: Symbolizing the Shoah in History and Memory* (New Brunswick, NJ: Rutgers University Press, 2015), 15.

99. Bosso and Gentile, *Alma doble*. "El fenómeno más importante de la resistencia a la dictadura."

100. While there is no documented proof, suspicion circulated that representatives of the military government started the fire in order to stop the festival from occurring. Graham-Jones, *Exorcising History*, 90.

101. Bosso and Gentile, *Alma doble*. "Conspiración del arte."

102. Ibid. "Como que se agarra también de una tradición."

103. Thank you to Jennifer Schaefer for this insight.

104. My descriptions of the Italian and Buenos Aires productions are based on video documentation from the Private Collection of Silvia Vladimivsky.

105. Taylor, *Paper Tangos*, 72.

CHAPTER 5

1. David Harvey, *A Brief History of Neoliberalism* (New York: Oxford University Press, 2005), 104.

2. Ibid., 105. For a book-length discussion of the political and economic roots and aftermath of the crisis, see Michael Cohen, *Argentina's Economic Growth and Recovery: The Economy in a Time of Default* (New York: Routledge, 2012).

3. For analysis of *piquetero* organizations, see Maristella Svampa and Sebastián Pereyra, *Entre la ruta y el barrio: La experiencia de las organizaciones piqueteras* (Buenos Aires: Biblos, 2003).

4. For detailed analyses of post-2001 political mobilization, see Sebastián Carassai, "The Noisy Majority: An Analysis of the Argentine Crisis of December 2001 from the Theoretical Approach of Hardt & Negri, Laclau and Žižek," *Journal of Latin American Cultural Studies* 16, no. 1 (2007): 45–62; Mónica Gordillo, *Piquetes y cacerolas . . . El "argentinazo" del 2001* (Buenos Aires: Sudamericana, 2010); and Cara Levey, Daniel Ozarow, and Christopher Wylde, eds., *Argentina Since the 2001 Crisis: Recovering the Past, Reclaiming the Future* (New York: Palgrave Macmillan, 2014). For focused analysis of women's organizing, see Sutton, *Bodies in Crisis*.

5. Marina Sitrin, *Horizontalism: Voices of Popular Power in Argentina* (Oakland, CA: AK Press, 2006), 3.

6. For a volume dedicated to the popular assembly and recuperated factory movements, see Ana María Fernández, *Política y subjetividad: Asambleas barriales y fábricas recuperadas* (Buenos Aires: Biblos, 2008).

7. The name Argentina Arde cites the 1968 multimedia art exhibition *Tucumán Arde* that critiqued the working conditions in sugar mills in the northern province of Tucumán.

8. For detailed discussions of these collectives mentioned in-text and the broader post-crisis artistic field, see Giunta, *Poscrisis: Arte argentino después de 2001* (Buenos Aires: Siglo XXI Editores, 2009), 54–64. For a discussion of the blurred lines between art, performance, and protest post-2001, see Marcela Alejandra Fuentes, "'Investments Towards Returns': Protest and Performance in the Era of Financial Crises," *Journal of Latin American Cultural Studies: Travesia* 21, no. 3 (2012): 449–68. For an overview of developments in the theater community, see Jean Graham-Jones, "Rethinking Buenos Aires Theater in the Wake of 2001 and Emerging Structures of Resistance and Resilience," *Theatre Journal* 66, no. 1 (2014): 37–54. Beyond the Argentine context, for a study of the role of self-management in socially engaged performance in Yugoslavia, see Branislav Jakovljevic, *Alienation Effects: Performance and Self-Management in Yugoslavia, 1945–91* (Ann Arbor: University of Michigan Press, 2016).

9. See Themis Chronopoulos, "The *cartoneros* of Buenos Aires, 2001–2005," *City* 10, no. 2 (2006): 167–82, and Mariano Daniel Perelman and Martín Boy, "Cartoneros en Buenos Aires: nuevas modalidades de encuentro," *Revista Mexicana de Sociología* 72, no. 3 (2010): 393–418.

10. Post-2011 dance initiatives centering on *horizontalidad* and social engagement are numerous. Between 2009 and 2011, the Cooperation Cultural Center's Programa Danza y Políticas (Dance and Politics Program, directed by Gabily Anadón) produced multiple concert works. The Cooperation Cultural Center, an institution dedicated to fostering cooperative intellectual and artistic work that identifies alternatives to neoliberal models, hosted the program. For an analysis of the Dance and Politics Program, see Fortuna, "Between the Cultural Center and the *Villa*," 371–94. Lucía Russo's c.a.s.a. colectivo artístico (c.a.s.a. artistic collective) focused on danced "co-laboración" (co-laboring), "c.a.s.a. colectivo artístico," last modified August 21, 2009, accessed December 12, 2012, https://casacolectivoartistico.wordpress.com/2009/08/21/c-a-s-a-colectivo-artistico/. Colectivo Siempre (Always Collective), based in the city of La Plata, combined site-specific work based on political themes with participation in political protests and rallies, see Estévez and Montequin, "Colectivo Siempre—Danza y activismo." Inés Sanguinetti founded the precrisis initiative Fundación Crear Vale la Pena (To Create Is Worth It Foundation) in 1993. The nonprofit organization works with young people across the Greater Buenos Aires region

in multiple movement genres, including contemporary, urban styles, and jazz. km29 (directed by Juan Onofri Barbato) also works with young people (particularly men) in the resource-scarce Greater Buenos Aires region.

11. Sutton, *Bodies in Crisis*, 43.
12. Judith Filc, "Desafiliación, extranjería y relato biográfico en la novela posdictadura," in *Lazos de familia: Herencias, cuerpos, ficciones*, ed. Ana Amado and Nora Dominguez (Buenos Aires: Paidós, 2004), 213. "Elementos de continuidad con las diversas modalidades de expulsión social producidas por el terrorismo de Estado."
13. Sutton, *Bodies in Crisis*, 39.
14. Nixon, *Slow Violence and the Environmentalism of the Poor*, 2. See also Clara Valverde Gefaell's consideration of neoliberal capitalism as "discrete" violence in *De la necropolítica neoliberal a la empatía radical* (Barcelona: Icaria Editorial, 2015).
15. Karen Ann Faulk, *In the Wake of Neoliberalism: Citizenship and Human Rights in Argentina* (Stanford, CA: Stanford University Press, 2013), 2.
16. During the early 2000s, the city of Buenos Aires established physical memory sites, including the conversion of the ESMA clandestine detention center into a museum and cultural center, and the construction of the public Memory Park. Concerns around the appropriation of memory discourse by the government have generated scholarly interest. For further discussion of the Kirchner administrations' relationship to memory of the last military dictatorship, see Lucas Manual Bietti, "Entre la cognición política y la cognición social: El discurso de la memoria colectiva en Argentina," *Discurso & Sociedad* 3, no. 1 (2009): 44–89, and Susana Kaiser, "Memory Inventory: The Production and Consumption of Memory Goods in Argentina," in *Accounting for Violence: Marketing Memory in Latin America*, ed. Ksenija Bilbija and Leigh A. Payne (Durham, NC: Duke University Press, 2011), 313–38.
17. For discussion of Argentina's recuperated factory movement within a broader consideration of Latin American social movements, see Raúl Zibechi, *Territories in Resistance: A Cartography of Latin American Social Movements*, trans. Ramor Ryan (Oakland, CA: AK Press, 2012), 91–108.
18. For a documentary on the Grissinopoli factory, see Darío Doria, *Grissinopoli: El país de los grisines* (A4FILMS, 2004), DVD.
19. Sutton, *Bodies in Crisis*, 161.
20. Bailarines Organizados, "Ballet del Terror" poster, Recoleta Cultural Center, July 2008. "¡¡¡Mirá quién baila . . .!!! En 9 meses 7 accidentes. En 6 meses 12 bailarines despedidos (desaparecidos). En 10 meses 6 funciones. El Ballet del Terror."
21. Ibid.
22. Ex-San Martín dancers Ariel Caramés, Ernesto Chacón Oribe, Silvina Cortés, Pablo Fermani, Guillermo Gonzáles Sevilla, Ana Clara Goswailer, Victoria Hidalgo, Bettina Quintá, Wanda Ramírez, and Jack Syzard helped launch Bailarines Organizados. See the organization's blog, *Bailarines Organizados*, last modified 2010, http://www.bailarinesorganizados.blogspot.com. An earlier example of a similar concert dance labor movement in Argentina dates to the 1960s, when members of the Argentine La Plata Theater Ballet organized. Alberto Somoza, interview by author, Buenos Aires, October 3, 2011.
23. Bettina Quintá, interview by author, Buenos Aires, July 31, 2009.
24. "Por ningún sueño: Despide de bailarines en el Teatro San Martín, un conflicto gremial oscurece el panorama del Ballet Contemporáneo," *Crítica de la Argentina*, August 8, 2008, 35.

25. "Ernesto Chacón Oribe," *YouTube*, last modified January 10, 2008, accessed May 15, 2017, https://www.youtube.com/watch?v=-YTkq89Yqvo. "Genocidio artístico." Chacón Oribe is at work on a book, tentatively titled *La danza de los invisibles (The Dance of the Unseen)*, that recounts the dancers' labor struggle and subsequent formation of the Compañía Nacional de Danza Contemporánea. Ernesto Chacón Oribe, email message to author, January 1, 2018.

26. Quoted in "Por ningún sueño," 35. "A raíz de recientes manifestaciones públicas de ex bailarines del Ballet Contemporáneo del Teatro San Martín, la Dirección General informa que se trata de personal artístico contratado bajo el régimen de 'locación de servicio', esto es contratos sin relación de dependencia, celebrados por tiempo determinado, sin cláusula de renovación, conforme lo establecido por el GCBA. A su vencimiento, el 30/6/08, automáticamente dos de esos contratos dejaron de tener vigencia en virtud de no haberse firmado con ellos nuevos contratos."

27. Lucía Russo, comment on, "Gracias por el apoyo," *Bailarines Organizados* (blog), last modified 2010, http://www.bailarinesorganizados.blogspot.com. "Pues el San Martín no es una empresa privada y los trabajadores tienen derecho a defender sus contractos y derechos laborales."

28. Faulk, *In the Wake of Neoliberalism*, 6.

29. See Wendy Brown, *States of Injury: Power and Freedom in Late Modernity* (Princeton: Princeton University Press, 1995).

30. "Volante difundido en el día del estreno 21 de Junio de 2008," *Bailarines Organizados* (blog), last modified 2010, http://www.bailarinesorganizados. blogspot.com. "Tenemos derecho a los derechos."

31. Quintá, interview by author. "En Argentina, puntualmente, es como que estamos educados a bailar, trabajar y gracias que podés bailar . . . . Es como que hay poco lugar donde trabajar y vos a la hora de decidir ser bailarín y vivir de eso tenés que fijarte bien todo, o si no te tenés que ir del país y desagregarte de todo tu familia y no sabés si afuera igual vas a conseguir trabajo. Entonces, qué sucede con eso, se cuida tanto el poco trabajo que hay, es como que todo el mundo tiene miedo y nadie se expresa realmente como quiere o si de repente hay algo que está mal en el trabajo, por miedo de perder el trabajo no decís nada. Y, los directores o los que tienen los cargos especulan y se aprovechan de eso en la mayoría de los casos. Encima, vienen de una línea de enseñanza vertical con la estructura del "El Director" que no podés hablar, tenés que respetar. Allí aparece el individualismo también, porque si yo mejor me callo, cuido mi lugar y si puedo hacer carrera, mejor. Entonces es re-difícil que los bailarines se puedan juntar para que la danza se respete, se logre en más espacios y se respete al bailarín como un trabajador."

32. For a discussion of the identification of media, communication, and cultural sectors by neoliberals as sites for potential market growth and job creation, see Greig de Peuter, "Creative Economy and Labor Precarity: A Contested Convergence," *Journal of Communication Inquiry* 31, no. 4 (2011): 417–25. For a study of the UK performance field see Jen Harvie, *Fair Play: Art, Performance and Neoliberalism* (New York: Palgrave Macmillan, 2013). For a consideration of neoliberalized labor and Indian classical dance, see Srinivasan, *Sweating Saris*, 141–64.

33. Quintá, interview by author.

34. Anusha Kedhar, "Flexibility and Its Bodily Limits: Transnational South Asian Dancers in an Age of Neoliberalism," *Dance Research Journal* 46, no. 1 (2014): 24.

35. Quintá, interview by author.

36. Giunta, *Poscrisis*, 31.

37. Quintá, interview by author, and Bailarines Organizados Protest, Photographs, 2008, Private Collection of Bettina Quintá.

38. Quintá, interview by author.

39. Martinez Heimann and Bousmpoura, *Trabajadores de la danza*.

40. Elizabeth Jelin, *State Repression and the Labors of Memory*, trans. Judy Rein and Marcial Godoy-Anativia (Minneapolis: University of Minnesota Press, 2003), 64.

41. See Sylvie Durmelat, "Yamina Benguigui as 'Memory Entrepreneur,'" in *Women, Immigration and Identities in France*, ed. Jane Freedman and Carrie Tarr (Oxford: Berg, 2000), 173.

42. Jelin, *State Repression*, 34–35.

43. Bailarines Organizados' memory entrepreneurship differs from the ways, as Jen Harvie points out, contemporary "artrepreneurs" reinforce neoliberal configurations. She identifies strategies such as crowd-sourced funding—itself a means of supporting art making in thin economic times—and a tendency to imagine spectators as consumers as characteristic of artrepreneurship. See Harvie, *Fair Play*, 62–107.

44. Ernesto Chacón Oribe, "¡Finalmente se logró la planta artística!," *La dignidad de ser artista* (blog), May 13, 2009, http://luchayrecompensa.blogspot.com.

45. Mauricio Wainrot, interview by author, Buenos Aires, July 26, 2011.

46. Quintá and Chacón Oribe's *Madre e hijo (historia de un pañuelo blanco)* (*Mother and Child (the story of a white headscarf)*, 2008) honored the work of the Madres de Plaza de Mayo and Jack Syzard's *In Memoriam* (2008) memorialized the lives lost in the dictatorship-era Malvinas conflict in 1982.

47. Original members were: Quintá, Chacón Oribe, Pablo Fermani, Victoria Hidalgo, Wanda Ramírez, and Jack Syzard.

48. Martinez Heimann and Bousmpoura, *Trabajadores de la danza*.

49. Luciana Benosilio's *Mujeres en movimiento-movimiento en mujer* (*Women's Movement*, 2010) remembers histories of feminist movements in Argentina. Eduardo Arguibel and Jorge Amarante's *La Patriótica* (2011), based on the poem by Argentine writer Leopoldo Marechal, questions how the nation is inscribed in, on, and through bodies and their movements. More recent repertory has been wide ranging in theme and stylistic approach. For a list of works, see "Compañía Nacional de Danza Contemporánea," *Ministerio de Cultura de la Nación*, accessed March 13, 2018, https://www.cultura.gob.ar/institucional/organismos/elencos/compania-nacional-de-danza-contemporanea/.

50. Daniel Payero Zaragoza, interview by author, Buenos Aires, March 16, 2011.

51. Ibid.

52. Ibid.

53. Daniel Payero Zaragoza, *Retazos pequeños de nuestra historia más reciente*, Compañía Nacional de Danza Contemporánea, Teatro Nacional Cervantes, Buenos Aires, November 28, 2010. My movement description here is supplemented by video documentation of the work from Zaragoza Payero's private collection.

54. For a complete description and extended choreographic analysis of this work, see Fortuna, "An Enormous Yearning for the Past."

55. Payero Zaragoza, *Retazos pequeños*. "En una visión así cristiana de los derechos humanos, el de la vida es fundamental, el de la libertad es importante, también los del trabajo, de la familia, de la vivienda, etc. etc etc. La Argentina atiende a los derechos humanos en esa omnicomprensión que el término de los derechos humanos significa. Pero yo hablo concretamente porque yo sé que usted hace

su pregunta no a esa visión omnicomprensiva de los derechos humanos sino concretamente al hombre que está detenido sin proceso, que es uno, o al desaparecido, que es otro. Frente al desaparecido, es una incógnita el desaparecido, si apareciera, bueno, tendrá un tratamiento X, y si la desaparición se convirtiera en certeza de su fallecimiento, tendrá un tratamiento Z. Pero mientras sea un desaparecido no, no, no puede tener ningún tratamiento especial, es una incógnita, es un desaparecido, no tiene entidad, no está, ni muerto ni vivo, está desaparecido." For the original footage, see "Pregunta a Videla sobre desaparecidos," *YouTube*, last modified April 25, 2013, accessed March 13, 2018, https://www.youtube.com/watch?v=3AlUCjKOjuc.

56. The dancers speak over each other, exaggerating the overlapping voices in the coverage itself. I have consolidated speakers' phrases for clarity based on the original recording. Slashes indicate a new speaker. "No nos dicen a nosotros si están vivos, si están muertos. ¿Por qué no nos dicen? Si buscamos eso nada más. Que nos respondan, nada más./[El gobierno] miente. ¡Miente!/Mi hija estaba embarazada de cinco meses cuando se la llevaron. Mi nieto tiene que haber nacido en agosto del año pasado. Hasta ahora, no he podido saber nada de él./Nosotros solamente queremos saber dónde están nuestros hijos, vivos o muertos. Angustia porque no sabemos si están enfermos, si tienen frío, si tienen hambre, no sabemos nada. Y desesperación, señor, porque ya no sabemos a quién recurrir." For the original footage, see "Entrevista a Madres de Plaza de Mayo en 1978," *YouTube*, last modified March 25, 2017, accessed March 3, 2018, https://www.youtube.com/watch?v=9dGNfGbI4Rc. See also, "Madres de Plaza de Mayo—Capítulo 3: La batalla por la imagen (1978), last modified March 25, 2015, accessed March 3, 2018, https://www.youtube.com/watch?v=4uM74BWrasc&list=PLxaulh35hPBvNm3yDkzcueBHMHPbxFVkZ&index=3.

57. Martinez Heimann and Bousmpoura, *Trabajadores de la danza*.

58. Ibid. "Conciencia grupal."

59. Ibid.

60. For a documentary on the group's genesis and creative process, see María Arcos, *Bailarines Toda la Vida: Los inicios de la danza comunitaria en Argentina* (Pamplona: Sonríe Que No Es Poco, 2011), DVD.

61. For a discussion of the main principles and objectives of Bailarines Toda la Vida, see Aurelia Chillemi, *Movimiento poético del encuentro: Danza comunitaria y desarrollo social* (Buenos Aires: Ediciones Artes Escénicas, 2015), 24–35.

62. Aurelia Chillemi, interview by author, Buenos Aires, August 6, 2009. Trained in classical and contemporary dance, psychology, and dance therapy, Chillemi developed an independent career in the contemporary dance world during the 1970s and 1980s.

63. For an overview of community theater in Argentina, see Marcela Bidegain *Teatro comunitario: Resistencia y transformación social* (Buenos Aires: Editorial Atuel, 2007) and Marcela Bidegain and Lola Proaño Gómez, eds., *El movimiento teatral comunitario: Reflexiones acerca de la experiencia en la última década (2001–2011)* (Buenos Aires: Ediciones del Centro Cultural de la Cooperación, 2014). For a discussion of newer community dance initiatives in Argentina, see Chillemi, *Movimiento poético del encuentro*, 245–58.

64. Bailarines Toda la Vida, *Identidad y La ruptura*, dir. Aurelia Chillemi, Espacio Cultural Nuestros Hijos, Buenos Aires, November 10, 2010. "Sistema alienante."

65. Ibid.

66. As of 2013, the estimate was around three hundred. See Chillemi, *Movimiento poético del encuentro*, 154–58.
67. Manning, *Ecstasy and the Demon*, 267. For book-length considerations of 1930s leftist modern dance in the United States, see Graff, *Stepping Left* and Franko, *The Work of Dance*. For consideration of the intersections of the leftist dance movements with race, see Manning, *Modern Dance/Negro Dance*, 57–114. For a focused discussion of choreographer Edith Segal's work with laborers, see Prickett, *Embodied Politics*, 11–53.
68. Beatriz Sarlo, *La ciudad vista: Mercancías y cultura urbana* (Buenos Aires: Siglo XXI, 2009), 202. "La 'fábrica-centro cultural' es fundamentalmente un concepto: allí donde hubo producción, los obreros vuelven a controlarla según los ideales cooperativos de una dirección tan horizontal como lo permita el proceso de trabajo, y a esa iniciativa de reorganización laboral . . . se suma la idea de una alianza entre lo cultural y lo productivo que forma parte de la imaginación socialista o libertaria. No se convierte a la fábrica en centro cultural porque la base de edificación industrial ofrece una escenografía atractiva para las actividades artísticas, sino porque el trabajo intelectual y el manual, separados por las formas capitalistas de producción, pueden encontrar en una isla urbana nuevas modalidades combinatorias. Como si fuera posible revitalizar una figura de obrero que estrecha la mano del artista, que pareció quebrarse varias veces en el siglo XX, comenzando por los desdichados avatares de la revolución en Rusia."
69. Ibid., 203. "Un instante reconciliado de la relación entre obreros y capas medias, acontecido en una época donde la culturalización es un estilo y una onda."
70. Ibid., 203–4.
71. Fuentes, "'Investments Toward Returns,'" 450.
72. In addition to my presence as a US-based researcher, during my time as a collective member a German participant, two Puerto Rican dancers, a Venezuelan participant, and many participants from provinces outside of Buenos Aires participated in weekly rehearsals and performances.
73. Fuentes, "'Investments Toward Returns,'" 450.
74. In addition to *La ruptura*'s references to labor, the group also choreographed ¡*Que se vayan todos!,* named after the post-2001 activist battle cry, in 2002.
75. During the early years of the project, the group made a concerted effort to invite workers to take part in weekly rehearsals. Chillemi recounted in an informal conversation that they did not account for the fact that the rehearsal schedule— Fridays from 6 to 9 p.m.—coincided with the end of a shift, after which workers were physically tired and eager to begin their weekend. Discussions with workers determined that social dances and barbeques offered better opportunities for dancers and workers to socialize. Furthermore, social dance, rather than Bailarines Toda la Vida's contemporary-influenced style, offered a more comfortable entry point for shared movement.
76. The Mutual Sentimiento is a community organization that was founded in 1998 by individuals who had been detained and exiled during the last military dictatorship. In addition to the Sexto Kultural (cultural center), the organization's initiatives have also included a community pharmacy, radio, and social programs for impoverished youth. See Ailín Bullentini, "Un Sentimiento en peligro," *Página/ 12*, June 15, 2009, accessed May 28, 2018, https://www.pagina12.com.ar/diario/ sociedad/3-126665-2009-06-15.html.
77. Aurelia Chillemi, email message to author, April 18, 2018.

78. For a comprehensive history of *expresión corporal*, see Kalmar, *Qué es la expresión corporal*. For a discussion of pedagogical approaches to teaching the practice, see Stokoe, *Expresión corporal*.

79. Stokoe, "Historia y antecedentes de esta corriente, según la experiencia de su creadora," 132. "La danza al alcance de todos."

80. Silvia Buschiazzo, "Las Artes del movimiento en la construcción de identidad individual y colectiva" (paper presented at the VI Jornadas de Sociología de la Universidad Nacional de la Plata, 2010), https://www.aacademica.org/000-027/646.pdf. "La necesidad de recomponer la red social fragmentada por un sistema político-social que no atendió las necesidades de la comunidad."

81. Aurelia Chillemi, "Danza Comunitaria: Movimiento, Comunicación, y Creatividad en Espacios No Convencionales" (paper presented at the Sexta Jornada de la Asociación de Psiquiatras Argentinos, Hospital Británico, Buenos Aires, September 23, 2007). "Cuando el movimiento circula, cuando alguien es capaz de recuperar *la gracia del movimiento*, la puede ir compartiendo, transmitiendo y retransmitiendo en forma de un rizoma . . . . Tomar prestados los movimientos en la improvisación grupal conduce a la construcción de un otro lenguaje de movimientos que enriquece el propio, ofreciendo nuevos matices. Este movimiento que circula es un bien común, que sostiene al individuo y le da soporte e identidad al grupo . . . . Cada improvisación grupal es un bien común . . . no hay que firmar escrituras ni convenios, simplemente estar, con el tácito acuerdo solidario del quehacer compartido, del encuentro."

82. Erin Manning, *Relationscapes: Movement, Art, Philosophy* (Boston: MIT, 2009), 31.

83. "Argentina makes arrests in 'flights of death' killings," *BBC*, May 11, 2011, accessed March 3, 2018, http://www.bbc.com/news/world-latin-america-13357301.

84. Manning, *Relationscapes*, 31.

85. For further description and analysis of this piece, see Chillemi, *Movimiento poético del encuentro*, 129–31.

86. Hamera, *Dancing Communities*, 73–74.

87. Adolfo Cabanchik, *Videodanza . . . Y el mar*, perf. Bailarines Toda la Vida (Buenos Aires: IUNA Movimiento, 2012), DVD. For description of the video dance, transcription of text used in the piece, and testimony from dancers that took part in its production, see Chillemi, *Movimiento poético del encuentro*, 131–44.

88. For discussion of the creation of the piece, see Chillemi, *Movimiento poético del encuentro*, 101–8.

89. Other works by Bailarines Toda la Vida include *La pluma del viento, metáfora de una locura* (*The Feather in the Wind, Metaphor of Madness*, 2007), *El baile* (*The Dance*, 2008), *La red* (*The Network*, 2009), and *Homenaje* (*Homage*, 2009).

90. Adolfo Cabanchik, *Videodanza La oscuridad*, perf. Bailarines Toda la Vida (Buenos Aires: IUNA Movimiento, 2009), DVD. See also Chillemi, *Movimiento poético del encuentro*, 116–17.

91. Cabanchik, *Videodanza La oscuridad*.

92. Ibid.

93. For a discussion of modern dance's broader relationship to shifting modes of embodiment in labor production, see Bojana Kunst, "Dance and Work: The Aesthetic and Political Potential of Dance," in *Emerging Bodies: The Performance of Worldmaking in Dance and Choreography*, ed. Gabriele Klein and Sandra Noeth (Bielefeld: Transcript Verlag, 2011), 47–60.

94. Harvey, *A Brief History*, 189.

95. Additional organizations dedicated to dancers' labor rights in Argentina include the Forum for Dance in Action (Foro Danza en Acción 2013–) and the Argentine Association of Dance Workers (Asociación Argentina de Trabajadores de la Danza 2015–). For a discussion of these groups, see Juan Ignacio Vallejos, "Articulations of the Political in Argentine Contemporary Dance" (lecture, Temple University, Philadelphia, PA, April 24, 2018), accessed April 25, 2018, https://livestream.com/accounts/1927261/events/8020705.

EPILOGUE

1. Alejandro Vassallo, email message to author, May 30, 2018.
2. For a collection of recent essays on race in Argentina, see Alberto and Elena, eds., *Rethinking Race in Modern Argentina*. For a concise historical overview of this history of erasure, see the book's introduction, "The Shades of the Nation," 5–9.
3. Ibid., 2. For further contextualization of Argentine dance history vis-à-vis past and present racial politics, see Fortuna, "Dancing Argentine Modernity."
4. "Oduduwá, las Madres y la Marcha," last modified November 21, 2011, accessed June 10, 2017, http://piedralibrepelicula.com.ar/oduduwa-las-madres-y-la-marcha/. "Una forma distinta de poner el cuerpo para evocar a otros cuerpos que ya no están y expresar lo que la voz muchas veces se cansó de gritar."
5. Anthropologist and Oduduwá member María Balmaceda has traced the emergence of secularized African diasporic dance practices in Buenos Aires to the early 1990s. A number of Brazilian, Cuban, and Uruguayan teachers—Isa Soares (teacher of several Oduduwá members), Claudio de Oliverira, Cidinha Fusan, and Evon Correira, among others—began offering classes at prominent cultural centers in Buenos Aires, including the Ricardo Rojas Cultural Center and Danzario Americano. Balmaceda marks the end of the 1990s as the time when Argentine dancers began their own artistic projects, among them Oduduwá, Buenos Aires Danza Afro, and Sambaires. See Balmaceda, "Recreaciones e identidades: Notas sobre arte afro en Buenos Aires," in *Emergencia: Cultura, música y política*, coord. Mariano Ugarte and comp. Luis Sanjurjo (Buenos Aires: Ediciones Centro Cultural de la Cooperación, 2008), 63–74.
6. Other political/student groups and private citizens also marched on March 24, but had to do so at designated times apart from the human rights march.
7. Alejandra Vassallo, interview by author, Buenos Aires, July 9, 2009. "Estamos construyendo historia, la historia de la memoria. Pero también me interesa porque hay mucho dicho, discutido y escrito acerca de qué es la memoria y qué es la historia reciente en Argentina . . . . Para mí, yo quería tratar de abrir el campo de esa discusión afuera de lo académico y decir bueno, hay ciertas cosas que también se hace que no pasan por un partido o agrupación, no pasan por una comunidad, sino que pasan por cosas mucho más puntuales y efímeras, o comunidades efímeras, como lo que pasa el 24 de marzo y cómo un grupo a través de una danza ancestral interviene en los discursos de la memoria."
8. For thorough consideration of the religious and secular practices that Orishá dance draws on as forms of embodied knowledge, see Yvonne Daniel's foundational study, *Dancing Wisdom: Embodied Knowledge in Haitian Vodou, Cuban Yoruba, and Bahian Candomblé* (Urbana: University of Illinois Press, 2005).
9. Balmaceda, "Recreaciones e identidades," 72.
10. See George Reid Andrews, *The Afro-Argentines of Buenos Aires, 1800–1900* (Madison: University of Wisconsin Press, 1980).

11. Lucía Dominga Molina and Mario Luis López, "Afro-Argentineans: 'Forgotten' and 'Disappeared'—Yet Still Present," in *African Roots/American Cultures: Africa in the Creation of the Americas*, ed. Sheila S. Walker (Lanham, MD: Rowman & Littlefield, 2001), 339.

12. Oduduwá Danza Afroamericana, email message to author, March 4, 2011. "Aunque viene llegando la justicia, sus tiempos deben acelerarse. Ya esperamos demasiado y a nuestras Madres y Abuelas se les acaba el largo tiempo de resistencia. También a los victimarios, a quienes corresponde, sin demoras, el juicio y castigo de toda la sociedad. Hay que acelerar los tiempos de la verdad. Ese avance se da sólo en movimiento, las idas y vueltas, los cambios de dirección que aparecen como contradictorios gestan en realidad el inicio de la acción, el empuje hacia adelante, la apertura de nuevos caminos que hasta ahora nos estaban vedados."

13. I have kept with the spelling of the Orishás that Oduduwá used in their communication with dancers. Oduduwá Danza Afroamericana, email message to author. Alternate spellings of Exú include Eshu, Echú, and Exu. Alternate spellings of Xangó include Chango, Changó, Shango, Shangó, and Xango.

14. Palmas testified in 2011 as part of a trial regarding human rights violations at the ESMA detention center. See Alejandra Dandan, "'Los cuerpos estaban muy deteriorados,'" *Página/12*, February 18, 2011, accessed March 3, 2018, https://www.pagina12.com.ar/diario/cartas/24-162563-2011-02-18.html.

15. La Chilinga is an open (*popular*) drumming school that was founded in Buenos Aires in 1995, and is dedicated to teaching and promoting Afro-Latin American musical traditions.

16. D. Soyini Madison, "Co-Performative Witnessing," in *Cultural Studies* 21, no. 6 (2007): 826. For Conquergood on co-performative witnessing as an embodied reimagination of ethnographic participant observation, see "Performance Studies: Interventions and Radical Research," in *TDR* 46, no. 2 (2002): 149.

17. Diana Taylor, "Performance and/as History," in *TDR* 50, no. 1 (2006): 67.

18. Rothberg, *Multidirectional Memory*, 17.

BIBLIOGRAPHY

ARCHIVES AND PRIVATE COLLECTIONS

Alejandro Cervera, Private Collection

Alicia Muñoz, Private Collection

Ana Deutsch, Private Collection

Ana Kamien, Private Collection

Aurelia Chillemi, Private Collection

Bettina Quintá, Private Collection

Biblioteca Nacional de la República de la Argentina (National Library of the Argentine Republic)

  Hemeroteca (Newspapers and Periodicals Collection)

Biblioteca Universidad Torcuato Di Tella (Torcuato Di Tella University Library)

  Archivos del Torcuato Instituto Di Tella (Torcuato Di Tella Institute Archives), Centro de Experimentación Audiovisual (Audiovisual Experimental Center)

Centro de Documentación (Documentation Center), Teatro Municipal General San Martín (General San Martín Municipal Theater)

  Colección Renate Schottelius (Renate Schottelius Collection)

  Hemeroteca (Newspapers and Periodicals Collection)

  Videoteca (Video Collection)

Centro de Documentación e Investigación de la Cultura de Izquierdas (Documentation and Research Center of Leftist Cultures)

Daniel Payero Zaragoza, Private Collection

Déborah Kalmar, Private Collection

Estela Maris, Private Collection

Jerome Robbins Dance Division, New York Public Library for the Performing Arts
  Miriam Winslow Papers

Luciana Acuña, Private Collection

Margarita Bali, Private Collection

Memoria Abierta

Nora Codina, Private Collection

Núcleo Audiovisual de Buenos Aires (Audiovisual Center of Buenos Aires), Centro Cultural General San Martín (General San Martín Cultural Center)

Oscar Araiz, Private Collection

Silvia Vladimivsky, Private Collection

Susana Tambutti, Private Collection

Susana Zimmermann, Private Collection

Vivan Luz, Private Collection

Note: Materials from additional private collections not directly cited in *Moving Otherwise* also informed the development of my analysis.

NEWSPAPERS AND MAGAZINES

(All Buenos Aires)
Clarín
Clarín Revista
Crítica de la Argentina
El Mundo
Estrella Roja
Gente
Kiné, La Revista de lo Corporal
La Causa Peronista
La Nación
La Opinión
La Prensa
La Razón
Mundo de la Danza
Panorama
Primera Plana
Talía
Teatro Popular
Tiempo Argentino
Página/12

INTERVIEWS CONDUCTED BY VICTORIA FORTUNA

Luciana Acuña
Norma Alcaide*
Osvaldo Aguilar
Gabily Anadón*
Oscar Araiz*
Margarita Bali
Adriana Barenstein
Luis Biasotto*
Alejandro Cervera
Aurelia Chillemi
Nora Codina
Fabio D'Aquila*
Catherine de la Trinidad*
Ana Deutsch
Patricia Dorin
Julieta Eskenazi*
Eugenia Estévez*
Laura Falcoff*
Mónica Fracchia
María Fux*
Román Ghilotti*
Silvia Kaehler
Carolina Herman*
Silvia Hodgers
Déborah Kalmar
Ana Kamien

Gerardo Litvak*
Vivan Luz
Estela Maris
Graciela Martínez*
Alicia Muñoz
Bettina Quintá
Claudio Pansera*
María José Patiño*
Salo Pasik*
Daniel Payero Zaragoza
Maralia Reca*
Gabriela Romero*
Mariela Ruggieri*
Lucía Russo*
Alicia Sanguinetti
Inés Sanguinetti*
Andrea Servera*
Ana María Stekelman
Alberto Somoza
Cuca Taburelli
Susana Tambutti
Milka Truol
Silvia Vainberg*
Alejandra Vassallo
Silvia Vladimivsky
Mauricio Wainrot
Susana Zimmermann

*These interviews are not directly cited in *Moving Otherwise*; however, I include them here because they inform the text, and I would like to acknowledge the time that these individuals took to speak with me.

BOOKS, ARTICLES, DISSERTATIONS, CONFERENCE PRESENTATIONS, AND FILMS

10 Años: Artes del movimiento. Buenos Aires: Instituto Universitario Nacional del Arte, 2008.

Aellig Régnier, Raphaëlle, and Norbert Wiedmer. *Juntos: Un Retour en Argentine*. Geneva: RaR and Biograph Film, 2001. https://www.artfilm.ch/juntos-un-retour-en-argentine.

Agamben, Giorgio. *Homo Sacer: Sovereign Power and Bare Life*. Translated by Daniel Heller-Roazen. Stanford, CA: Stanford University Press, 1998.

Agosín, Marjorie. "The Dance of Life: Women and Human Rights in Chile." In *Dance, Human Rights, and Social Justice: Dignity in Motion*, edited by Naomi M. Jackson and Toni Shapiro-Phim, translated by Janice Molloy, 296–303. Lanham, MD: Scarecrow, 2008.

Alberto, Paulina L., and Eduardo Elena. "Introduction: The shades of the nation." In *Rethinking Race in Modern Argentina*, edited by Paulina L. Alberto and Eduardo Elena, 1–23. New York: Cambridge University Press, 2016.

Alberto, Paulina L., and Eduardo Elena, eds. *Rethinking Race in Modern Argentina*. New York: Cambridge University Press, 2016.

Albright, Ann Cooper. *Choreographing Difference: The Body and Identity in Contemporary Dance*. Middletown, CT: Wesleyan University Press, 1997.

Amado, Ana. *La imagen justa: Cine argentino y política, 1980–2007*. Buenos Aires: Ediciones Colihue SRL, 2009.

Amado, Ana, and Nora Domínguez, eds. *Lazos de familia: Herencias, cuerpos, ficciones*. Buenos Aires: Paidós, 2004.

Anadón, Gabily, ed. *El milagro al borde del estado: Discursividades políticas de danza*. Buenos Aires: Centro Cultural de la Cooperación, 2011.

Andrews, George Reid. *The Afro-Argentines of Buenos Aires, 1800–1900*. Madison: University of Wisconsin Press, 1980.

Andújar, Andrea. Prologue to *De minifaldas, militancias y revoluciones: Exploraciones sobre los 70 en la Argentina*, edited by Andrea Andújar, Débora D'Antonio, Fernanda Gil Lozano, Karin Grammático and María Laura Rosa, 9–16. Buenos Aires: Ediciones Luxemburg, 2009.

Andújar, Andrea, Débora D'Antonio, Fernanda Gil Lozano, Karin Grammático, and María Laura Rosa, eds. *De minifaldas, militancias y revoluciones: Exploraciones sobre los 70 en la Argentina*. Buenos Aires: Ediciones Luxemburg, 2009.

Arancibia, Juana A., and Zulema Mirkin, eds. *Volumen II: Teatro argentino durante el Proceso (1976–1983): ensayos críticos-entrevistas*. Buenos Aires: Instituto Literario y Cultural Hispánico, 1992.

Arcos, María. *Bailarines Toda La Vida: Los inicios de la danza comunitaria en Argentina*. Pamplona: Sonríe Que No Es Poco, 2011. DVD.

Arendt, Hannah. *The Origins of Totalitarianism*. San Diego: Harcourt, 1973.

Arruti, Mariana. *Trelew: La fuga que fue masacre*. Buenos Aires: Fundación Alumbrar, 2004. DVD.

Avelar, Idelber. *The Untimely Present: Postdictatorial Latin American Fiction and the Task of Mourning*. Durham, NC: Duke University Press, 1999.

Babic, Karolina. "Todavía Bailamos la cueca sola: From Local Protest Practice against Chile's Dictatorship to (Trans)national Memory Icon." PhD diss., University at Albany, State University of New York, 2014.

Balmaceda, María. "Recreaciones e identidades: Notas sobre arte afro en Buenos Aires." In *Emergencia: Cultura, música y política*, coordinated by Mariano Ugarte and compiled by Luis Sanjurjo, 63–74. Buenos Aires: Ediciones Centro Cultural de la Cooperación, 2008.

Banes, Sally. *Democracy's Body: Judson Dance Theater, 1962–1964*. Durham, NC: Duke University Press, 1993.

Banes, Sally. "Terpsichore in Combat Boots." *TDR: The Drama Review* 33, no. 1 (1989): 13–16.

Beguán, Viviana, ed. *Nosotras, presas políticas*. Buenos Aires: Nuestra America, 2006.

Benjamin, Walter. "On the Concept of History." Translated by Dennis Redmond. *Marxists Internet Archive*, 2005. https://www.marxists.org/reference/archive/benjamin/1940/history.htm.

Bialet, Graciela, and Ángel Luis Luján. "Censura y LIJ durante la dictadura argentina de 1976–1983." In *Censuras y literatura infantil y juvenil en el siglo XX (En España y 7 países latinoamericanos)*, edited by Pedro C. Cerrillo and M.ª Victoria Sotomayor, 271–328. Cuenca: Ediciones de la Universidad de Castilla-Mancha, 2016.

Bidegain, Marcela. *Teatro comunitario: Resistencia y transformación social*. Buenos Aires: Editorial Atuel, 2007.

Bidegain, Marcela, and Lola Proaño Gómez, eds. *El movimiento teatral comunitario: Reflexiones acerca de la experiencia en la última década (2001–2011)*. Buenos Aires: Ediciones Centro Cultural de la Cooperación, 2014.

Bietti, Lucas Manual. "Entre la cognición política y la cognición social: El discurso de la memoria colectiva en Argentina." *Discurso & Sociedad* 3, no. 1 (2009): 44–89.

Blanco Borelli, Melissa. *She Is Cuba: A Genealogy of the Mulata Body*. New York: Oxford University Press, 2015.

Bosso, Ivana, and Francesca Gentile. *Alma doble*. Turin: La Sarraz Pictures, 2007. DVD.

Brown, Wendy. *States of Injury: Power and Freedom in Late Modernity*. Princeton: Princeton University Press, 1995.

Browning, Barbara. *Samba: Resistance in Motion*. Bloomington: Indiana University Press, 1995.

Buch, Esteban. *The Bomarzo affair: Ópera, perversión y dictadura*. Buenos Aires: Adriana Hidalgo Editora, 2003.

Burt, Ramsay. *The Male Dancer: Bodies, Spectacle, Sexualities*. New York: Routledge, 1995.

Burt, Ramsay. *Ungoverning Dance: Contemporary European Theatre Dance and the Commons*. New York: Oxford University Press, 2017.

Buschiazzo, Silvia. "Las artes del movimiento en la construcción de identidad individual y colectiva." Paper presented at the VI Jornadas de Sociología de La Universidad Nacional de La Plata, 2010. https://www.aacademica.org/000-027/646.pdf.

Cabanchik, Adolfo. *Videodanza La oscuridad*. Performed by Bailarines Toda La Vida. Buenos Aires: IUNA Movimiento, 2009. DVD.

Cabanchik, Adolfo. *Videodanza . . . Y el mar*. Performed by Bailarines Toda La Vida. Buenos Aires: IUNA Movimiento, 2012. DVD.

Cadús, María Eugenia. "La consolidación de la práctica de la danza escénica durante el primer peronismo." *Revista Afuera: Estudio de crítica cultural*. 17–18 (2016–17), http://revistaafuera17-18.blogspot.com.ar/p/blog-page.html.

Cadús, María Eugenia. "La danza escénica durante el primer Peronismo: Formación y práctica de la danza y políticas del estado." PhD diss., University of Buenos Aires, 2017.

Cadús, María Eugenia. "'¿Dejarás el baile por mí?': La representación de la bailarina como trabajadora en *Mujeres que bailan* de Manuel Romero." *Cultura: Debates y perspectivas de un mundo en cambio* 9 (2015): 49–65.

Candelario, Rosemary. *Flowers Cracking Concrete: Eiko & Koma's Asian/American Choreographies*. Middletown, CT: Wesleyan University Press, 2016.

Cara, Ana. "Entangled Tangos: Passionate Displays, Intimate Dialogues." *The Journal of American Folklore* 122, no. 486 (2009): 438–65.

Carassai, Sebastián. *The Argentine Silent Majority: Middle Classes, Politics, Violence, and Memory*. Durham, NC: Duke University Press, 2014.

Carassai, Sebastián. "The Noisy Majority: An Analysis of the Argentine Crisis of December 2001 from the Theoretical Approach of Hardt & Negri, Laclau and Žižek." *Journal of Latin American Cultural Studies* 16, no. 1 (2007): 45–62.

Caruth, Cathy. *Unclaimed Experience: Trauma, Narrative, and History*. Baltimore: Johns Hopkins University Press, 1996.

Chasteen, John Charles. *National Rhythms, African Roots: The Deep History of Latin American Popular Dance*. Albuquerque: University of New Mexico Press, 2004.

Chatterjea, Ananya. "On the Value of Mistranslations and Contaminations: The Category of 'Contemporary Choreography' in Asian Dance." *Dance Research Journal* 45, no. 1 (2013): 7–21.

Chillemi, Aurelia. "Danza comunitaria: Movimiento, comunicación, y creatividad en espacios no convencionales." Paper presented at the Sexta Jornada de la Asociación de Psiquiatras Argentinos, Hospital Británico, Buenos Aires, September 23, 2007.

Chillemi, Aurelia. *Movimiento poético del encuentro: Danza comunitaria y desarrollo social.* Buenos Aires: Artes Escénicas, 2015.

Chronopoulos, Themis. "The Cartoneros of Buenos Aires, 2001–2005." *City* 10, no. 2 (2006): 167–82.

Citro, Silvia. *Cuerpos significantes: Travesía de una etnografía dialéctica.* Buenos Aires: Biblos, 2009.

Citro, Silvia, and Patricia Aschieri, eds. *Cuerpos en movimiento: Antropología de y desde las danzas.* Buenos Aires: Biblos, 2012.

Clayton, Michelle. "Modernism's Moving Bodies." *Modernist Cultures* 9, no. 1 (2014): 27–45.

Cohen, Michael A. *Argentina's Economic Growth and Recovery: The Economy in a Time of Default.* New York: Routledge, 2012.

Collier, Simon. "The Birth of the Tango." In *The Argentina Reader: History, Culture, Politics*, edited by Gabriela Nouzeilles and Graciela R. Montaldo, 196–202. Durham, NC: Duke University Press, 2002.

Collier, Simon, Artemis Cooper, María S. Azzi, and Richard Martin. *Tango!: The Dance, the Song, the Story.* London: Thames & Hudson, 1995.

Conquergood, Dwight. "Performance Studies: Interventions and Radical Research." *TDR* 46, no. 2 (2002): 145–56.

Copel, Melinda. "The 1954 Limón Company Tour to South America: Goodwill Tour or Cold War Cultural Propaganda?" In *José Limón: The Artist Re-viewed*, edited by June Dunbar, 97–112. New York: Routledge, 2003.

Coscia, Jorge. *Danza contemporánea argentina: Nucleodanza, 1974–1993.* Buenos Aires: Filmes de Colección Blakman, 1994. DVD.

Cosse, Isabella. "Infidelities: Morality, Revolution, and Sexuality in Left-Wing Guerilla Organizations in 1960s and 1970s Argentina." *Journal of the History of Sexuality* 23, no. 3 (2014): 415–50.

Cosse, Isabella. *Pareja, sexualidad y familia en los años sesenta: Una revolución discreta en Buenos Aires.* Buenos Aires: Siglo XXI Editores, 2010.

Croft, Clare. *Dancers as Diplomats: American Choreography in Cultural Exchange.* New York: Oxford University Press, 2015.

Cvejić, Bojana. *Choreographing Problems: Expressive Concepts in European Contemporary Dance and Performance.* Hampshire, UK: Palgrave Macmillan, 2015.

Daly, Ann. *Done Into Dance: Isadora Duncan in America.* Bloomington: Indiana University Press, 1995.

Daniel, Yvonne. *Dancing Wisdom: Embodied Knowledge in Haitian Vodou, Cuban Yoruba, and Bahian Candomblé.* Urbana: University of Illinois Press, 2005.

De Peuter, Greig. "Creative Economy and Labor Precarity: A Contested Convergence." *Journal of Communication Inquiry* 31, no. 4 (2011): 417–25.

De Toro, Fernando. "Ideología y teatro épico en Santa Juana de América." *Latin American Theatre Review* 14, no. 1 (1980): 55–64.

Del Priore, Oscar, and Irene Amuchástegui. *Cien tangos fundamentales.* Buenos Aires: Aguilar, 2011. E-book.

Delgado, Celeste Fraser, and José Esteban Muñoz, eds. *Everynight Life: Culture and Dance in Latin/o America.* Durham, NC: Duke University Press, 1997.

Desmond, Jane. "Dancing Out the Difference: Cultural Imperialism and Ruth St. Denis's 'Radha' of 1906." *Signs: Journal of Women in Culture and Society* 17, no. 1 (1991): 28–49.

Destaville, Enrique Honorio. "Mirada sobre el siglo XIX y el siglo XX en sus primeros años." In *Historia general de la danza en la Argentina*, edited by Beatriz Durante, 13–49. Buenos Aires: Fondo Nacional de las Artes, 2008.

Diana, Marta. *Mujeres guerrilleras: La militancia de los setenta en el testimonio de sus protagonistas.* Buenos Aires: Planeta, 1996.

Doria, Darío. *Grissinopoli: El país de los grisines.* Buenos Aires: A4FILMS, 2004. DVD.

Dorin, Patricia. "Legados y continuidades: Derivaciones de una danza de expresión en Argentina." In *Pensar con la danza*, edited by Carlos Eduardo Sanabria Bohóriquez and Ana Carolina Ávila Pérez, 119–130. Bogotá: Ministerio de Cultura de Colombia, Universidad de Bogotá Jorge Tadeo Lozano, Facultuad de Ciencias Sociales, Departamento de Humanidades, 2014.

Doumerc, Beatriz, and Ayax Barnes. *La línea.* Digitized by Roberto Boote. Buenos Aires: Ediciones del Eclipse, 2003. https://www.youtube.com/watch?v=vbR_ l1VnKm4.

Durmelat, Sylvie. "Yamina Benguigui as 'Memory Entrepreneur.'" In *Women, Immigration, and Identities in France*, edited by Jane Freedman and Carrie Tarr, 171–88. Oxford: Berg, 2000.

Estévez, Mariana, and Diana Montequin. "Colectivo Siempre—Danza y activismo." *Universidad Nacional de La Plata* (blog). August 2013. http://blogs.unlp.edu.ar/ arteaccionlaplataxxi/files/2014/05/2013-colectivo-Siempre.pdf.

Falcoff, Laura. "La danza moderna y contemporánea." In *Historia general de la danza en la Argentina*, 231–321, edited by Beatriz Durante. Buenos Aires: Fondo Nacional de las Artes, 2008.

Falicov, Tamara L. *The Cinematic Tango: Contemporary Argentine Film.* London: Wallflower Press, 2007.

Faulk, Karen. *In the Wake of Neoliberalism: Citizenship and Human Rights in Argentina.* Stanford, CA: Stanford University Press, 2013.

Felitti, Karina. "Poner el cuerpo: Género y sexualidad en la política revolucionaria de Argentina en las décadas de los sesenta y setenta." In *Political and Social Movements During the Sixties and Seventies in the Americas and Europe*, edited by Avital H. Bloch, 69–93. Colima: University of Colima, 2010.

Fernández, Ana María. *Política y subjetividad: Asambleas barriales y fábricas recuperadas.* Buenos Aires: Biblos, 2008.

Filc, Judith. "Desfiliación, extranjería y relato biográfico en la novela postdictadura." In *Lazos de familia: Herencias, cuerpos, ficciones*, edited by Ana Amado and Nora Domínguez, 197–230. Buenos Aires: Paidós, 2004.

Fortuna, Victoria. "Araiz, Oscar (1940–)." *The Routledge Encyclopedia of Modernism.* New York: Taylor and Francis, 2016. https://www.rem.routledge.com/articles/ araiz-oscar-1940.

Fortuna, Victoria. "Between the Cultural Center and the *Villa*: Dance, Neoliberalism, and Silent Borders in Buenos Aires." In *The Oxford Handbook of Dance and Politics*, edited by Rebekah J. Kowal, Gerald Siegmund, and Randy Martin, 371–94. New York: Oxford University Press, 2017.

Fortuna, Victoria. "A Dance of Many Bodies: Moving Trauma in Susana Tambutti's *La puñalada.*" *Performance Research* 16, no. 1 (2011): 43–51.

Fortuna, Victoria. "Dancing Argentine Modernity: Imagined Indigenous Bodies on the Buenos Aires Concert Stage (1915–1966)." *Dance Research Journal* 48, no. 2 (2016): 44–60.

Fortuna, Victoria. "Danza, historia, memoria." In *VI Jornadas de investigación en danza 2012*, edited by María Eugenia Cadús, 20–45. Buenos Aires: Universidad Nacional de las Artes, 2016.

Fortuna, Victoria. "An Enormous Yearning for the Past: Movement/Archive in Two Contemporary Dance Works." *e-misférica* 9, nos. 1-2 (2012). http://hemisphericinstitute.org/hemi/en/e-misferica-91/fortuna.

Fortuna, Victoria. *"Poner el cuerpo*: Buenos Aires Contemporary Dance and the Politics of Movement." PhD diss., Northwestern University, 2013.

Fortuna, Victoria. "Schottelius, Renate (1921–1998)." *The Routledge Encyclopedia of Modernism*. New York: Taylor and Francis, 2016. https://www.rem.routledge.com/articles/schottelius-renate-1921-1998.

Foster, Susan Leigh. "Choreographing History." In *Choreographing History*, edited by Susan Leigh Foster, 3–21. Bloomington: Indiana University Press, 1995.

Foster, Susan Leigh. "Worlding Dance—An Introduction." In *Worlding Dance*, edited by Susan Leigh Foster, 1–13. New York: Palgrave Macmillan, 2009.

Foster, Susan Leigh, ed. *Worlding Dance*. New York: Palgrave Macmillan, 2009.

Foucault, Michel. *"Society Must Be Defended" Lectures at the Collège de France 1975–1976*. Translated by David Macey. New York: Picador, 2003.

Franco, Jean. *Cruel Modernity*. Durham, NC: Duke University Press, 2013.

Franko, Mark. "Dance and the Political: States of Exception." *Dance Research Journal* 38, no. 1-2 (2006): 3–18.

Franko, Mark. *The Work of Dance: Labor, Movement, and Identity in the 1930s*. Middletown, CT: Wesleyan University Press, 2002.

Freeman, Elizabeth. "Packing History, Count(er)ing Generations." *New Literary History* 31, no. 4 (2002): 727–44.

Fuentes, Marcela Alejandra. "'Investments Towards Returns': Protest and Performance in the Era of Financial Crises." *Journal of Latin American Cultural Studies: Travesia* 21, no. 3 (2012): 449–68.

Fusco, Coco. "The Tango of Esthetics and Politics: An Interview with Fernando Solanas." *Cineaste* 16, nos. 1–2 (1987–88): 57–59.

Fux, María. *Primer encuentro con la danzaterapia*. Buenos Aires: Paidós, 1982.

Garafola, Lynn, ed. *Rethinking the Sylph: New Perspectives on the Romantic Ballet*. Middletown, CT: Wesleyan University Press, 1997.

Garaño, Santiago, and Werner Pertot, eds. *Detenidos-aparecidos: presas y presos políticos desde Trelew a la dictadura*. Buenos Aires: Biblos, 2007.

Getino, Aldo, Laura Lagar, and Mónica Simoncini. *Gaviotas blindadas: historias del PRT-ERP*. Córdoba: Mascaró Cine Americano, 2007.

Giersdorf, Jens Richard. *The Body of the People: East German Dance Since 1945*. Madison: University of Wisconsin Press, 2013.

Giunta, Andrea. *Avant-Garde, Internationalism, and Politics: Argentine Art in the Sixties*. Translated by Peter Kahn. Durham, NC: Duke University Press, 2007.

Giunta, Andrea. *Poscrisis: Arte argentino después de 2001*. Buenos Aires: Siglo XXI Editores, 2009.

Goldman, Danielle. *I Want to Be Ready: Improvised Dance as a Practice of Freedom*. Ann Arbor: University of Michigan Press, 2010.

Gordillo, Mónica. *Piquetes y cacerolas . . . El "argentinazo" del 2001*. Buenos Aires: Sudamericana, 2010.

Gorelik, Adrián. *Miradas sobre Buenos Aires*. Buenos Aires: Siglo XXI Editores, 2004.

Graff, Ellen. *Stepping Left: Dance and Politics in New York City, 1928–1942*. Durham, NC: Duke University Press, 1997.

Graham-Jones, Jean. *Exorcising History: Argentine Theater Under Dictatorship*. Cranbury, NJ: Bucknell University Press, 2000.

Graham-Jones, Jean. "Rethinking Buenos Aires Theater in the Wake of 2001 and Emerging Structures of Resistance and Resilience." *Theatre Journal* 66, no. 1 (2014): 37–54.

Graziano, Frank. *Divine Violence: Spectacle, Psychosexuality, and Radical Christianity in the Argentine "Dirty War."* Boulder, CO: Westview Press, 1992.

Green, James N. "'Who Is the Macho Who Wants to Kill Me?' Male Homosexuality, Revolutionary Masculinity, and the Brazilian Armed Struggle of the 1960s and 1970s." *Hispanic American Historical Review* 92, no. 3 (2012): 437–69.

Guevara, Ernesto. *El socialismo y el hombre en Cuba*. Atlanta: Pathfinder Press, 1992.

Guy, Donna J. "Life and the Commodification of Death in Argentina: Juan and Eva Perón." In *Death, Dismemberment and Memory: Body Politics in Latin America*, edited by Lyman Johnson, 245–72. Albuquerque: University of New Mexico Press, 2004.

Halperín Donghi, Tulio. *Proyecto y construcción de una nación (1846–1880)*. Buenos Aires: Emecé, 2007.

Hamera, Judith. "Becoming-Other-Wise: Conversational Performance and the Politics of Experience." *Text and Performance Quarterly* 18, no. 34 (1998): 273–99.

Hamera, Judith. *Dancing Communities: Performance, Difference, and Connection in the Global City*. New York: Palgrave, 2007.

Harvey, David. *A Brief History of Neoliberalism*. New York: Oxford University Press, 2005.

Harvie, Jen. *Fair Play: Art, Performance and Neoliberalism*. New York: Palgrave Macmillan, 2013.

Hazzard-Gordon, Katrina. *Jookin': The Rise of Social Dance Formations in African American Culture*. Philadelphia: Temple University Press, 2010.

Hellier-Tinoco, Ruth. *Embodying Mexico: Tourism, Nationalism & Performance*. New York: Oxford University Press, 2011.

Hewitt, Andrew. *Social Choreography: Ideology as Performance in Dance and Everyday Movement*. Durham, NC: Duke University Press, 2005.

Isse Moyano, Marcelo. "Argentina–Modern Dance," edited by Selma Jean Cohen. *The International Encyclopedia of Dance*. Oxford Reference Online, 2005. http://www.oxfordreference.com/view/10.1093/acref/9780195173697.001.0001/acref-9780195173697.

Isse Moyano, Marcelo, ed. *Cuadernos de Danza III*. Buenos Aires: Facultad de Filosofía y Letras UBA, 2002.

Isse Moyano, Marcelo. *La danza moderna argentina cuenta su historia*. Buenos Aires: Ediciones Artes del Sur, 2006.

Jackson, Naomi M. *Converging Movements: Modern Dance and Jewish Culture at the 92nd Street Y*. Middletown, CT: Wesleyan University Press, 2000.

Jackson, Naomi, and Toni Shapiro-Phim, eds. *Dance, Human Rights, and Social Justice: Dignity in Motion*. Lanham, MD: Scarecrow Press, 2008.

Jakovljevic, Branislav. *Alienation Effects: Performance and Self-Management in Yugoslavia, 1945–91*. Ann Arbor: University of Michigan Press, 2016.

Jelin, Elizabeth. *State Repression and the Labors of Memory*. Translated by Judy Rein and Marcial Godoy-Anativia. Minneapolis: University of Minnesota Press, 2003.

John, Suki. *Contemporary Dance in Cuba: Técnica Cubana as Revolutionary Movement.* Jefferson: McFarland & Company, Inc., Publishers, 2012.

Kaehler, Silvia. *Asociación Amigos de la Danza 1962–1966.* Buenos Aires: Eudeba, 2013.

Kaiser, Susana. "Memory Inventory: The Production and Consumption of Memory Goods in Argentina." In *Accounting for Violence: Marketing Memory in Latin America,* edited by Ksenija Bilbija and Leigh A. Payne, 313–38. Durham, NC: Duke University Press, 2011.

Kalmar, Déborah. *Qué es la expresión corporal: A partir de la corriente de trabajo creada por Patricia Stokoe.* Buenos Aires: Lumen, 2005.

Katzenstein, Inés, and Andrea Giunta, eds. *Listen, Here, Now! Argentine Art of the 1960s: Writings of the Avant-Garde.* New York: The Museum of Modern Art, 2004.

Kedhar, Anusha. "Flexibility and Its Bodily Limits: Transnational South Asian Dancers in an Age of Neoliberalism." *Dance Research Journal* 46, no. 1 (2014): 23–40.

King, John. *El Di Tella y el desarrollo cultural argentino en la década del sesenta.* Buenos Aires: Asunto Impreso Ediciones, 2007.

Kolb, Alexandra. "Cross-Currents of Dance and Politics: An Introduction." In *Dance and Politics,* edited by Alexandra Kolb, 1–36. Bern: Peter Lang, 2011.

Kowal, Rebekah J. *How To Do Things with Dance: Performing Change in Postwar America.* Middletown, CT: Wesleyan University Press, 2010.

Kowal, Rebekah J., Gerald Siegmund, and Randy Martin. Introduction to *The Oxford Handbook of Dance and Politics,* edited by Rebekah J. Kowal, Gerald Siegmund, and Randy Martin, 1–24. New York: Oxford University Press, 2017.

Kraut, Anthea. *Choreographing Copyright: Race, Gender, and Intellectual Property Rights in American Dance.* New York: Oxford University Press, 2016.

Kunst, Bojana. "Dance and Work: The Aesthetic and Political Potential of Dance." In *Emerging Bodies: The Performance of Worldmaking in Dance,* edited by Gabriele Klein and Sandra Noeth, 47–60. Bielefeld: Transcript Verlag, 2011.

Larasati, Rachmi Diyah. *The Dance That Makes You Vanish: Cultural Reconstruction in Post-Genocide Indonesia.* Minneapolis: University of Minnesota Press, 2013.

Larvin, Asunción. "Juana Azurduy de Padilla (c. 1780–1862)." *The Oxford Encyclopedia of Women in World History.* Oxford Reference Online, 2008. http://www. oxfordreference.com/view/10.1093/acref/9780195148909.001.0001/ acref-9780195148909-e-71?rskey=PFy5U4&result=61.

Lepecki, André. "Choreopolice and Choreopolitics: or, the task of the dancer." *TDR: The Drama Review* 57, no. 4 (2013): 13–27.

Lepecki, André. *Exhausting Dance: Performance and the Politics of Movement.* New York: Routledge, 2005.

Lepecki, André. *Singularities: Dance in the Age of Performance.* New York: Routledge, 2016.

Levey, Cara, Daniel Ozarow, and Christopher Wylde, eds. *Argentina Since the 2001 Crisis: Recovering the Past, Reclaiming the Future.* New York: Palgrave Macmillan, 2014.

Levine, Annette. *Cry For Me, Argentina: The Performance of Trauma in the Short Narratives of Aida Bortnik, Griselda Gambaro, and Tununa Mercado.* Madison, NJ: Fairleigh Dickinson University Press, 2008.

Lizárraga, Andrés. *Santa Juana de América.* Havana: Casa de las Américas, 1968.

Longoni, Ana. "El FATRAC, frente cultural del PRT/ERP." *Lucha Armada en la Argentina* 4 (2006): 20–33.

Longoni, Ana. *Vanguardia y revolución: Arte e izquierdas en la Argentina de los sesenta-setenta.* Buenos Aires: Ariel, 2014.

Longoni, Ana, and Gustavo A. Bruzzone, eds. *El Siluetazo*. Buenos Aires: Adriana Hidalgo Editora, 2008.

Longoni, Ana, and Mariano Mestman. *Del Di Tella a "Tucumán Arde": Vanguardia artística y política en el 68 argentino*. Buenos Aires: Eudeba, 2010.

Lozano, Ezequiel. *Sexualidades disidentes en el teatro: Buenos Aires, años 60*. Buenos Aires: Editorial Biblos, 2015.

Maccarini, Manuel. *Teatro de identidad popular: los géneros sainete rural, circo criollo y radioteatro argentino*. Buenos Aires: Inteatro, 2006.

Madison, D. Soyini. *Acts of Activism: Human Rights as Radical Performance*. Cambridge: Cambridge University Press, 2010.

Madison, D. Soyini. "Co-Performative Witnessing." *Cultural Studies* 21, no. 6 (2007): 826–31.

Malinow, Inés. *Desarrollo del ballet en la Argentina*. Buenos Aires: Ediciones Culturales Argentinas, 1963.

Manning, Erin. *Politics of Touch: Sense, Movement, Sovereignty*. Minneapolis: University of Minnesota Press, 2007.

Manning, Erin. *Relationscapes: Movement, Art, Philosophy*. Boston: MIT Press, 2009.

Manning, Susan. "Dance History." In *The Bloomsbury Companion to Dance Studies*, edited by Sherril Dodds. London: Bloomsbury, Forthcoming 2019.

Manning, Susan. *Ecstasy and the Demon: Feminism and Nationalism in the Dances of Mary Wigman*. Berkeley: University of California Press, 1993.

Manning, Susan. *Modern Dance/Negro Dance: Race in Motion*. Minneapolis: University of Minnesota Press, 2004.

Manning, Susan. "Modernist Dogma and Post-modern Rhetoric: A Response to Sally Banes' Terpsichore in Sneakers." *TDR: The Drama Review* 44, no. 4 (1988): 32–39.

Manso, Carlos. "Cuatro décadas del cuerpo de baile del Teatro Colón." In *Historia General de la danza en la Argentina*, edited by Beatriz Durante, 41–51. Buenos Aires: Fondo Nacional de las Artes, 2008.

Manzano, Valeria. *The Age of Youth in Argentina: Culture, Politics, and Sexuality from Perón to Videla*. Chapel Hill: The University of North Carolina Press, 2014.

Martin, Randy. *Critical Moves: Dance Studies in Theory and Politics*. Durham, NC: Duke University Press, 1998.

Martin, Randy. *Knowledge LTD: Toward a Social Logic of the Derivative*. Philadelphia: Temple University Press, 2015.

Martínez, Paola. *Género, política y revolución en los años setenta: Las mujeres del PRT-ERP*. Buenos Aires: Imago Mundi, 2009.

Martínez, Tomás Eloy. *La pasión según Trelew*. Buenos Aires: Granica Editor, 1973.

Martinez Heimann, Julia, and Konstantina Bousmpoura. *Trabajadores de la danza*. Buenos Aires and Athens: Kinsi, 2016.

Masiello, Francine. "La Argentina durante el Proceso: Las múltiples resistencias de la cultura." In *Ficción y política: la narrativa argentina durante el proceso militar*, edited by Daniel Balderston, 11–29. Buenos Aires: Alianza Editorial, 1987.

Masiello, Francine. *The Art of Transition: Latin American Culture and Neoliberal Crisis*. Latin America Otherwise. Durham, NC: Duke University Press, 2001.

Mbembe, Achille. "Necropolitics." Translated by Libby Meintjes. *Public Culture* 15, no. 1 (2003): 11–40.

Melgar, Analía, ed. *Puentes y atajos: Recorridos por la danza en Argentina*. Buenos Aires: Editorial De Los Cuatro Vientos, 2005.

Merritt, Carolyn. *Tango Nuevo*. Gainesville: University of Florida Press, 2012.

Mills, Dana. *Dance & Politics: Moving Beyond Boundaries*. Manchester: Manchester University Press, 2017.

Molina, Lucía Dominga, and Mario Luis López. "Afro-Argentineans: 'Forgotten' and 'Disappeared'—Yet Still Present." In *African Roots/American Cultures: Africa in the Creation of the Americas*, edited by Sheila S. Walker, 332–47. Lanham, MD: Rowman & Littlefield, 2001.

Molinero, Carlos, and Pablo Vila. "A Brief History of the Militant Song Movement in Argentina." In *The Militant Song Movement in Latin America: Chile, Uruguay, and Argentina*, edited by Pablo Vila, 193–228. Lanham, MD: Lexington Books, 2014.

Montez, Noe. *Memory, Transitional Justice, and Theater in Postdictatorship Argentina*. Carbondale: Southern Illinois University Press, 2017.

Mora, Ana Sabrina. "El cuerpo en la danza desde la antropología. Prácticas, representaciones y experiencias durante la formación en danzas clásicas, danza contemporánea y expresión corporal." PhD diss., National University of La Plata, 2010.

Morris, Gay, and Jens Richard Giersdorf, eds. *Choreographies of 21st Century Wars*. New York: Oxford University Press, 2016.

Mouján, Lucía Fernández. "Danza Abierta: Open Dance against Oppression in Buenos Aires." MA Thesis, University of Amsterdam, 2003.

Narbed, Sofie. "The Cultural Geographies of Contemporary Dance in Quito, Ecuador." PhD diss., Royal Holloway, University of London, 2016.

Naser Rocha, Lucía. "La Politización de la danza a la dancificación de la política." PhD diss., University of Michigan, 2017.

Negroni, María. *Ciudad gótica*. Rosario: Bajo la luna nueva, 1994.

Nixon, Rob. *Slow Violence and the Environmentalism of the Poor*. Cambridge: Harvard University Press, 2011.

Nunca más: Informe de la Comisión Nacional sobre la Desaparición de Personas. Buenos Aires: Eudeba, 2009.

Olivera-Williams, María Rosa. "The Twentieth Century as Ruin: Tango and Historical Memory." In *Telling Ruins in Latin America*, edited by Michael J. Lazzara and Vicky Unruh, 95–106. New York: Palgrave Macmillan, 2009.

O'Nan, Stewart. "Songs." In *The Vietnam Reader: The Definitive Collection of American Fiction and Nonfiction on the War*, edited by Stewart O'Nan, 279–98. New York: Anchor Books, 1998.

Padín, Luis, comp. *El vuelco latinoamericano: De Cristóbal Colón a Juana Azurduy*. Buenos Aires: Ediciones de la UNLa, 2015.

Page, Philippa. *Politics and Performance in Post-Dictatorship Argentine Film and Theater*. Woodbridge, UK: Tamesis, 2011.

Papa, Laura Noemí. "La danza como una instancia de construcción de la memoria." *Colectivo Siempre–Lecturas* (blog). July 23, 2009. http://cslecturaspapa.blogspot.com/2009/07/la-danza-como-una-instancia-de.html.

Patricia Stokoe "Con los ojos del corazón . . . " (imágenes y recuerdos). Produced by Estudio Kalmar Stokoe, n.d. DVD.

Pellarolo, Sirena. "Queering Tango: Glitches in the Hetero-National Matrix of a Liminal Cultural Production." *Theatre Journal* 60, no. 3 (2008): 409–31.

Perelman, Mariano Daniel, and Martín Boy. "Cartoneros en Buenos Aires: nuevas modalidades de encuentro." *Revista Mexicana de Sociología* 72, no. 3 (2010): 393–418.

Petruzzi, Herminia. *Teatro por la identidad: antología*. Buenos Aires: Ediciones Colihue SRL, 2009.

Pinta, María Fernanda. "Pop! La puesta en escena de nuestro 'folklore urbano.'" *Caiana: Revista de Historia del Arte y Cultural Visual del Centro Argentino de Investigadores de Arte* 4 (2014): 1–15. http://caiana.caia.org.ar/resources/uploads/4-pdf/PINTA%20PDF.pdf.

Pinta, María Fernanda. *Teatro expandido en el Di Tella*. Buenos Aires: Biblos, 2013.

Podalsky, Laura. *Specular City: Transforming Culture, Consumption, and Space in Buenos Aires, 1955–1973*. Philadelphia: Temple University Press, 2004.

Portela, Edurne M. *Displaced Memories: The Poetics of Trauma in Argentine Women's Writing*. Lewisburg, PA: Bucknell University Press, 2009.

Prickett, Stacey. *Embodied Politics: Dance, Protest and Identities*. Alton, UK: Dance Books, 2013.

Puga, Ana Elena. "The Abstract Allegory of Griselda Gambaro's Stripped (*El Despojamiento*)." *Theatre Journal* 56, no. 3 (2004): 415–28.

Puga, Ana Elena. *Memory, Allegory, and Testimony in South American Theater: Upstaging Dictatorship*. New York: Routledge, 2008.

Purkayastha, Prarthana. *Indian Modern Dance, Feminism and Transnationalism*. New York: Palgrave Macmillan, 2014.

Rancière, Jacques. *Dissensus: On Politics and Aesthetics*. Translated by Steven Corcoran. London: Bloomsbury, 2010.

Reca, Maralia. *Tortura y trauma: Danza/movimiento terapia en la reconstrucción del mundo de sobrevivientes de tortura por causas políticas*. Buenos Aires: Editorial Biblos, 2011.

Reinhart, Stephanie. "Renate Schottelius: Dance at the Bottom of the World in Argentina." In *Dancing Female: Lives and Issues of Women in Contemporary Dance*, edited by Sharon E. Friedler and Susan Glazer, 45–58. London: Taylor & Francis, 1997.

"Report on an Amnesty International Mission to Argentina 6–15 November 1976." Middlesex: Amnesty International, 1977. https://www.amnesty.org/en/documents/amr13/083/1977/en/.

Reynoso, Jose Luis. "Racialized Dance Modernisms in Lusophone and Spanish-Speaking Latin America." In *The Modernist World*, edited by Stephen Ross and Allana C. Lindgren, 392–400. New York: Routledge, 2015.

Rivera-Servera, Ramón H. *Performing Queer Latinidad: Dance, Sexuality, Politics*. Ann Arbor: University of Michigan Press, 2012.

Rock, David. *Authoritarian Argentina: The Nationalist Movement, Its History, and Its Impact*. Berkeley: University of California Press, 1993.

Rodríguez, Paula. "Danza y 'más allá.' Una crónica reflexiva-analítica sobre el Proyecto de la Ley Nacional de Danza." In *VI Jornadas de investigación en danza 2012*, edited by María Eugenía Cadús, 198–216. Buenos Aires: Universidad Nacional de las Artes, 2016.

Rosa, Cristina F. *Brazilian Bodies and Their Choreographies of Identification: Swing Nation*. New York: Palgrave Macmillan, 2015.

Rossen, Rebecca. *Dancing Jewish: Jewish Identity in American Modern and Postmodern Dance*. New York: Oxford University Press, 2014.

Rot, Gabriel. "Entrevista a Alicia Sanguinetti." In *El Devotazo: Alicia Sanguinetti Fotografías*, compiled by Gabriel Rot, 13–16. Buenos Aires: El Topo Blindado, 2013.

Rothberg, Michael. *Multidirectional Memory: Remembering the Holocaust in the Age of Decolonization*. Stanford, CA: Stanford University Press, 2009.

Rovner, Eduardo, ed. *Ballet Contemporáneo: 25 años en el San Martín.* Buenos Aires: Teatro Municipal General San Martín, 1993.

Sagaseta, Julia Elena, and Perla Zayas de Lima, comps. *El teatro-danza.* Conference proceedings of the III Encuentro de Estudios del Teatro, Instituto de Artes del Espectáculo, Facultad de Filosofía y Letras, University of Buenos Aires, September 17–20, 1992.

Salessi, Jorge. "Medics, Crooks and Tango Queens: The National Appropriation of a Gay Tango." In *Everynight Life: Culture and Dance in Latin/o America,* edited by Celeste Fraser Delgado and José Esteban Muñoz, translated by Celeste Fraser Delgado, 141–74. Durham, NC: Duke University Press, 1997.

Sarlo, Beatriz. *La ciudad vista: Mercancías y cultura urbana.* Buenos Aires: Siglo XXI Editores, 2009.

Sarlo, Beatriz. *La pasión y la excepción: Eva, Borges y el asesinato de Aramburu.* Buenos Aires: Siglo XXI Editores, 2003.

Savigliano, Marta. *Tango and the Political Economy of Passion.* Boulder, CO: Westview Press, 1995.

Savigliano, Marta. "Worlding Dance and Dancing Out There in the World." In *Worlding Dance,* edited by Susan Leigh Foster, 163–90. New York: Palgrave Macmillan, 2009.

Schaefer, Jennifer L.. "Rebels, Martyrs, Heroes: Authoritarianism and Youth Culture in Argentina, 1966–1983." PhD diss., Emory University, 2015.

Schottelius, Renate. "Renate Schottelius habla sobre 'Paisaje de gritos.'" In *Ballet Contemporáneo: 25 años en el San Martín,* edited by Eduardo Rovner, 32–33. Buenos Aires: Teatro Municipal General San Martín, 1993.

Schwall, Elizabeth. "Dancing With the Revolution: Cuban Dance, State, and Nation, 1930–1960." PhD diss., Columbia University, 2016.

Scolieri, Paul A. *Dancing the New World: Aztecs, Spaniards, and the Choreography of Conquest.* Austin: University of Texas Press, 2013.

Shea Murphy, Jacqueline. *The People Have Never Stopped Dancing: Native American Modern Dance Histories.* Minneapolis: University of Minnesota Press, 2007.

Sherman, Stephanie. "(Dis)Plazas and (Dis)Placed Danzas: Space, Trauma, and Moving Bodies in Mexico City." PhD diss., University of California, Berkeley, 2016.

Siegmund, Gerald, and Stefan Hölscher. Introduction to *Dance, Politics & Co-Immunity,* edited by Gerald Siegmund and Stefan Hölscher, 7–18. Zürich: Diaphanes, 2013.

Sitrin, Marina. *Horizontalism: Voices of Popular Power in Argentina.* Oakland, CA: AK Press, 2006.

Sosa, Cecilia. *Queering Acts of Mourning in the Aftermath of Argentina's Dictatorship: The Performances of Blood.* Rochester, NY: Tamesis, 2014.

Spinelli, María Estela. *Los vencedores vencidos: El antiperonismo y la "revolución libertadora."* Buenos Aires: Editorial Biblos, 2005.

Srinivasan, Priya. *Sweating Saris: Indian Dance as Transnational Labor.* Philadelphia: Temple University Press, 2011.

Stier, Oren Baruch. *Holocaust Icons: Symbolizing the Shoah in History and Memory.* New Brunswick, NJ: Rutgers University Press, 2015.

Stokoe, Patricia. *Expresión Corporal: Arte-Salud-Educación.* Buenos Aires: ICSA-Hvmanitas, 1987.

Stokoe, Patricia. "Grupo Aluminé, antecedentes e historia." Appendix in *Qué es la expresión corporal: A partir de la corriente de trabajo creada por Patricia Stokoe,* by Déborah Kalmar, 137–40. Buenos Aires: Lumen, 2005.

Stokoe, Patricia. "Historia y antecedentes de esta corriente, según la experiencia de su creadora." Appendix in *Qué es la expresión corporal: A partir de la corriente de trabajo creada por Patricia Stokoe*, by Déborah Kalmar, 131–38. Buenos Aires: Lumen, 2005.

Sutton, Barbara. *Bodies in Crisis: Culture, Violence, and Women's Resistance in Neoliberal Argentina*. New Brunswick, NJ: Rutgers University Press, 2010.

Svampa, Maristella, and Sebastian Pereyra. *Entre la ruta y el barrio: La experiencia de las organizaciones piqueteras*. Buenos Aires: Biblos, 2003.

Szuchmacher, Rubén, comp. *Archivo Itelman*. Buenos Aires: Eudeba, 2002.

Taburelli, Cuca. *Una valija de vida: cuarenta años de danzateatro*. Bogotá: Goethe-Institut Kolumbien, 2010.

Tambutti, Susana. "100 años de la danza en Buenos Aires." *Funámbulos: Revista bimestral de teatro y danza alterativos* 12, no. 3 (2000): 23–32.

Tambutti, Susana. "Miriam Winslow como nexo entre la danza moderna norteamericana y el surgimiento de la danza moderna en Argentina." Course text. Reflexiones sobre la danza escénica en Argentina Siglo XX. Facultad de Filosofía y Letras, Universidad de Buenos Aires, 2011.

Tambutti, Susana. "El 'nosotros' europeo." Course text. Reflexiones sobre la danza escénica en Argentina Siglo XX. Facultad de Filosofía y Letras, Universidad de Buenos Aires, 2011.

Tambutti, Susana. *La puñalada*. In *Nucleodanza and Monica Valenciano Presented by ADF 23 June*. Durham: American Dance Festival, 1992. VHS. American Dance Festival Reference Collection, Duke University Archives, David M. Rubenstein Rare Book & Manuscript Library, Duke University.

Taylor, Diana. *The Archive and the Repertoire: Performing Cultural Memory in the Americas*. Durham, NC: Duke University Press, 2003.

Taylor, Diana. *Disappearing Acts: Spectacles of Gender and Nationalism in Argentina's "Dirty War."* Durham, NC: Duke University Press, 1997.

Taylor, Diana. "Performance and/as History." *TDR* 50, no. 1 (2006): 67–86.

Taylor, Julie. "Death Dressed As a Dancer: The Grotesque, Violence, and the Argentine Tango." *TDR: The Drama Review* 57, no. 3 (2013): 117–31.

Taylor, Julie. *Paper Tangos*. Durham, NC: Duke University Press, 1998.

Thompson, Robert Farris. *Tango: The Art History of Love*. New York: Vintage Books, 2006.

Tomé, Lester. "'Music in the Blood': Performance and Discourse of Musicality in Cuban Ballet Aesthetics." *Dance Chronicle* 36, no. 2 (2013): 218–42.

Tsing, Anna. *Friction: An Ethnography of Global Connection*. Princeton: Princeton University Press, 2005.

Urondo, Francisco. *La patria fusilada*. Buenos Aires: Ediciones de Crisis, 1973.

Vallejos, Juan Ignacio. "Articulations of the Political in Argentine Contemporary Dance." Lecture presented at Temple University, Philadelphia, PA, April 24, 2018. https://livestream.com/accounts/1927261/events/8020705.

Vallejos, Juan Ignacio. "Dance, Sexuality, and Utopian Subversion Under the Argentine Dictatorship of the 1960s: The Case of Oscar Aráiz's *The Rite of Spring* and Ana Itelman's *Phaedra*." *Dance Research Journal* 48, no. 2 (2016): 61–79.

Vallejos, Juan Ignacio. "Danza, política y posdictadura: acerca de *Dirección obligatoria* de Alejandro Cervera." *Revista Afuera: Estudios de crítica cultural* 15 (2015). http://www.revistaafuera.com/articulo.php?id=328&nro=15.

Valverde Gefaell, Clara. *De la necropolítica neoliberal a la empatía radical*. Barcelona: Icaria Editorial, 2015.

Varela, Gustavo. *Tango y política: Sexo, moral burguesa y revolución en Argentina*. Buenos Aires: Ariel, 2016.

Vassallo, Marta. "Militancia y transgresión." In *De minifaldas, militancias y revoluciones: Exploraciones sobre los 70 en la Argentina*, edited by Andrea Andújar, Débora D'Antonio, Fernanda Gil Lozano, Karin Grammático, and María Laura Rosa, 19–32. Buenos Aires: Ediciones Luxemburg, 2009.

Verbitsky, Horacio. *Ezeiza*. Buenos Aires: Editorial Planeta Argentina, 1995.

Verzero, Lorena. *Teatro militante: Radicalización artística y política en los años 70*. Buenos Aires: Editorial Biblos, 2013.

Vezzetti, Hugo. *Pasado y presente: Guerra, dictadura, y sociedad en Argentina*. Buenos Aires: Siglo XXI Editores, 2002.

Vezzetti, Hugo. *Sobre la violencia revolucionaria: memorias y olvidos*. Buenos Aires: Siglo XXI Editores, 2009.

Vila, Pablo, ed. *The Militant Song Movement in Latin America: Chile, Uruguay, and Argentina*. Lanham, MD: Lexington Books, 2014.

Vila, Pablo, ed. *Music, Dance, Affect and Emotions in Latin America*. Lanham, MD: Lexington Books, 2017.

Vila, Pablo, and Paul Cammack. "Rock Nacional and Dictatorship in Argentina." *Popular Music* 6, no. 2 (1987): 140–43.

Wainerman, Catalina H., and Rebeca Barck de Raijman. *Sexismo en los libros de lectura de la escuela primaria*. Buenos Aires: IDES, 1987.

Weber, Jody. *The Evolution of Aesthetic and Expressive Dance in Boston*. Amherst, NY: Cambria Press, 2009. Kindle edition.

Werth, Brenda. *Theater, Performance, and Memory Politics in Argentina*. New York: Palgrave Macmillan, 2010.

Wexler, Berta. *Juana Azurduy y las mujeres en la revolución altoperuana*. Sucre: Centro "Juana Azurduy," 2002.

Wilcox, Emily E. "When place matters: Provincializing the 'global.'" In *Rethinking Dance History: Issues and Methodologies*, 160–72. New York: Routledge, 2018.

Wilcox, Emily E. "Women Dancing Otherwise: The Queer Feminism of Gu Jiani's Right & Left." In *Queer Dance: Meanings & Makings*, edited by Clare Croft, 67–82. New York: Oxford University Press, 2017.

Wong, Yutian. *Choreographing Asian America*. Middletown, CT: Wesleyan University Press, 2010.

Zaldívar, Saúl Domínguez. *La música de nuestra tierra la zamba: Historia, autores, y letras*. Buenos Aires: Imaginador, 1998.

Zandstra, Dianne Marie. *Embodying Resistance: Griselda Gambaro and the Grotesque*. Lewisburg, PA: Bucknell University Press, 2007.

Zayas de Lima, Perla. *El universo mítico de los argentinos en escena: Tomo 2*. Buenos Aires: Inteatro, 2010.

Zibechi, Raúl. *Territories in Resistance: A Cartography of Latin American Social Movements*. Translated by Ramor Ryan. Oakland, CA: AK Press, 2012.

Zimmermann, Susana. *Cantos y exploraciones: caminos de teatro-danza*. Buenos Aires: Editorial Balletin Dance, 2007.

Zimmermann, Susana. *El laboratorio de danza y movimiento creativo*. Buenos Aires: Editorial Hvmanitas, 1983.

INDEX

AADA. *See* Friends of Dance Association
Abuelas de Plaza de Mayo
  (Grandmothers of the Plaza
  de Mayo), xi, 92, 114, 124,
  141, 148–49, 164, 174–75,
  181n3(FM), 211n22
activism, x. *See also* militancy; *poner*
  el cuerpo
  agitprop and, 159
  alleged shortcomings of contemporary
  dance as, x–xi, 181n3(FM)
  against censorship, 34
  criticism of Di Tella Institute
  and, 195n67
  desaparecidos (disappeared persons)
  and, 68
  mobility and, 31–53
  tradition of, 3
Acts of Activism: Human Rights as Radical
  Performance (Madison), 24
Acuña, Luciana, 19–22, 115
Aellig Régnier, Raphaëlle, 124
African diaspora, 28, 172, 223n5
Afro-Argentines, 28, 117, 173–74
Afro Dance Collective (Colectivo Danza
  Afro), 172
Agamben, Giorgio, 7, 183n17
agitprop, 159
Agosti, Orlando Ramón, 76, 209n2
Aguerreberry, Rodolfo, 113
Aguilar, Osvaldo, 90, 165
Aida (Verdi), 39
Akihito (Japanese Prince), 194n51
Alberdi, Juan Bautista, 187n52
Alfonsín, Raúl, 4, 27, 102, 109
Alianza Anticomunista Argentina.
  See Argentine Anti–Communist
  Alliance

allegory, 46–48, 81, 97–105,
  132, 209n6
  Holocaust as (*see* Holocaust)
Allende, Salvador, 55–56, 66
Alma doble (Double Soul) (Bosso and
  Gentile), 129–36
Althusser, Louis, 7
Amábile, Beatriz, 191n21
Amazonas, 71
American Dance Festival
  (ADF), 17, 122
Amor humano (Human Love)
  (Zimmermann), 35
Anadón, Gabily, 1, 216n10
Ana Kamien (Kamien), 34, 48–53, 71,
  158–59, 178, 190n10, 197n4
Andean Impressions (Ballet Winslow),
  15–16, 19
Andújar, Andrea, 43
Anne Frank (Wainrot), 209n6
Antechamber Workshop, The (L'Atelier
  de l'Antichambre), 124
Antígona furiosa (Gambaro), 213n49
Araiz, Oscar, 60, 71, 85, 191n16,
  191n21, 192n36, 193n45, 194n51,
  195n69, 202n10, 208n109
Aramburu, Pedro Eugenio, 52,
  197n4, 197n99
Areco, Jorge Pacheco, 60
Arendt, Hannah, 5
Argentina Arde (Argentina Is Burning),
  140, 216n7
Argentine Anti–Communist Alliance
  (Alianza Anticomunista Argentina,
  aka Triple A), 67–68, 76, 202n3
Argentine Association of Dance
  Workers (Asociación Argentina de
  Trabajadores de la Danza), 223n95

Argentine Metalwork and Plastics Industries (Industrias Metalúrgicas y Plásticas Argentina, IMPA), 164

Argentine Revolution, 25, 32, 53, 56, 202n10. *See also* OnganíaJuan Carlos

Argentine Workers Central Union (Central de Trabajadores de la Argentina, CTA), 143

Arrigone, Guillermo, 86

Asociación Amigos de la Danza. *See* Friends of Dance Association

Asociación Argentina de Trabajadores de la Danza (Argentine Association of Dance Workers), 223n95

Asociación Trabajadores del Estado (ATE, Association of State Workers), 143

Associated Contemporary Choreographers-Independent Dance Theater (Coreógrafos Contemporáneos Asociados-Danza Teatro Independiente), 1

Association of State Workers (Asociación Trabajadores del Estado, ATE), 143

Astudillo, Carlos, 63, 65

attire, 38, 74, 80, 192n34

autogestión (self-management), 140

Avelar, Idelber, 128–29, 209n5

Aventures (Ligeti), 116

Azurduy, Juana, 26, 71–75. See also *Juana Azurduy* (Maris)

Bach, Johann Sebastian, 101

Bailarines Organizados (Organized Dancers), 28, 141–51, 154–56, 159, 164, 168–69, 174, 179, 217n22, 219n43

Bailarines Toda la Vida (Dancers for Life), 25, 28, 141–42, 156–69, 175, 178–79, 221n66, 221n72, 221n74, 221n75, 222n89

baile, El (The Dance) (Bailarines Toda la Vida), 222n89

Bakhtin, Mikhail, 96

Bali, Margarita, 17, 82–83, 86, 115–16, 207n97, 212n29, 212n30

Ballet Contemporáneo (Contemporary Ballet), ix, 141–51, 155. *See also* Grupo de Danza Contemporánea

Ballet de Hoy (Ballet of Today), 193n45

Ballet del San Martín (San Martín Ballet), 85, 195n69

Ballet Nacional Danza (Dance National Ballet), 155

Ballet of Terror, 142–43, 147, 149, 152

Ballets Jooss, 14, 187n56

Ballet Winslow, 13, 15

Balmaceda, María, 173–74, 223n5

Bambalinas Theater, 93, 95, 179

Baño (Bathroom) (Plate), 42

Baños, Héctor Fernández, 68, 123–24, 128, 200n52

Barco, Susana, 199n39

Barenstein, Adriana, 97, 106

Barnes, Ayax, 90

Barretta, Claudia, 181n3(FM)

Baryshnikov, Mikhail, 95

Bases y puntos de partida para la organización de la República Argentina (Alberdi), 187n52

Bausch, Pina, 116

Beethoven, Ludwig von, 50

Béjart, Maurice, 44, 60

Belgrano, Manuel, 71, 73

Bendahan, Marta Sol, 71

benefits, workers', 144

Benjamin, Walter, 133

Berger, María Antonia, 66, 200n48

Beytelmann, Gustavo, 130–31, 134

Binaghi, Norma, 86

biopolitics, 7, 183n17

Biósfera (Biosphere) (Bali), 207n97

blacklisting, 82, 93

Blanca Podestá Theater, 93

body. See *expresión corporal;* movement; *poner el cuerpo*

Bomarzo (Ginastera), 194n51

Bosso, Ivana, 132

Bousmpoura, Konstantina, 154

Bowling, o el orden establecido (Bowling, or the Established Order) (Barenstein), 97–98, 106

Brief History of Neoliberalism, A (Harvey), 168

Brodsky, Lisu, 86

Brown, Wendy, 145

Bullaude, Cecilia, 191n21

Bunster, Patricio, 187n56

Burela, Luis, 63, 65, 73

Buschiazzo, Silvia, 161
Buti, Carlo, 119

Cabanchik, Adolfo, 165
Cadús, María Eugenia, 16
Camarero, Pedro Cazes, 60
Cámpora, Héctor José, 66–68
Camps, Alberto Miguel, 66, 200n48
Cara, Ana C., 112–13, 129, 130
Caramés, Ariel, 217n22
Carassai, Sebastián, 103
Carlos Gardel Cultural Center, 164
Carlotto, Estela de, 124
Caruth, Cathy, 111, 117, 133
casa de Bernarda Alba, La (The House of Bernarda Alba) (Lorca), 207n97
Casa de las Américas Prize, 72, 90
Casa de puertas (House of Doors) (Itelman), 207n97
Cascaflores (Flowercracker) (Kamien), 193n43
Castro, Fidel, 55
Catalinas Theater, 93
Cavallo, Domingo, 139
CCGSM. *See* General San Martín Cultural Center
censorship, 132, 215n95
    activism against, 33–34
    under last military dictatorship, 4, 82–83, 86–89, 93, 95, 106, 202n10
    under Onganía, 33–34, 41–47, 52–53, 194n51, 202n10
Central de Trabajadores de la Argentina (CTA, Argentine Workers Central Union), 143
Centro Cultural de la Cooperación. *See* Cooperation Cultural Center
Centro Cultural General San Martín. *See* General San Martín Cultural Center
Centro Cultural Recoleta (Recoleta Cultural Center), 106, 142
Centro Cultural Ricardo Rojas (Ricardo Rojas Cultural Center), 106, 223n5
Ceremonias (Zimmermann), 47, 59
Cervantes National Theater (Teatro Nacional Cervantes), 151–52
Cervera, Alejandro, 9, 27, 81, 98–99, 102–6, 208n111, 210n14
chacarera, 63
Chacón Oribe, Ernesto, 144, 154–55, 217n22, 218n35, 219n46, 219n47

Chatterjea, Ananya, 19
children, 17, 136. *See also* H.I.J.O.S.
    Abuelas de Plaza de Mayo and, 211n22
    Madres de Plaza de Mayo and, 92
    militancy and, 74
    youth theater and, 206n65
Chilean National Ballet, 35
Chilinga, La, 176, 224n15
Chillemi, Aurelia, 142, 156–57, 160–63, 220n62, 221n75
choreopolicing, 7–9, 103
choreopolitics, 7
Chwojnik, Gabriel, 20
Cine Abierto (Open Film), 206n65
circo criollo (Podestá brothers), 17–18, 188n70
civilización occidental y cristiana, La (Western Christian Civilization) (Ferrari), 38
Clarín, 77, 99–100
Clarín Award, 144
Clarín Revista, 88, 95
classical ballet, 22, 50, 93, 146, 155, 181n2, 203n17
    Friends of Dance Association and, 35–36, 191n19, 191n22
    history in Argentina of, 14, 16, 187n51 (Intro)
CNDC. *See* Compañía Nacional de Danza Contemporánea
Codina, Nora, xii, 94–95, 127–28, 209n6
Cold War, 4, 36, 55
Colectivo Danza Afro (Afro Dance Collective), 172
Colectivo Siempre, 209n6
Coliseo Theater, 13
Collage (Grupo Aluminé), 205n54
Colón Theater, 14, 34, 36, 146, 194n51, 202n10
community, Danza Abierta (Open Dance) festival and, 4, 81, 92, 95, 97
compadrito, 114–22, 125
Compañía Nacional de Danza Contemporánea (National Contemporary Dance Company, CNDC), 28, 141–45, 149–56, 164, 168–69, 178, 219n47
Con los restos (With the Remains) (Hodgers), 214n57

consagración de la primavera, La (The
    Rite of Spring) (Araiz), 147–48,
    194n51, 202n10
constitutional rule, ix, 187n52
Contemporary Ballet. See Ballet
    Contemporáneo
contemporary dance, 190n10. See also
    expresión corporal; modern dance;
    moving otherwise
  as activism (see activism)
  alleged shortcomings of, x–xi,
    181n3(FM)
  Argentina's role in development of, xii
  crisis of 2001 and, 136–69
  Cuban Revolution and, 195n62
  defined, 10–12
  gender and, 55
  history of, 12–23
  independent, 1, 181n2(Intro)
  during last military dictatorship,
    79–107, 202n3, 205n54
  memory and, 140–69,
    217n16, 219n43
  militancy and, 55–77, 198n6, 198n14,
    198n18, 198n20, 199n27, 201n83
  mobility and, 31–53
  neoliberalism and, 139–69
  rise of, 3
  support for, 196n90
  violence and, x
Contemporary Dance Group. See Grupo
    de Danza Contemporánea
Contemporary Dance Workshop. See
    Taller de Danza Contemporánea
Cooperation Cultural Center (Centro
    Cultural de la Cooperación), 1
cooperative labor, 136, 139–69. See also
    labor movement
Cordobazo uprising, 48–52
Coreógrafos Contemporáneos Asociados-
    Danza Teatro Independiente
    (Contemporary Choreographers
    Associated-Independent Dance
    Theater), 1
"Corporeal Expression, the New Fever of
    the Porteños," 88
Correira, Evon, 223n5
Cortés, Silvina, 217n22
Cossa, Roberto, 206n65
Cosse, Isabella, 74

Crash (Araiz), 192n36
creole culture. See circo criollo (Podestá
    brothers); criollo (creole) culture;
    grotesco criollo
criollo (creole) culture, 17–18, 63, 118–
    21, 136, 188n70
critique, political. See activism
Croft, Clare, 36
Cuban Revolution, 22, 195n62
  contemporary dance and, 195n62
  militancy and, 55, 72
  new man and, 43, 53, 90, 194n61
Cuello, Leonardo, 131
Cultural Workers Anti–Imperialist
    Front (Frente Antiimperialista
    de Trabajadores de la Cultura,
    FATRAC), 59, 69, 198n14
culture
  appropriation of, 15, 17–19, 188n64
  criollo (creole), 17–18, 63, 118–21,
    136, 188n70
  gaucho, 17, 19, 63
  isolationism and, 38
  marginal space and, 81–88
  politics and, 16
  transmission of memory and,
    110, 210n9
Cunningham, Merce, 191n14
Currier, Ruth, 207n97

Dance for Identity (Danza por la
    Identidad) festival, xi, 181n3(FM)
Dance Laboratory. See Laboratorio
    de Danza
Dance National Ballet (Ballet Nacional
    Danza), 155
Dancers for Life. See Bailarines Toda
    la Vida
Dance That Makes You Think, The: Cultural
    Reconstruction in Post–Genocide
    Indonesia (Larasati), 9
dance theater. See specific group; specific
    theater; specific work
Danse Bouquet (Kamien and Marini),
    38–40, 69, 193n38
Dantón, Rodolfo, 16, 191n21, 201n66
Danza Abierta (Open Dance) festival,
    26–27, 130, 179, 206n65, 206n73
  under last military dictatorship, 4,
    7–8, 81, 92–99, 102, 105–6

"Danza Abierta: Freedom's New Paths," 95, 99

danza contemporánea. *See* contemporary dance

danza moderna. See modern dance

Danza por la Identidad (Dance for Identity) festival, xi, 181n3(FM)

Danza ya (Dance Now) (Zimmermann), 41–42, 58–62, 65, 70, 77

death squads, 67–68, 76, 202n3

De Mille, Agnes, 204n39

. . . *de nudos y desnudos* (Barretta), 181n3(FM)

de Oliverira, Claudio, 223n5

de San Martín, José, 73

Derp, Clotilde von, 14

desaparecido (disappeared person), ix, 3, 27, 206n64. *See also* kidnapping
economic, 140–49, 161, 164–67
under last military dictatorship, 79–81, 85, 92, 95, 99, 104, 107, 202n3
memory and, 140–56, 161–67, 217n16, 219n43
militancy and, 69, 200n48, 200n64
under Juan Domigo Perón, 68
use of tango themes to address trauma of, 109–36, 209n6

Descueve, El, 107

Detenidos–aparecidos: presas y presos políticos desde Trelew a la dictadura (Re–appeared Detainees: Political Prisoners from Trelew to the Dictatorship) (Garaño and Pertot), 64

de Toro, Fernando, 72

Deutsch, Ana, 82, 86–87, 212n29

de Vos, Catherine, 204n39

Devotazo, El, 67

día del campeón, El (The Day of the Champion) (Vladimivsky), 96–98, 130

Día Nacional de la Memoria por la Verdad y la Justicia. *See* National Day of Memory for Truth and Justice

Diary of Anne Frank, The, 99

Dies Irae (Penderecki), 44–45

Dirección obligatoria (One Way) (Cervera), 9, 98–99, 102–6, 208n111

"Dirty War." *See* last military dictatorship

disappeared. *See desaparecido* (disappeared person); kidnapping

Disappearing Acts: Spectacles of Gender and Nationalism in Argentina's "Dirty War" (Taylor), 80, 83

Discépolo, Armando, 118

Discépolo, Enrique Santos, 118

Di Tella Institute (Instituto Torcuato Di Tella), 52–53, 179
Audiovisual Experimentation Center of, 38
militancy and, 58–59, 69
mobility and, 31–34, 37–41
Onganía regime and, 41–52, 194n51, 195n67, 196n81

Dolentango (Zimmermann), 210n14

"Don't Cry For Me, Argentina" (Lloyd Webber), 122

Doors, The, 50

Dorin, Patricia, 88, 97

Doumerc, Beatriz, 90

Dragún, Osvaldo, 206n65

Due Obedience Law, 27, 209n3, 209n5

Duncan, Isadora, 13–14, 88, 188n64

Dunham, Katherine, 198n11

economy/economic violence, x–xi, 3–5, 27. *See also* socioeconomic standing
crisis of 2001 and, 136–69
desaparecido (disappeared person) and, 140–49, 161, 164–67
isolationism and, 38
middle–class consumption and, 33
modernization and, 36
uprisings over, 48–52

Ejército Revolucionario del Pueblo. *See* People's Revolutionary Army

Eloísa Cartonera publishing cooperative, 140

ERP. *See* People's Revolutionary Army

escraches (public shaming), 113, 147, 149, 164

Escuela Nacional de Danzas (National Dance School), 88, 90

Escuela Superior de Mecánica de la Armada. *See* Navy Petty–Officers School of Mechanics

Eskenazi, Julieta, 181n3(FM)

ESMA. *See* Navy Petty–Officers School of Mechanics

Espacio Cultural Nuestros Hijos
    (ECuNHi, Our Children Cultural
    Space), 156
Esta ciudad de Buenos Aires (This City of
    Buenos Aires) (Itelman), 210n7
Este es nuestro canto (This Is Our Song)
    (Grupo Aluminé), 205n54
Estrella Roja (Red Star), 73
Etchecolatz, Miguel, 164
European diaspora, 47
Evita (Lloyd Webber), 122
executions. See also political violence
    death squads and, 67–68, 76, 202n3
    Ezeiza Massacre and, 67
    of Pedro Eugenio Aramburu, 52,
        197n4, 197n99
    Tlatelolco massacre and, 55
    Trelew Massacre and, 26, 57, 62,
        66–70, 75, 123
Experiencias 42, 68
experimentalism of the 1960s, 31–53
Expodanza, 48, 51
expresión corporal, 26, 160–63. See also
    contemporary dance; movement;
    moving otherwise
    under last military dictatorship, 81,
        87–93, 106, 204n41, 205n47
Ezeiza Massacre, 67

Facio, Carmelo, 62, 65
Facundo o civilización y barbarie en la
    pampas argentinas (Sarmiento),
    14, 187n52
Falzone, Juan, 47, 49, 71, 191n21
Fantastic Theater of Buenos Aires (Teatro
    Fantástico de Buenos Aires), 130
"Fantastic War of the Human Body
    Against Its Enemies, The," 79
FAP (Peronist Armed Forces, Fuerzas
    Armadas Peronistas), 56
FAR. See Revolutionary Armed Forces
FATRAC. See Cultural Workers
    Anti–Imperialist Front
Faulk, Karen Ann, 140, 145
Feldenkrais, Moshé, 88
Felitti, Karina, 182n15
feminism. See gender
Fermani, Pablo, 153, 155,
    217n22, 219n47
Fernandes, Augusto, 130

Ferrari, León, 38
festivals. See specific festival
Fiesta (Celebration) (Wainrot), 100
fiesta, La (The Party) (Kamien and
    Marini), 40, 69
Filc, Judith, 140
Filomena, Karina, 131–34
Fitz–Simons, Foster, 13–15
Five Pulse Dance Theater (Pulso Cinco
    Danza Teatro), 69–70, 75–76
flamenco, 93, 125–26
Flores, Julio, 113
folkloric dance/music, 1, 10–22,
    62–65, 84, 91, 93, 122, 151,
    181n2, 199n31
Folkwang Schule, 35
forced disappearance. See desaparecido
    (disappeared person); kidnapping
Foro Danza en Acción (Forum for Dance
    in Action), 223n95
"For the Disappearance of Almost All
    Their Groups, the Dancers Ask for
    Help" (Muñoz), 77
Forum for Dance in Action (Foro Danza
    en Acción), 223n95
Foster, Susan Leigh, 189n82
Foucault, Michel, 7, 183n17
Fracchia, Mónica, 86
Frank, Anne, 99
Franko, Mark, 9
Freeman, Elizabeth, 116–17
Freixá, Ricardo, 49, 196n90
Frente Antiimperialista de Trabajadores
    de la Cultura. See Cultural Workers
    Anti–Imperialist Front
Freud, Sigmund, 111
friction, 13, 19–20
Friends of Dance Association (Asociación
    Amigos de la Danza, AADA)
    militancy and, 59, 71
    mobility and, 31, 34–41, 52–53,
        191n22, 193n45
    Onganía regime and, 41–42, 47
Fuentes, Marcela A., 160
Fuerzas Armadas Peronistas (FAP,
    Peronist Armed Forces), 56
Fuerzas Armadas Revolucionarias. See
    Revolutionary Armed Forces
Full Stop Law, 27, 209n3, 209n5
"Funeral March" (Beethoven), 50

Fusan, Cidinha, 223n5
Fux, María, 35, 49, 95–97, 99, 191n14, 191n18, 198n17

Gadea, Hilda, 60
Galanta, Ekaterina de, 35
Galli, Emilio, 60
Gambaro, Griselda, 119, 206n65, 213n49
Garaño, Santiago, 199n40
gaucho culture, 17, 19, 63
Gaucho War, 63, 73
gender, 29, 40, 55, 182n15
    Amazonas and, 71
    militancy and, 55–77, 201n83
    moving otherwise and, 83–84, 203n14, 203n17
    Name Law and, 33
    in performance, 114–15
    sexual assault and, 61, 125, 127, 136
    shifting cultural practices and, 33
    tango and, 114–22, 125
    torture and, 110–11
General San Martín Cultural Center (Centro Cultural General San Martín, CCGSM), 31, 34, 47–52, 71
General San Martín Municipal Theater (Teatro Municipal General San Martín), ix, 23, 179, 196n90
    labor dispute at, 28, 141–51, 155, 217n22
    under last military dictatorship, 27, 81, 85–87, 90, 97–105
    mobility and, 35, 38, 47–48
Gente, 79, 81, 105
Gentile, Francesca, 132
German diaspora, 47
German expressionism, 14, 35, 42, 100, 208n106
Giachero, Roberto, 35
gimnasia, 62, 64–65
Ginastera, Alberto, 194n51, 196n81
Goldfinger, 38
Gonzáles Sevilla, Guillermo, 217n22
Gorelik, Adrián, 14
Goswailer, Ana Clara, 217n22
graffiti, 42
Graham, Martha, 10, 35, 48, 100, 188n64, 191n14

Graham-Jones, Jean, 203n15, 215n95, 215n100, 216n8
Grandmothers of the Plaza de Mayo. *See* Abuelas de Plaza de Mayo
Green Table, The (Jooss), 35
Grigorieva, Tamara, 35
Grinberg, Luisa, 16
Grissinopoli factory, 141, 156–60, 164–68, 179
grotesco criollo, 118–21, 136
Grupo Aluminé, 89–92, 106, 205n54
Grupo de Arte Callejero (Street Art Group), 140
Grupo de Danza Contemporánea (Contemporary Dance Group), 81, 85–87, 90, 93, 98–105. *See also* Ballet Contemporáneo
Grupo Krapp, 20
Güemes, Martín Miguel de, 71
Guevara, Ernesto "Che," 55, 60, 201n83
    new man and, 43, 53, 90, 194n61
    writings of, 69
Guevarism, 34, 56
Gutiérrez, Eduardo, 188n70
Guzzetti, César Augusto, 79–80

hadas, Las (The Fairies) (Orfila), 100
Haidar, Ricardo René, 66, 200n48
Halbwachs, Maurice, 148
Hamera, Judith, 83, 163
Handel, George Frideric, 148
Hanson, Laura, 18
Harvey, David, 168
Harvie, Jen, 219n43
Hazzard–Gordon, Katrina, 64
Heinrich, Annemarie, 59, 198n11
Hello, Dolly!, 192n36
Hewitt, Andrew, 7
Hidalgo, Victoria, 155, 217n22, 219n47
H.I.J.O.S. (Hijos e Hijas por la Identidad y la Justicia contra el Olvido y el Silencio [Sons and Daughters for Identity and Justice Against Forgetting and Silence]), xi, 113–14, 147, 173, 211n22
Hodgers, Silvia, 26–27, 43, 107, 178
    addressing trauma through tango and, 112–14, 123–33, 135–36, 214n57
    militancy and, 57–66, 68, 70–71, 76–77, 198n20, 199n27

Holocaust, 29, 34, 46–47, 58, 98–102, 105, 133, 178, 209n6
Homenaje (Homage) (Bailarines Toda la Vida), 222n89
homosexuality. *See* sexual norms
hora de los hornos, La (The Hour of the Furnaces) (Solanas and Getino), 195n67
horizontalidad, 140–41, 150, 155–56, 159, 216n10
Horst, Louis, 191n14
Hoyer, Dore, 35, 191n15, 191n21
Huis Clos (No Exit) (Zimmermann), 35
human rights march of 2006, ix–x, xii, 25, 28, 171–79, 223n6
Humphrey, Doris, 207n97

Ilusiones de grandeza (Illusions of Grandeur) (Cervera), 98
immigration, 14, 32, 110, 117–18, 221n72
inclusion, 2, 4, 84, 87–98, 141, 156, 206n73
independence struggle
    militancy and, 63, 72–73
    wars of, 68
Independence Day plan, 59–60, 198n18
indigenous peoples, 15, 28, 71–73, 186n40, 187n55
Indignados, 168
Indonesian national troupe, 9–10, 59, 87, 91
Industrias Metalúrgicas y Plásticas Argentina (IMPA, Argentine Metalwork and Plastics Industries), 164
Ingenieros, Cecilia, 16
In Memoriam (Syzard), 219n46
Instituto Torcuato Di Tella. *See* Di Tella Institute
Instituto Universitario Nacional del Arte. *See* National University Institute of the Arts
International Day of Dance, 2
International Monetary Fund (IMF), 139
Isse Moyano, Marcelo, 11, 83, 185n36
Itelman, Ana, 16, 116, 130, 191n21, 207n97, 210n7
IUNA. *See* National University Institute of the Arts

jazz, 91, 93, 216n10
Jelin, Elizabeth, 148–49, 154
Jewish diaspora, 47
Jooss, Kurt, 35, 187n56
Jorge Donn Dance School No. 2, 84, 164
José Limón Dance Company, ix
Juana Azurduy (Maris), 57, 68, 71–76, 90, 178, 201n66, 201n83. *See also* AzurduyJuana
Juan Moreira (Gutiérrez), 188n70
Judson Memorial Church, 31, 40
Jugamos en la bañera? (Martínez), 192n36
Juntos: Un Retour en Argentine (Together: A Return to Argentina) (Régnier and Wiedemer), 123–31, 136

Kaehler, Silvia, 48
Kalmar, Déborah, 4–5, 7, 24, 26, 81, 89, 182n13
Kamien, Ana, xi, 25–26, 52–53, 69, 71, 115, 158–59, 178–79, 181n3(FM)
    mobility and, 32–41, 190n10, 191n18, 193n43
    moving otherwise and, 81, 83–85, 87–88, 90, 95–97, 99, 203n14
    Onganía regime and, 33–34, 41–42, 47–52, 197n4, 197n99
Karkoff, Maurice, 99
Kedhar, Anusha, 146–47
Kennedy, Robert, 44
Kexel, Guillermo, 113
kidnapping, 3, 52, 113–14, 211n22. *See also desaparecido* (disappeared person)
kinestheme, 183n23
Kirchner, Cristina Fernández de, 3, 21, 140–41, 150, 162, 177–78
Kirchner, Néstor, 129, 140–41, 162, 177–78
Kisselgoff, Anna, 122–23
Kowal, Rebekah J., 36

Laban, Rudolf Von, 88
Labat, Ana, 191n16, 191n21, 193n45
Laboratorio de Danza (Dance Laboratory), 33, 40–48, 53, 58, 195n62

laboratorio de danza y movimiento creativo, El (*The Dance Laboratory and Creative Movement*) (Zimmermann), 42
labor movement, 28, 48–52
  Ballet Contemporáneo and, 141–51, 155
  benefits and, 144
  cooperative labor and, 136, 139–69
  escraches (public shaming) and, 147, 149, 164
  service agreements and, 144
"Landschaft aus Schreien" (Sachs), 99, 101
Lanusse, Alejandro Agustín, 55, 60, 66
La Plata Argentine Theater (Teatro Argentino de La Plata), 35, 217n22
Larasati, Rachmi Diyah, 9–10, 59, 87, 91
last military dictatorship, 26–27, 59
  censorship under, 4, 82–83, 86–87, 89, 93, 95, 106, 202n10
  commemoration of (*see* National Day of Memory for Truth and Justice)
  contemporary dance during, 79–107, 202n3, 205n54
  "Dirty War" and, 182n10
  expresión corporal under, 81, 87–93, 106, 205n54
  marginal space and, 81–88
  National Reorganization Process of, 79–80, 83–85, 202n3
"Latin Lovers, Lethal Props" (Probber), 122–23
Law of Due Obedience, 27
Leeder, Sigurd, 204n39
Lepecki, André, 7, 103
Lesgart, Gustavo, 18
Levingston, Roberto M., 52
Ley Nacional de Danza. *See* National Dance Law
Ligeti, György, 116
Limón, José, 35, 192n32
línea, La (*The Line*) (Grupo Aluminé), 90–92, 106, 205n54
Lizárraga, Andrés, 72–75, 90, 201n83
Lloyd Webber, Andrew, 122
Locardi, Élide, 16
London Contemporary Dance School, 60
Longoni, Ana, 43
López, Jorge Julio, 164
López Rega, José, 67–68

Lorca, Federico García, 207n97
Lozano, Amalia, 35, 191n22
"Luis Burela," 63, 65, 73
Luz, Vivian, 25, 69–70, 95, 200n54

Macri, Maurico, 150, 155, 168
Madison, D. Soyini, 24, 178, 224n16
Madre e hijo (historia de un pañuelo blanco) (*Mother and Child (the story of a white headscarf)*) (Quintá and Chacón Oribe), 219n46
Madres (Rúpolo), 181n3(FM)
Madres de Plaza de Mayo (Mothers of the Plaza de Mayo), xi, 92, 101, 113, 135, 141, 148–54, 162–64, 173–77, 209n4, 210n14, 211n19, 219n46
Malambo, 63
Malvinas, 102, 103, 219n46
Manning, Erin, 8, 127, 162
Manning, Susan A., 12–13, 188n64, 191n15
Manzano, Valeria, 33, 182n15
Maoism, 34, 56
Marco, Martín, 60
marginal space, 81–88
María Mar (Hodgers), 112, 123–36
Marin, Maguy, 20
Marini, Marilú, 36, 38–40, 69
Maris, Estela, 26, 48, 57, 68–76, 90, 178, 191n16, 191n21, 201n66
... mar, Y el (... And the Sea) (Bailarines Toda la Vida), 141, 162–65, 168, 175
Martin, Randy, 183n23
Martínez, Graciela, 192n36
Martínez de Perón, María Estela, 76
Martinez Heimann, Julia, 154
Martinoli, Lida, 34, 39
Marxism–Leninism, 34, 43, 56, 123
Masiello, Francine, 81–82, 96–97
Massera, Emilio, 76, 109, 209n2
Mater dolorosa (Ossona), 181n3(FM)
Maucieri, María Elena, 57–61, 198n17, 198n20, 199n25
Mbembe, Achille, 7, 183n17
Memorias (Stekelman), 207n97
memory. *See also* trauma, aftermath of
  contemporary dance and, 140–69, 217n16, 219n43
  national day of, ix–x, 25, 171
  transmission of, 110, 210n9

Menem, Carlos, 4, 109, 111, 139, 209n4
Merello, Tita, 198n11
Mesías, El (The Messiah)
    (Wainrot), 147–48
Mestman, Mariano, 43
Michiko (Japanese Princess), 194n51
militancy, 4, 9, 26, 83. See also
    specific group
    contemporary dance and, 55–77,
        198n6, 198n14, 198n18, 198n20,
        199n27, 200n48, 201n83
    defined, 57, 69
    Di Tella Institute and, 41
    gender and, 55–77, 201n83
    mobility and, 32, 34
    under Onganía, 43, 52–53
    sexual norms and, 201n83
    social change and, 74–75, 201n83
military dictatorships. See last military
    dictatorship; trials of military
    leaders; specific dictator
milonga, 117–18, 129, 131, 136
Minujín, Marta, 38
Miriam Winslow School of Dance, 13
mobility, 31–53
modern dance, 190n10. See also
    contemporary dance
    defined, 10–12, 36, 185n36
    history of, 12–23
modernism, 11, 14, 188n57, 208n106
    modernization and, 34–36, 40
Moguillansky, Alejo, 19–22
Monti, Ricardo, 206n65
Montoneros, 52–53, 56, 63, 66, 73, 166,
    197n4, 197n99
Mores, Mariano, 126
Mothers of the Plaza de Mayo. See
    Madres de Plaza de Mayo
movement. See also expresión corporal;
    moving otherwise
    under last military dictatorship, 80
    National Dance Law and, 1–2
    normative patterns of, 7
    stabilizing bodies and, 5, 95–96
Movimiento Nacional de Fábricas
    Recuperadas (National Movement
    of Worker Recuperated Factories),
    141, 157
moving otherwise. See also contemporary
    dance; expresión corporal; movement

addressing trauma through, 109–36,
    140, 178, 209n6, 210n7, 210n8,
    210n14, 212n30
    crisis of 2001 and, 136–69
    defined, xii, 4–10, 182n13
    human rights march of 2006 and,
        ix–x, xii, 25, 28, 171–79, 223n6
    during last military dictatorship,
        79–107, 202n3, 205n54
    marginal space and, 81–88
    memory and, 140–69,
        217n16, 219n43
    militancy and, 55–77, 198n6, 198n14,
        198n18, 198n20, 199n27, 201n83
    mobility and, 31–53
moving trauma, 111, 136. See also
    trauma, aftermath of
Mugnani, Filiberto, 200n54
Muller, Jennifer, ix
Muñoz, Alicia, 26, 77, 84–85, 87, 90,
    94–95, 164
murga, 1
Música Siempre (Music Always), 206n65
Music for 18 Musicians (Reich), 102
Mutual Sentimiento's Sexto Kultural,
    160, 221n76

Name Law, 33
National Commission on the
    Disappearance of Persons, 109
National Congress, 1–2, 181n3(Intro)
National Contemporary Dance Company.
    See Compañía Nacional de Danza
    Contemporánea
National Dance Law (Ley Nacional
    de Danza), 1–3, 155, 168,
    181n1(Intro), 182n9
National Dance School (Escuela Nacional
    de Danzas), 88, 90
National Day of Dance, 2
National Day of Memory for Truth and
    Justice (Día Nacional de la Memoria
    por la Verdad y la Justicia), ix–x,
    25, 171
National Genetic Bank, xi, 114, 211n22
National Movement of Worker
    Recuperated Factories (Movimiento
    Nacional de Fábricas Recuperadas),
    141, 157
National Music Institute, 181n1(Intro)

National Music Law, 181n1(Intro)
National Reorganization Process, 79–80, 83–85, 202n3. *See also* last military dictatorship
National Theater Institute, 181n1(Intro)
National Theater Law, 181n1(Intro)
National University Institute of the Arts (Instituto Universitario Nacional del Arte, IUNA), ix–x, xii. *See also* National University of the Arts
National University of the Arts (Universidad Nacional de las Artes, UNA), ix, 107. *See also* National University Institute of the Arts
Navy Petty–Officers School of Mechanics (Escuela Superior de Mecánica de la Armada, ESMA), 156, 209n4, 217n16, 224n14
necropolitics, 183n17
Negroni, María, 122
neoliberalism, 4–5, 19, 27, 168, 209n5, 216n10, 219n43
    crisis of 2001 and, 136–37, 139–42
    contemporary dance and, 139–69
New Dance (Humphrey), 207n97
New Hope, The. *See* Nueva Esperanza, La
new man, 43, 53, 90, 194n61
New York Times, 13
Night of the Long Sticks (La Noche de los Bastones Largos), 33
Nixon, Rob, 5
Noche de los Bastones Largos, La. *See* Night of the Long Sticks
Noiriel, Gérard, 148–49
nombre, otros tangos, El (The Name, Other Tangos) (Vladimivsky), 112, 129–36, 215n91
Nucleodanza, 17, 19–20, 22, 27, 209n6
    under last military dictatorship, 82, 94, 107, 207n97
    tango and, 113, 115, 122, 127, 212n30
Nueva Esperanza, La (The New Hope), 141, 156–57, 160, 164–65
nueva tierra, La (The New World) (Lozano), 191n22
Nuevos Rumbos (New Waves), 141, 150
Nunca Más (Never Again) report, 109
Nutcracker, The (Tchaikovsky), 193n43

Occupy Wall Street, 168
Oduduwá Danza Afroamericana (Oduduwá Afro–American Dance), 25, 28, 171–79, 223n5, 224n13
Oh! Casta Diva (Kamien), 40, 69, 193n43
Olivera–Williams, María Rosa, 117, 133
Onganía, Juan Carlos, 25, 32–33, 40–42, 46–47, 50–53, 58, 101, 178. *See also* Argentine Revolution
    censorship under, 33–34, 41–47, 52–53, 194n51, 202n10
Open Dance. *See* Danza Abierta (Open Dance) festival
Open Theater. *See* Teatro Abierto (Open Theater)
Orfila, Elena, 100
Organized Dancers. *See* Bailarines Organizados
organized labor. *See* cooperative labor; labor movement; *specific organizations*
Orgelbüchlein (Little Organ Book) (Bach), 101
Orishá, 172–75, 178–79, 224n13
Ortega, Palito, 39
Osatinsky, Marcos, 65
oscuridad, La (The Darkness) (Bailarines Toda la Vida), 141, 164–68
Ossona, Paulina, 16, 181n3(FM)
Our Children Cultural Space (Espacio Cultural Nuestros Hijos, ECuNHi), 156
Oye, humanidad (Listen, Humanity) (Scaccheri), 192n36

Pachamama, 74
Padilla, Manuel, 71, 73
Pais, Ernestina, 200n64
Pais, Federica, 200n64
Pais, José Miguel, 69, 200n64
Paisaje de gritos (Landscape of Screams) (Schottelius), 29, 98–102, 105–6, 133, 178
Palmas, Oscar Santiago, 175, 224n14
Panorama, 33, 47, 55–56, 76
Partido Revolucionario de los Trabajadores. *See* Workers' Revolutionary Party
Pasik, Salo, 130

Patagonia trío/Patagonia Song and Dance Team (Tambutti), 17–20
patria fusilada, La (The Executed Nation) (Urondo), 66
Payero Zaragoza, Daniel, 141, 150–56, 162, 168, 220n56
Pellarolo, Sirena, 117
Penderecki, Krzysztof, 44, 196n81
People's Revolutionary Army (Ejército Revolucionario del Pueblo, ERP), 43, 56–60, 63, 68, 73, 123–24, 128, 200n52
Pepino el 88 (Podestá brothers), 188n70
percepticide, 8
Perfiles (Profiles) (Maris), 71, 201n66
Perón, Eva, 52, 198n11
Perón, Isabel, ix
Perón, Juan Domingo
   cultural politics under, 16
   death of, 4, 76
   Lanusse government and, 66
   overthrow of, 4, 10
   return of, 4, 67–68
   state-centered populism of, 36
Peronism/Peronists, 34, 56
   infighting amongst, 67–68
   Montoneros and, 52–53, 56, 63, 66, 73, 166, 197n4, 197n99
Peronist Armed Forces (Fuerzas Armadas Peronistas, FAP), 56
Perpoint, Matthieu, 20
Pertot, Werner, 199n40
Petroni, Doris, 191n16, 191n21
physical self-sacrifice. See *poner el cuerpo*
Picadero Theater (Teatro Picadero), 134–35, 215n100
Piedra Libre: Women Dance Memories (Vassallo), 173
Pinochet, Augusto, 187n56, 206n64
Pintos, Norma, 157
Plate, Roberto, 42
pluma del viento, metáfora de una locura, La (The Feather in the Wind, Metaphor of Madness) (Bailarines Toda la Vida), 222n89
Podestá brothers, 17–18, 188n70
Poesía Abierta (Open Poetry), 206n65
police harassment, 41, 96–97, 110, 132, 215n95
political dance *vs.* politics of dance, 8–9

political statement. See activism; militancy; *poner el cuerpo*
political violence, 55–56. See also executions; Ezeiza Massacre; Trelew Massacre
   allegories of, 98–105, 207n97
   death squads and, 67–68, 76, 202n3
   "laws of movement" and, 5
   middle-class anxiety re, 55
   performance of, 135
   spectatorship and, 8, 95–98
politics of dance, 8–9, 48–49
Pollarolo, Patrizia, 131
Polymorphia (Penderecki), 44
Polymorphias (Zimmermann), 29, 34, 40–48, 58–60, 101, 133, 178, 190n10, 196n81
poner el cuerpo (to put the body on the line), 3, 5–6, 26, 43, 182n15. See also activism
   labor movement and, 142
   Oduduwá Danza Afroamericana (Oduduwá Afro-American Dance) and, 171–79, 223n5, 224n13
Por el dinero (Acuña/ Moguillansky), 19–22
power dynamics, xi–xii, 9
Powers, Rhea, 188n62
Preludio para un final (Prelude for an Ending) (Taburelli), 57, 68–71, 75–76
Primera Plana, 39–40
Probber, Jonathan, 122–23
Prodanza, 182n4
protest. See also activism
   crisis of 2001 and, 139
   danced representation of, 69–70, 105, 135, 210n14, 219n46
   escraches (public shaming) and, 147, 149, 164
   human rights march of 2006 and, ix–x, xii, 25, 28, 171–79, 223n6
   labor movement and, 48–49. See also Bailarines Organizados
   Madres de Plaza de Mayo (Mothers of the Plaza de Mayo) and, 92, 101, 113, 135, 148–54, 173–77, 211n19
PRT. See Workers' Revolutionary Party
public gatherings, 4, 8, 80, 95–98
public shaming, 113, 147, 149, 164

Pulso Cinco Danza Teatro (Five Pulse Dance Theater), 69–70, 75–76
puñalada, La (The Stab) (Tambutti), 19, 27, 112–36, 213n50, 213n53
putting one's body on the line. See *poner el cuerpo*

¡Que se vayan todos! (Bailarines Toda la Vida), 221n74
Quintá, Bettina, 145–47, 155, 217n22, 219n46, 219n47
Quintana, Mercedes, 34

race/racism, 117
  Argentina national identity and, 14, 28, 117, 174, 187n54
  classical ballet and, 187n55
  cultural appropriation and, 15, 17–19, 188n64
  slavery and, 28, 64, 172, 178
Ramirez, Olkar, 200n54
Ramírez, Wanda, 217n22, 219n47
Rancière, Jacques, 7
Rawson Penitentiary, 9, 26, 57, 61–68, 73, 76, 123, 179
Raznovich, Diana, 206n65
Reca, Maralia, 205n47
Recoged, esta voz (Pick Up, This Voice) (Grupo Aluminé), 205n54
Recoleta Cultural Center (Centro Cultural Recoleta), 106, 142
red, La (The Network) (Bailarines Toda la Vida), 222n89
Red Star (Estrella Roja), 73
Red Sudamerica de Danza (South American Dance Network), 189n80
Reich, Steve, 102
resistive force, dance as, xi–xii
Restos de oscuras (Eskenazi), 181n3(FM)
Retazos pequeños de nuestra historia más reciente (Small Pieces of Our Recent History) (Payero Zaragoza), 141, 150–56, 162, 168, 220n56
Revolutionary Armed Forces (Fuerzas Armadas Revolucionarias, FAR), 56, 63, 65–66
Ricardo Rojas Cultural Center (Centro Cultural Ricardo Rojas), 106, 223n5
Río de la Plata, 124, 128, 154
Rivera–Servera, Ramón H., 85

Rodriguez, Mario, 60
"Romanina, La" (Buti), 119
Romero, Gabriela, 209n6
Romero Brest, Jorge, 47
Rosariazo uprising, 48–52
Rothberg, Michael, 178–79
Rúa, Fernando de la, 4, 139
Ruanova, María, 59–60
Ruggieri, Mariela, 1
Rúpolo, Vilma Emilia, 181n3(FM)
ruptura, La (The Rupture) (Bailarines Toda la Vida), 157, 221n74
Russo, Lucía, 145

Sachs, Nelly, 99, 101
St. Denis, Ruth, 13, 188n64
Sakharoff, Alexander, 14
Salazar, António de Oliveira, 44, 60
Salessi, Jorge, 117
Sanguinetti, Alicia, 26, 43, 57–71, 76, 178, 198n17, 198n18, 198n20, 199n27
Sanguinetti, Inés, 18
Sanguinetti, Ricardo, 66–67
San Martín. See General San Martín Cultural Center; General San Martín Municipal Theater
Santa Juana de América (Saint Juana of America) (Lizárraga), 72–75, 90, 201n83
Santucho, Mario Roberto, 63–64
Sario, Agustina, 20
Sarlo, Beatriz, 159–60
Sarmiento, Domingo Faustino, 14, 187n52
Savigliano, Marta, 112, 117, 119, 130
Scaccheri, Iris, 191n16, 192n36
Scarlet Letter, The (Winslow), 15
scenery, 44, 103, 133
Schottelius, Renate, 14, 16, 27, 29, 34–35, 37, 60, 71, 81, 98–102, 105–6, 133, 178, 208n106, 208n111
Schvartzman, Eugenia, 1
self–management (*autogestión*), 140
self–sacrifice, physical. See *poner el cuerpo*
Senderos de la memoria (Paths of Memory) (Romero), 209n6
set design, 44, 103, 133
sexual assault, 61, 125, 127, 136
  in performance, 115, 125–27

sexual norms, 40, 182n15. *See also* gender
immigration and, 117
militancy and, 201n83
moving otherwise and, 83–84, 203n17
sexual assault and, 61
shifting cultural practices and, 33
tango and, 114–22, 125
Shawn, Ted, 13
Siempre (Always) (Colectivo Siempre), 209n6
Siluetazo, 113
Sitrin, Marina, 140
slavery, 28, 64, 172, 178
"slow violence," 5
Soares, Isa, 223n5
social change
attire and, 38, 74, 80, 192n34
militancy and, 74–75, 201n83
mobility and, 31–53
socioeconomic standing. *See also* economy/economic violence
crisis of 2001 and, 139
middle–class consumption and, 33
political violence and, 55
tango and, 117–19
Solanas, Fernando, 116, 195n67, 212n30
Sonnino, Leone, 83
Sons and Daughters for Identity and Justice Against Forgetting and Silence. *See* H.I.J.O.S.
Sosa, Luis Emilio, 66, 200n48
Sosa, Mercedes, 198n11, 205n54
South American Dance Network (Red Sudamerica de Danza), 189n80
spectatorship, 8, 95–98
Staiff, Kive, 85–86, 98, 102, 142, 204n28
Stekelman, Ana María, 26, 80–81, 87, 99, 107, 130, 207n97
Stokoe, Patricia, 88–91, 161, 204n39, 205n54
Stravinsky, Igor, 148
Streger, Eduardo, 60
Suharto, H. Muhammad, 87
Suicida (Codina), 128, 209n6
Sujoy, Liana, 86
surveillance, xii, 41, 84–85, 90, 92
Sutton, Barbara, 5–6, 140
Swan Lake (Tchaikovsky), 50
Syzard, Jack, 217n22, 219n46, 219n47

Taburelli, Cuca, 26, 57, 68–71, 77
Talia, Marta Inés, 72
Taller de Danza Contemporánea (Contemporary Dance Workshop), 85, 102, 151, 204n28
Taller Popular de Serigrafía (Popular Silkscreen Workshop), 140
Tambutti, Susana, 17–19, 26–27, 178, 185n36
addressing trauma through tango and, 112–36, 212n29, 212n30, 213n50, 213n53
moving otherwise and, 81–83, 87, 94, 96–97, 107
tango, 1, 11–12, 27, 84, 93, 191n22
addressing trauma through, 107–36, 140, 178, 209n6, 210n7, 210n8, 210n14, 212n30
Tango and the Political Economy of Passion (Savigliano), 112
Tango Argentino, 112
Tangokinesis, 107
Tango para una ciudad (Tango for the City) (Lozano), 191n22
Tangos: El exilio de Gardel (Tangos: The Exile of Gardel) (Solanas), 116, 212n30
Tangos golpeados (Coup Tangos) (Cervera), 210n14
"Taquito militar" ("Military Heel") (Mores), 126–27
Taylor, Diana, 8, 80, 83, 102, 111, 120, 178, 210n9
Taylor, Julie, 118–19, 133
Tchaikovsky, Pyotr Ilyich, 50, 193n43
Teatro Abierto (Open Theater), xi, 81, 93, 98, 130, 134, 206n65
Teatro Argentino de La Plata (La Plata Argentine Theater), 35, 217n22
Teatro Fantástico de Buenos Aires (Fantastic Theater of Buenos Aires), 130
Teatro Municipal General San Martín. *See* General San Martín Municipal Theater
Teatro Nacional Cervantes (Cervantes National Theater), 151–52
Teatro Picadero (Picadero Theater), 134–35, 215n100

Teatro por la Identidad (Theater for
    Identity), xi, 114, 134, 211n22
Thatcher, Margaret, 102
Theater for Identity. *See* Teatro por la
    Identidad
Tlatelolco massacre, 55
Toccaceli, Liliana, ix
Torcuato Di Tella Institute. *See* Di Tella
    Institute
torture, 3
    gender and, 110–11
    under last military dictatorship,
        79–84, 202n3
    militancy and, 56, 58, 60–61, 66, 68
    use of tango themes to address trauma
        of, 109–10, 113, 120–28, 131,
        135–36, 209n6
*Trabajadores de la danza (Working
    Dancers)* (Martinez Heimann and
    Bousmpoura), 154–55
trauma, aftermath of, 107–36, 140,
    178, 209n6, 210n7, 210n8,
    210n14, 212n30
Traviata, La (Verdi), 39
*Trelew: La fuga que fue masacre
    (Trelew: The Jailbreak That Was a
    Massacre)*, 62, 199n27
Trelew Massacre, 26, 57, 62, 66–70,
    75, 123
trials of military leaders, 4, 27, 109,
    113, 141, 147, 162, 209n2,
    209n3, 209n5
Triple A. *See* Argentine Anti–Communist
    Alliance
Trotskyism, 34, 56
Truol, Milka, 69, 200n54, 200n64
Tsing, Anna, 13
Tucumán Arde (Tucumán is Burning), 34, 43

UNA. *See* National University of
    the Arts
*Unclaimed Experience: Trauma, Narrative,
    and History* (Caruth), 111
United States
    counterculture movements in, 31, 50
    dance forms in, 64
    Occupy Wall Street and, 168
    State Department of, on modern
        dance, 36
Universidad Nacional de las Artes. *See*
    National University of the Arts

University of Buenos Aires
    Night of the Long Sticks and, 33
    Ricardo Rojas Cultural Center and,
        106, 223n5
"Unknown Soldier" (The Doors), 50
Urondo, Francisco, 66
US. *See* United States

Vaca Narvaja, Fernando, 63–64
Valenzuela, Juan Gregorio, 66
Vallejos, Juan Ignacio, 103–4
Vassallo, Alejandra, 173–74
Vassallo, Marta, 74
Verdi, Giuseppe, 39
Verzero, Lorena, 57, 69
Vestida de novia (Dressed as a Bride)
    (Marini), 39–40
Vezzetti, Hugo, 56, 57, 76, 194n61
Videla, Jorge Rafael, 76, 109, 142–43,
    152–54, 209n2
Vietnam War, 38, 50
Villa Devoto prison, 60–61, 65–68, 76,
    123, 198n20, 199n25, 199n39
Villaflor, Azucena, 162–64, 175
Villanueva, Roberto, 41, 192n34
violence. *See* economy/economic
    violence; political violence
Vivos (Alive) (Codina), 128, 209n6
Vladimivsky, Silvia, 27, 96–97, 107,
    112–14, 129–36, 178, 215n91

Wainrot, Mauricio, 86, 100, 142,
    147–49, 209n6
Wallmann, Margarete, 14
"Waltz of the Flowers"
    (Tchaikovsky), 193n43
War of the Triple Alliance, 173–74
Weber, Jody, 15
Weber, Max, 148
welfare state, 4, 32
Werberg, Otto, 14
Wexler, Berta, 74
Wiedmer, Norbert, 124
Wigman, Mary, 10, 35
Wilcox, Emily E., 12
Winslow, Miriam, 13–17, 19, 22, 35,
    188n58, 188n62, 191n21
Workers' Revolutionary Party (Partido
    Revolucionario de los Trabajadores,
    PRT), 43, 56–60, 63, 68, 73,
    123–24, 128, 200n52

"Works That Cry for Argentina"
(Kisselgoff), 122–23

Y ella lo visitaba (She Was a Visitor)
(Itelman), 207n97
Yoruba, 28, 172
youth theater, 156, 206n65

zamba, 63, 199n31
Zemma, Alfredo, 93

Zibell, Carlos, 86
Zimmermann, Susana, 25, 29, 52–53,
90, 95, 101, 106–7, 133, 178,
181n2(Intro), 210n14. *See also*
Laboratorio de Danza
militancy and, 58–60, 77
mobility and, 32–38, 40–41,
190n10, 193n45
Onganía regime and, 33–34, 41–47,
195n62, 195n69